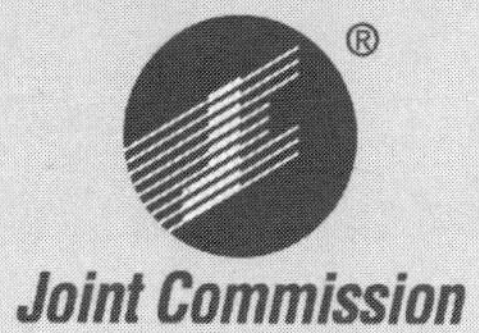

Accreditation Manual for Office-Based Surgery Practices

2nd Edition

Standards

Rationales

Elements of Performance

Scoring

Joint Commission Mission

The mission of the Joint Commission on Accreditation of Healthcare Organizations is to continuously improve the safety and quality of care provided to the public through the provision of health care accreditation and related services that support performance improvement in health care organizations.

Joint Commission Resources, Inc. (JCR), a not-for-profit affiliate of the Joint Commission on Accreditation of Healthcare Organizations (Joint Commission), has been designated by the Joint Commission to publish publications and multimedia products. JCR reproduces and distributes these materials under license from the Joint Commission.

Printed in the U.S.A. 5 4 3 2 1

ISBN: 0-86688-869-1
ISSN: 1552-8235

For more information about the Joint Commission on Accreditation of Healthcare Organizations, please visit http://www.jcaho.org.

Contents

Foreword

The year 2005 will be round two for the Joint Commission's new accreditation process. So far, so good. The new standards format, the opportunity for a structured mid-cycle self-assessment, the patient-centered on-site review process are all—thus far—being well-received by health care organizations. More to the point, a growing number of organizations are coming to view the standards as highly relevant to and supportive of their day-to-day operations. From the Joint Commission's perspective, "continuous standards compliance" should be a by-product of effective organization management. We seem closer now to achieving that ideal than ever before.

But the new standards and the new accreditation process are very much works in progress. When continuous quality improvement (CQI) concepts were introduced into the standards requirements in 1994, the Joint Commission made a commitment to apply CQI concepts to itself on a going-forward basis as well. The new accreditation process is a product of that commitment, and the commitment to continuing improvement is ongoing.

No change better reflects this promise than the complete reformulation of the content and presentation of the Joint Commission's standards. The process began with an intense effort to do the following:

- Eliminate redundancies in standards requirements
- Retire standards whose intents are now reflected in the basic operations of virtually all health care organizations
- Simplify and clarify the expressions of standards expectations
- Reduce the documentation burden on accredited organizations
- Sharpen the focus of the standards on patient safety and health care quality
- Assure that standards compliance is measurable in a consistent fashion
- Make the process for assessing standards compliance entirely transparent

These changes set the stage for the creation of a completely new standards format. Each standard is now followed by a series of elements of performance and, where appropriate, a rationale for the standard is provided. The elements of performance, once buried in the now defunct intent statements, are what the surveyors use to assess standards compliance. Now they are available to you as well. Indeed, we expect organizations to use these new tools to monitor their performance on a continuing basis. To support this effort, the scoring scale for measuring standards compliance has also been simplified, and each element of performance can now be scored in an objective, quantifiable basis.

Health care is, of course, in continuous change. The challenge to the standard setter is to select priorities for new performance expectations. While we are mindful of the resource limitations facing many health care organizations, neither the Joint Commission nor its accredited organizations can afford to fall behind in meeting the needs and expectations of America's communities.

In the 2005 manual we introduce a substantially revised "Surveillance, Prevention, and Control of Infection" chapter. The chapter has been reframed in response to growing public concerns about health care–associated (formerly "nosocomial") infections. This standards initiative expands the expectations of the performance of organization leaders.

More change is afoot. Most notable is the shift to totally unannounced surveys in 2006. This change was actually suggested by leaders in the hospital field and the early experience with volunteer organizations that are undergoing unannounced surveys in 2004 and 2005 has been remarkably positive thus far. But this will be a challenging transition for all of us. For its part, the Joint Commission is committed to assisting health care organizations adapt to this new process, just as it has done and is continuing to do, with the launch of the new accreditation process.

If change is difficult, these are at least constructive changes, and they are changes that accredited organizations have asked the Joint Commission to make. This accreditation manual reflects a major down payment by the Joint Commission on its promise to provide a state-of-the-art accreditation process that truly helps accredited organizations improve their performance on an ongoing basis.

As always, we rely on your feedback to help us continuously improve our standards, our accreditation manuals, and our accreditation process. As the sophomore year of this new accreditation process begins, please know that the Joint Commission truly values your partnership in our shared vision for continuous improvement in patient safety and health care quality.

Dennis S. O'Leary, M.D.
President
Joint Commission on Accreditation of Healthcare Organizations
July 2004

How to Use This Manual

The "How to Use This Manual" chapter is designed to help office-based surgery practices understand both the purpose and the content of their program's accreditation manual. This chapter highlights new and updated initiatives about the evolving accreditation process and orients readers to the structure of their accreditation manual.

The *Accreditation Manual for Office-Based Surgery Practices* (*AMOBS*) is designed to facilitate an office-based surgery practice's continuous operational improvement, as well as the self-assessment of its performance against Joint Commission office-based surgery standards. The *AMOBS* includes all the information an office-based surgery practice needs for continuous operational improvement: standards, rationales, elements of performance (EPs), scoring, decision rules, and accreditation policies and procedures. The standards are provided in a new, user-friendly format that fosters a better understanding of each standard, its rationale (when applicable), and its EPs. Additional chapters that support ongoing accreditation efforts provide guidance on how to use the standards-related information found throughout the manual.

What Is the Purpose of the Manual?

The *AMOBS* is designed to provide office-based surgery practices with information about the accreditation process. The *AMOBS* includes more than the latest standards and compliance information; it also includes material that supports an office-based surgery practice's continuous operational improvement and its accreditation efforts.

The *AMOBS* also provides a better understanding of the connection between safety and quality-focused standards, day-to-day activities, and the accreditation process. In essence, the manual is a one-stop resource for office-based surgery practices accreditation and continuous standards compliance.

When Does This Manual Become Effective?

The standards and EPs are effective for accreditation purposes beginning January 1, 2005, and remain in effect until the next edition of the *AMOBS*, unless otherwise announced in *Joint Commission Perspectives*®. *Perspectives* is the official Joint Commission monthly newsletter sent complimentary to practice administrators and chief executive officers.

Office-based surgery practices are responsible for meeting the requirements of the standards and EPs in effect at the time of the survey. Thus, all office-based surgery practice surveys conducted after January 1, 2005, will be based on this manual; any changes will be noted in *Perspectives*.

What's New in the *AMOBS*?

Shared Visions–New Pathways®

The Joint Commission implemented its new initiative, Shared Visions–New Pathways, in January 2004. This initiative stemmed from the Joint Commission's critical look at its services, which included significant input from health care organizations, to dramatically redesign and improve the value of the accreditation process. Shared Visions–New Pathways represents a paradigm shift away from a focus on survey preparation to one of continuous operational improvement.

Specifically, this initiative does the following:

- Focuses the survey to a greater extent on the actual delivery of care, treatment, and services
- Increases the value of and the satisfaction with accreditation among accredited office-based surgery practices and their staff

- Shifts the accreditation-related focus from survey preparation and scores to continuous operational improvement
- Makes the accreditation process more continuous
- Increases the public's confidence that office-based surgery practices continuously comply with standards that emphasize patient safety and health care quality

See "The New Joint Commission Accreditation Process" chapter for more detailed information about this initiative.

Changes to the *AMOBS* are made in response to suggestions from accredited office-based surgery practices and relate to important issues that clearly support high-quality care, treatment, and services. Since the last edition, many chapters have been revised and improved to include additional information requested by customers. Table 1, page HM-3, summarizes the major revisions that have occurred since publication of the previous manual.

What Does This Manual Include?

"The New Joint Commission Accreditation Process" chapter explains the Joint Commission's new accreditation process. This chapter includes a description of the components of the new accreditation process, a sample timeline, and the new decision categories and decision rules for this edition of the manual.

The "Accreditation Policies and Procedures" chapter includes current information on accreditation policies and procedures relevant to all health care organizations. This chapter, which has been updated to reflect the new accreditation process, details the types of surveys and provides in-depth discussions of, for example, the Joint Commission's Information Accuracy and Truthfulness Policy and its Public Information Policy. This chapter contains updated information about the accreditation and appeals procedures. Specific links to the "Accreditation Participation Requirements" (APR) chapter are provided to facilitate understanding of the policies that appear in both chapters.

The "Sentinel Events" chapter contains background information on the Joint Commission's Sentinel Event Policy, including the definition of a sentinel event, the goals of the policy, which adverse events constitute sentinel events, sentinel event–related standards, definitions of what occurrences are reviewable under the policy, and the various activities that surround the policy.

The new "National Patient Safety Goals" chapter details the Joint Commission's 2005 National Patient Safety Goals for office-based surgery practices.

The "Accreditation Participation Requirements" chapter addresses the ongoing requirements for continued participation in the accreditation process. These requirements are scorable.

The central portion of the manual is divided into two sections—Patient-Focused Functions and Practice Functions. The two sections contain the 11 functional chapters of the safety and quality-focused standards, rationales, EPs, and scoring that apply to office-based surgery practices.

Section 1 includes patient functions directly related to the provision of care, treatment, and services. Patient-focused standards appear in the following four functional chapters:

1. "Practice Ethics, and Patient Rights and Responsibilities" (RI)
2. "Provision of Care, Treatment, and Services" (PC), a new chapter including requirements from the former "Surgical and Invasive Procedures, Sedation, Anesthesia, and Recovery" (PC), "Clinical Support Services" (SU), and "Education" (PF) chapters
3. "Medication Management" (MM), a new chapter including medication requirements that previously appeared in the "Clinical Support Services" (SU) chapter
4. "Surveillance, Prevention, and Control of Infection" (IC), a new chapter that addresses infection control practices in an office-based surgery practice setting.

HM

Table 1. Summary of Major Revisions to *AMOBS*

Chapter	Summary of Major Revisions
Foreword	New Foreword for the Second Edition.
How to Use This Manual	This chapter has been revised to include information about Shared Visions–New Pathways as it relates to using the accreditation manual. It provides a description of the reformatted standards chapters and information on EPs.
The New Joint Commission Accreditation Process	This **new** chapter details the Joint Commission's new accreditation process and explains the new decision categories and decision rules.
Accreditation Policies and Procedures	Formerly found in the appendix and titled "Official Accreditation Policies and Procedures," this chapter has been updated to reflect changes resulting from Shared Visions–New Pathways. This chapter also references the "Accreditation Participation Requirements" chapter to facilitate understanding of the policies that appear in both chapters.
Sentinel Events	This chapter has been revised and contains extensive information on the Joint Commission's Sentinel Events Policy.
National Patient Safety Goals	This **new** chapter details the Joint Commission's 2005 National Patient Safety Goals for office-based surgery practices.
Accreditation Participation Requirements	This chapter has been modified for Shared Visions–New Pathways to address the ongoing requirements for continued participation in accreditation.
Surgical and Invasive Procedures, Sedation, Anesthesia, and Recovery (PC)	This chapter is being **eliminated,** effective January 1, 2005. Many of the requirements have been moved to the new "Provision of Care, Treatment, and Services" (PC) chapter. *See* the "Crosswalks of Previous OBS Standards to New OBS Standards" chapter for information on where requirements from this chapter appear in the new PC chapter.
Clinical Support Services (SU)	This chapter is being **eliminated,** effective January 1, 2005. Many of the requirements have been moved to the new "Provision of Care, Treatment, and Services" (PC) chapter. *See* the "Crosswalks of Previous Standards to New Standards" chapter for information on where requirements from this chapter appear in the new PC chapter.
Education (PF)	This chapter is being **eliminated**, effective January 1, 2005. Many of the requirements have been moved to the new "Provision of Care, Treatment, and Services" (PC) chapter. *See* the "Crosswalks of Previous Standards to New Standards" chapter for information on where requirements from this chapter appear in the new PC chapter.

continued on next page

HM

Table 1. Summary of Major Revisions to *AMOBS* (continued)

Practice Ethics, and Patient Rights and Responsibilities (RI)	This chapter was formerly called "Patient Rights and Practice Ethics." This chapter includes reformatted standards, rationales, and EPs. For detailed information about the changes, please *see* the "Crosswalks of Previous Standards to New Standards" chapter.
Provision of Care, Treatment, and Services (PC)	This is a **new** chapter that includes requirements from the "Surgical and Invasive Procedures, Sedation, Anesthesia, and Recovery," "Clinical Support Services," and "Education" chapters. *See* the "Crosswalks of Previous Standards to New Standards" chapter for more information on where requirements from the previous chapters appear in the PC chapter.
Medication Management (MM)	This **new** chapter includes requirements from the "Clinical Support Services" chapter. *See* the "Crosswalks of Previous Standards to New Standards" chapter for more information on where requirements from the previous chapter appear in the MM chapter.
Surveillance, Prevention, and Control of Infection (IC)	This **new** chapter details the Joint Commission's Surveillance, Prevention, and Control of Infection (IC) standards, rationales, and EPs.
Improving Practice Performance (PI)	This chapter includes reformatted standards, rationales, and EPs. For detailed information about the changes in this chapter, please *see* the "Crosswalks of Previous Standards to New Standards" chapter.
Practice Leadership (LD)	Formerly titled "Planning and Directing Practice Services," this chapter includes reformatted standards, rationales, and EPs. For detailed information about the changes in this chapter, please *see* the "Crosswalks of Previous Standards to New OBS Standards" chapter.
Management of the Environment of Care (EC)	This chapter includes reformatted standards, rationales, and EPs. For detailed information about the changes in this chapter, please *see* the "Crosswalks of Previous Standards to New Standards" chapter.
Management of Human Resources (HR)	Formerly titled "Staff Development, Training, and Competence," this chapter includes reformatted standards, rationales, and EPs. For detailed information about the changes in this chapter, please *see* the "Crosswalks of Previous Standards to New Standards" chapter.
Management of Information (IM)	This chapter includes reformatted standards, rationales, and EPs. For detailed information about the changes in this chapter, please *see* the "Crosswalks of Previous Standards to New Standards" chapter.

continued on next page

Table 1. Summary of Major Revisions to *AMOBS (continued)*

Crosswalks of Previous Standards to New Standards	This **new** chapter includes crosswalks that identify where the previous standards requirements appear in the reformatted chapters for the second edition.
Appendix A: *2005 Comprehensive Accreditation Manual for Ambulatory Care* Crosswalk to the *Accreditation Manual for Office-Based Surgery Practices, Second Edition*	This **updated** appendix includes crosswalks that identify where similar standards requirements appear in both the *2005 Comprehensive Accreditation Manual for Ambulatory Care* and the *Accreditation Manual for Office-Based Surgery Practices, Second Edition.*
Appendix B: Required Written Policies and Documentation	This **new** appendix provides examples of documentation to have readily accessible during the different elements of an accreditation survey.
Glossary	The Glossary has been updated to include key terminology related to Shared Visions–New Pathways.
Index	A comprehensive, updated index appears at the end of the book.

Section 2 contains practice functions that, although not directly experienced by the patient, are vital to the office-based surgery practice's ability to provide high-quality care, treatment, and services. Practice standards appear in the following five functional chapters:

1. "Improving Practice Performance" (PI)
2. "Practice Leadership" (LD)
3. "Management of the Environment of Care" (EC)
4. "Management of Human Resources" (HR)
5. "Management of Information" (IM)

Immediately following the functional chapters is the new "Crosswalks of Previous Standards to New Standards" chapter, which identifies where the previous standards requirements appear in the reformatted standards chapters for the updated edition of this manual. The crosswalks list the current standards and the corresponding reformatted standards, if applicable, and identify what changes have occurred between the current standards and the reformatted standards.

Appendix A: "*2005 Comprehensive Accreditation Manual for Ambulatory Care* Crosswalk to the *Accreditation Manual for Office-Based Surgery Practices, Second Edition*" includes crosswalks that identify where similar standards requirements appear in both the *2005 Comprehensive Accreditation Manual for Ambulatory Care* and the *Accreditation Manual for Office-Based Surgery Practices, Second Edition.*

Appendix B: "Required Written Policies and Documentation" provides examples of documentation to have readily accessible during the different elements of an accreditation survey.

The Glossary provides definitions of many terms used throughout the manual. In addition, the first page of every functional chapter includes a special box with key terms to recognize. These terms are highlighted so that readers know to access the Glossary for the Joint Commission definition and use of these terms. Please note that not all terms defined in the Glossary appear in these boxes, only those terms for which readers are encouraged to look up the unique Joint Commission definitions.

A comprehensive Index appears at the end of the manual.

The endsheets, "Joint Commission Resources Educational Products," list current Joint Commission Resources (JCR) publications, videotapes, audiotapes, software, and educational programs that might be of interest to office-based surgery practices. Visit JCR's Web site at http://www.jcrinc.com/infomart to find the most current product catalog and information about education seminars, consulting services, and continuous service readiness (CSR).

What Do the Reformatted Functional Chapters Include?

One goal of the Shared Visions–New Pathways initiative is to ensure and enhance the relevance of the Joint Commission standards to critical patient safety and health care quality issues.

Through the Standards Review Task Force, the Joint Commission has streamlined standards and reduced documentation burdens to do the following:

- Ensure the relevance of standards to safety and quality
- Reduce redundancy
- Improve the clarity of standards
- Reduce the associated paperwork and the documentation of compliance burden

As a result of this review, the standards are displayed in a new format, which includes the following:

- Each chapter has an Overview that provides background and explanatory information.
- **Standards** are statements that define the performance expectations and/or structures or processes that must be in place for an office-based surgery practice to provide safe, high-quality care, treatment, and services. An office-based surgery practice compliance with a standard is either "compliant" or "not compliant," as reflected by the check boxes in the margin by the standard:

❏ Compliant
❏ Not Compliant

Accreditation decisions are based on simple counts of the standards that are determined to be "not compliant."

- A **rationale** is background, justification, or additional information about a standard. A rationale is included for those standards needing additional text describing the purpose of the standard. In some cases, the rationale for a standard is self-evident. Therefore, not every standard has a written rationale. A rationale is *not* scored.
- **Elements of performance (EPs)** are statements that detail the specific performance expectations and/or structures or processes that must be in place for an organization to provide high-quality care, treatment, and services. EPs are scored and determine an office-based surgery practice's overall compliance with a standard. EPs are evaluated by the following scale:

0 Insufficient compliance
1 Partial compliance
2 Satisfactory compliance
NA Not applicable

Some EPs have a measure of success (MOS) associated with them, which is indicated by an MOS icon—Ⓜ—next to the EP. A measure of success needs to be developed for certain EPs when a standard is judged to be out of compliance through the on-site survey. An MOS is defined as a quantifiable measure, usually related to an audit, that can be used to determine whether an action has been effective and is being sustained.*

- A self-assessment grid (otherwise known as a scoring grid) provided in the margins helps your practice assess its performance and mark its scores for the EPs and standards. The grid identifies the EP's scoring category (a sample grid follows). **Note:** *You are not required to complete this scoring grid. It is provided for your convenience to assess your own performance.*

B	0	1	2	NA

* For more information about MOS, see the "The New Joint Commission Accreditation Process" chapter in this manual.

- Scoring helps you determine your compliance with the requirements in the functional chapters. Two components are scored for each EPs: (1) Compliance with the actual requirement itself, and (2) Compliance with the track record* for that requirement. Scoring has been simplified from past editions of the manual, and track record achievements, which have always been part of the scoring, have been appropriately modified. The functional chapters in this manual have been designed to help you assess your compliance with the EPs. To do so, take the steps described on HM-7 to HM-10.

Note: *Some standards and EPs in the* AMOBS *do not apply to office-based surgery practices; these standards and EPs are marked "not applicable" and the related text is not included. Your practice does not have to comply with standards and EPs marked "not applicable."*

In addition, some standards and EPs that do apply to office-based surgery practices might not apply to the specific care, treatment, and services that your individual practice provides. Although these standards and EPs are included in the manual, you are not expected to comply with them. If you are unsure about the standards or EPs that apply to your practice, please contact the Joint Commission's Standards Interpretation Group at 630/792-5900.

Step 1: Score Your Compliance with Each Element of Performance

Before you can determine your compliance with the standards, you must score your compliance with each EP. First, look at the **EP scoring criteria category** listed immediately preceding the scoring scale in the margin next to the EP. There are three scoring criteria categories: **A, B, and C** (described in the following sections). Please note that for each EP scoring criteria category, your practice must meet the performance requirement itself **and** the track record achievements.

Category A

These EPs relate to the presence or absence of the requirement(s) and are scored either yes (2) or no (0); however, a score of 1 for partial compliance is also possible based on track record achievements (*see* below).

If an A EP has multiple components designated by bullets, your practice must be compliant with all the bullets to receive a score of 2. If your practice does not meet one or more requirements in the bullets, you receive a score of 0.

Your organization's compliance is scored in accordance with the following track record achievements:

Score	Initial Survey	Full Survey
2	4 months or more	12 months or more
1	2 to 3 months	6 to 11 months
0	Fewer than 2 months	Fewer than 6 months

Category B

Category B EPs are scored in two steps:

1. As with category A EPs, category B EPs relate to the presence or absence of the requirement(s). If your practice *does not meet* the requirement(s), the EP is scored 0; there is no need to assess your compliance with the principles of good process design (*see* step 2).
2. If your practice *does meet* the requirement(s), but there is concern about the quality or comprehensiveness of the effort, then and only then should you assess the qualitative aspect of the EP. That is, review the applicable principles of good process design and ask how the principles were applied in the situation under discussion. Good process design has the following characteristics:
   - Is consistent with your practice's mission, values, and goals
   - Meets the needs of patients

---

* **Track record** The amount of time that an office-based surgery practice has been in compliance with a standard, EP, or other requirement.

HM

- Reflects the use of currently accepted practices (doing the right thing, using resources responsibly, using practice guidelines)
- Incorporates current safety information such as sentinel event data and National Patient Safety Goals
- Incorporates relevant performance improvement results

This two-part evaluation applies to both simple and bulleted B EPs. First, the EPs are assessed to determine whether the requirements are present. If the EP has multiple components designated by bullets, as with the category A EPs, your practice must meet the requirements in *all* the bulleted items to get a score of 2. If your practice meets *none* of the requirements in the bullets, it receives a score of 0. If your practice meets *at least one, but not all,* of the bulleted requirements, it receives a score of 1 for the EPs.

Use the following rules to determine your EP score:

- Your EP score is 0 if your practice does not meet the requirement(s); you *do not* need to assess your compliance with the preceding applicable principles of good process design.
- Your EP score is 1 if your practice does meet the requirement(s), but considered only *some* of the preceding applicable principles of good process design.
- Your EP score is 2 if your practice does meet the requirement(s) *and* considered *all* the preceding principles of good process design.

Category C

C EPs are scored 0, 1, or 2 based on the number of times your practice does not meet the EP. These EPs are frequency based and require totaling the number of occurrences (that is, results of performance or non performance) related to a particular EP. Each event discovered by a surveyor(s) is counted as a separate occurrence.

Note: *Multiple events of the same type related to a single patient and single practitioner/staff member are counted as* one occurrence only.

Use the following rules to determine your EP score:

- Your EP score is 2 if you find one or fewer occurrences of noncompliance with the EP
- Your EP score is 1 if you find two occurrences of noncompliance with the EP
- Your EP score is 0 if you find three or more occurrences of noncompliance with the EP

If an EP in the C category has multiple requirements designated by bullets, the following scoring guidelines apply:

- If there are fewer than two findings in all bullets, the EP is scored 2.
- If there are three or more findings in all bullets, the EP is scored 0.
- In all other combinations of findings, the EP is scored 1.

Track Record Achievements

In addition to meeting the requirement(s) in each EP, regardless of category, your practice must also meet the following track record achievements:

Score	Initial Survey	Full Survey
2	4 months or more	12 months or more
1	2 to 3 months	6 to 11 months
0	Fewer than 2 months	Fewer than 6 months

Sample Sizes

If during an on-site survey, your practice has been found not compliant with one or more standards, you must demonstrate Evidence of Standards Compliance (ESC) for each standard that is not compliant. The ESC must address compliance at the EP level; when an EP within a not compliant standard requires an MOS, your practice must demonstrate achievement with the MOS when completing the ESC.

Note: *Not every EP requires an MOS. EPs that do require an MOS are clearly marked in this chapter. Practices are required to demonstrate achievement with an MOS* only *for EPs within a not compliant standard that require an MOS. Practices* do not *need to demonstrate achievement with an MOS for any EP within a compliant standard.*

When demonstrating achievement with an MOS during the ESC process, your practice is **required** to use the following sample sizes, which were established because of their statistical significance, their relative simplicity in application, and their sensitivity to an organization's population size:

- For a population size of fewer than 30 cases,* sample 100% of available cases.
- For a population size of 30 to 100 cases, sample 30 cases.
- For a population size of 101 to 500 cases, sample 50 cases.
- For a population size greater than 500 cases, sample 70 cases.

When demonstrating ESC, use the following percentages to determine your EP score: 90% through 100% (zero or one instance of noncompliance) of your sample size is in compliance = score 2; 80% through 89% (two instances of noncompliance) of your sample size is in compliance = score 1; less than 80% (three or more instances of noncompliance) of your sample size is in compliance = score 0.

In addition, the following information should govern your practice's selection of samples:

- The appropriate sample size should be determined by the specific population related to the survey findings.
- The sampling approach should involve either systematic random sampling (for example, your practice selects every second or third case for review) or simple random sampling (for example, your practice uses a series of random numbers generated by a computer to identify the cases to be reviewed).
- When submitting clarifying ESC, if your practice selects records as part of its sample, the records should be from a period of no more than three months before the last date of the survey.
- Assessment of MOS compliance is conducted for a four-month period following the date of ESC approval. Your practice should select records as a part of your sample following the date of ESC approval.

Step 2: Use Your EP Scores to Gauge Your Compliance with the Standards

Now that you have evaluated and scored each EP for a particular standard, use these simple rules to determine your compliance with the standard itself:

- Your practice is not compliant with the standard if any EP is scored 0.
- Otherwise, your practice is compliant with a standard if 65% or more of the EPs are scored 2.

Note: *For easy reference, information about how to understand the reformatted standards and how to manually assess your practice's compliance with the EPs is also included at the beginning of each functional chapter.*

The new format for the functional chapters in this manual separates the rationale for the standard (explanatory or educational background) and its scorable requirements (EPs) that were previously combined in the standards' intent statement. Health care organizations now know exactly what surveyors are looking for when scoring compliance with the standards.

In addition, a revised standard numbering system is being used with the reformatted standards. The first standard in each chapter begins with 1.10, and then increases in increments of either 1.0 or .10. This revised numbering system allows for more flexibility to add standards while maintaining the current number for each standard.

---

* Case refers to a single instance in which a situation related to a survey finding occurs. For example, if a survey finding is related to **pain assessment,** a case is any patient record. If a survey finding is related to **pain management,** a case is any patient record for patients receiving pain management.

A sample of a reformatted standard follows.

HM

❑ Compliant
❑ Not Compliant

Standard PI.2.10
Data are systematically aggregated and analyzed.

Rationale for PI.2.10
Aggregating and analyzing data means transforming data into information. Aggregating data at points in time enables the organization to judge a particular process's stability or a particular outcome's predictability in relation to performance expectations. Accumulated data are analyzed in such a way that current performance levels, patterns, or trends can be identified.

Elements of Performance for PI.2.10

1. Not applicable.
2. Data are aggregated at the frequency appropriate to the activity or process being studied. (B | 0 | 1 | 2 | NA)
3. Not applicable.
4. Data are analyzed and compared internally over time and externally with other sources of information when available. (B | 0 | 1 | 2 | NA)
5. Comparative data are used to determine whether there is excessive variability or unacceptable levels of performance when available. (B | 0 | 1 | 2 | NA)

Figure 1, page HM-11, shows a typical section from a previous functional chapter, and Figure 2, page HM-12, shows a section from a newly formatted functional chapter. These figures point out the components of each chapter so that you can *see* and understand the relationship among the standards, rationales, EPs, scoring categories, and MOS.

What Is *Not* Included in the Reformatted Functional Chapters?

To streamline the functional chapters and focus only on scorable elements, the following components have been removed from the functional chapters:

- Practical applications
- Examples of evidence of performance
- Compliance tips
- Suggested readings and other resources

What Are Some Tips for Success?

The following tips are intended as helpful suggestions for using this manual to successfully achieve continuous compliance with the standards:

- Make the *AMOBS* available to staff by keeping a complete copy or multiple copies of the manual in a resource center. Let staff and others know that the manual is available and how they can access it.
- Read all parts of each chapter in this manual.
- Turn the manual into a scrapbook of ideas, strategies, questions, and answers. Keep a record of calls to the Joint Commission's Standards Interpretation Group (630/792-5900), including both questions and answers, for future reference and to avoid duplicate calls by other staff members.
- Focus on the concepts described and the points made in all standards and EPs. Concentrate on incorporating the frameworks and concepts of standards and EPs into day-to-day work, rather than on viewing the concepts as rules that must be followed just for Joint Commission survey purposes.

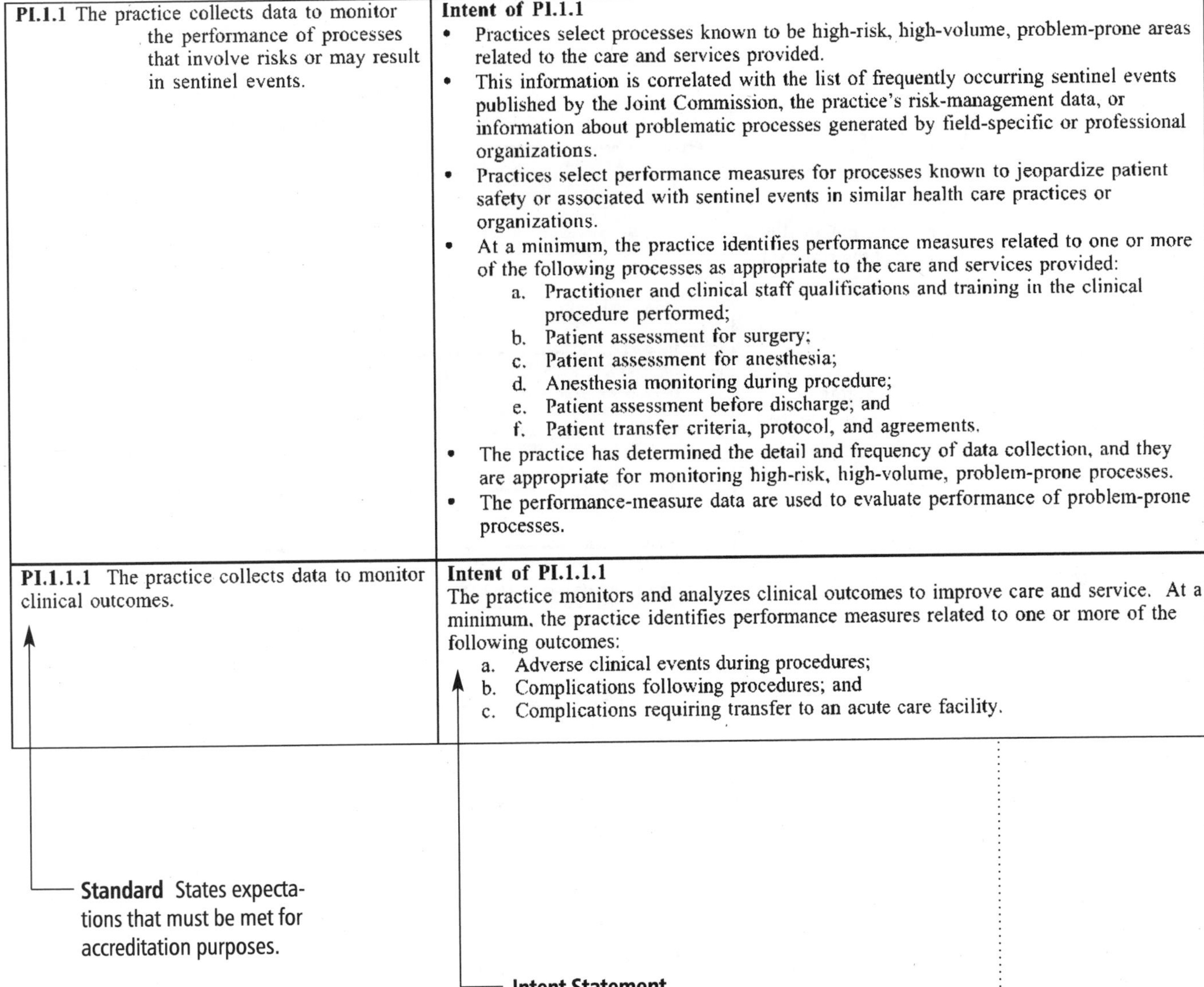

PI.1.1 The practice collects data to monitor the performance of processes that involve risks or may result in sentinel events.	**Intent of PI.1.1** • Practices select processes known to be high-risk, high-volume, problem-prone areas related to the care and services provided. • This information is correlated with the list of frequently occurring sentinel events published by the Joint Commission, the practice's risk-management data, or information about problematic processes generated by field-specific or professional organizations. • Practices select performance measures for processes known to jeopardize patient safety or associated with sentinel events in similar health care practices or organizations. • At a minimum, the practice identifies performance measures related to one or more of the following processes as appropriate to the care and services provided: a. Practitioner and clinical staff qualifications and training in the clinical procedure performed; b. Patient assessment for surgery; c. Patient assessment for anesthesia; d. Anesthesia monitoring during procedure; e. Patient assessment before discharge; and f. Patient transfer criteria, protocol, and agreements. • The practice has determined the detail and frequency of data collection, and they are appropriate for monitoring high-risk, high-volume, problem-prone processes. • The performance-measure data are used to evaluate performance of problem-prone processes.
PI.1.1.1 The practice collects data to monitor clinical outcomes.	**Intent of PI.1.1.1** The practice monitors and analyzes clinical outcomes to improve care and service. At a minimum, the practice identifies performance measures related to one or more of the following outcomes: a. Adverse clinical events during procedures; b. Complications following procedures; and c. Complications requiring transfer to an acute care facility.

Standard States expectations that must be met for accreditation purposes.
Intent Statement Explains the rationale, meaning, and significance of the standard(s); also states expectations that must be met for accreditation purposes.

Figure 1. *A typical section from a previous functional chapter.*

HM

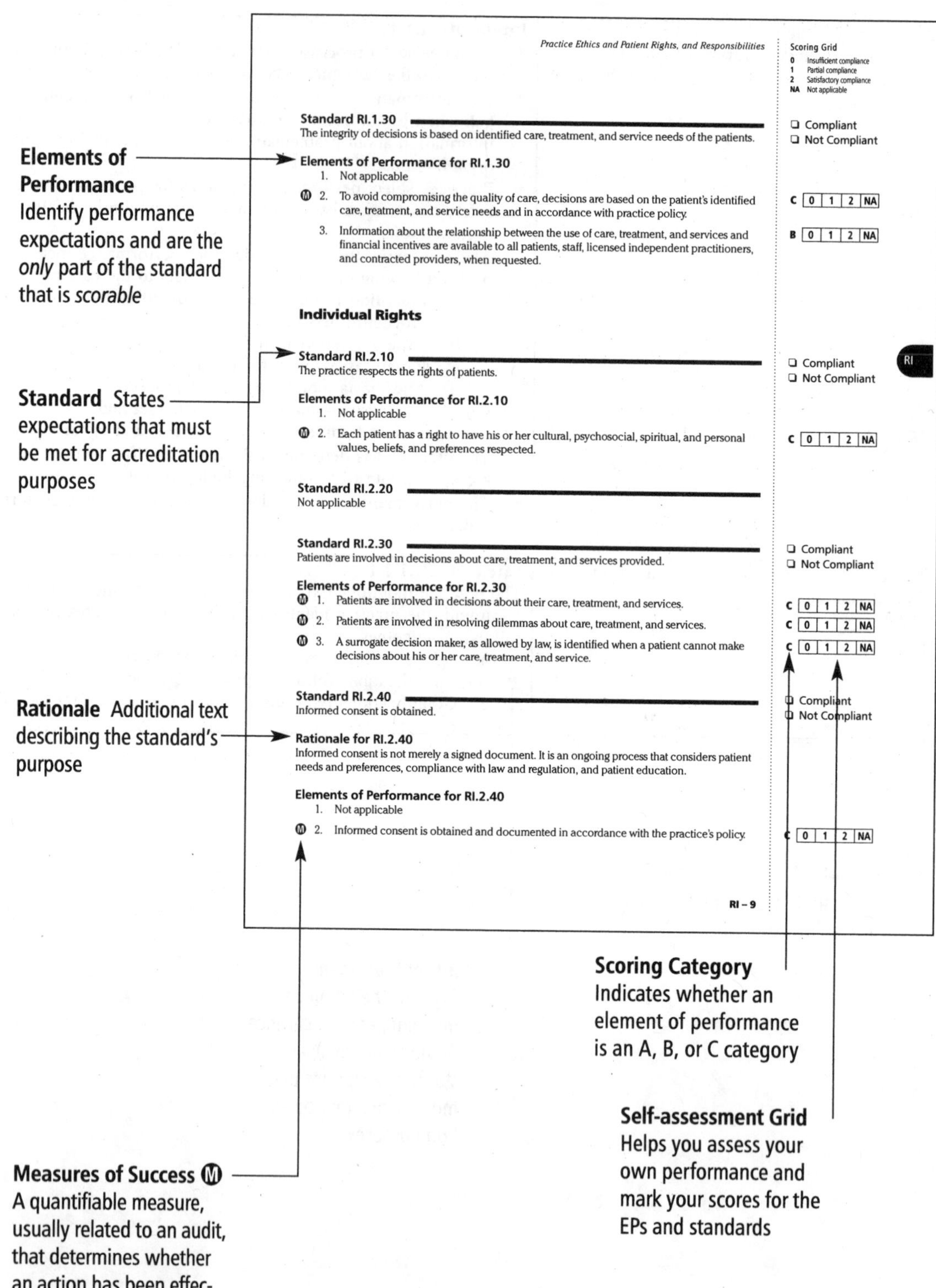

Figure 2. *A typical section from a newly reformatted functional chapter.*

- Keep up with *AMOBS* changes as they occur instead of waiting until your survey is near. Read *Perspectives*, the official monthly Joint Commission newsletter, to find new scoring, standard interpretations, and other useful information as the year progresses. File all significant changes in the *AMOBS*.
- View changes to requirements under the "Joint Commission Requirements" page on the *Perspectives* Web site for free access to standards and policy revisions and requirements that are specific to your organization. Look for the *"Joint Commission" Requirements* page at http://www.jcrinc.com/2815.
- Check the Joint Commission's Web site (*www.jcaho.org*) for any revisions to office-based surgery standards.
- Go to http://www.jcaho.org/accredited+organizations/standards+faqs.htm for Standards Frequently Asked Questions. You can also use the online form for submitting standards questions to the Joint Commission at http://www.jcaho.org/onlineform/onlineform.asp.
- Keep a year's track record of evidence of implementation on hand. Data from the preceding 12 months is reviewed and assessed during an on-site accreditation survey.
- Develop a team responsible for creating innovative ways to achieve and maintain continuous operational improvement and standards compliance, such as the following:
  - Question of the week or month
  - Standards-related posters
  - Column in a weekly all-staff newsletter

Where Should I Go if I Still Have Questions?

If you still have questions about how to use this manual, *see* Table 2 (page HM-14), "Whom Do I Call?" which includes Joint Commission staff to whom specific questions can be directed. Consult the endsheets, "Joint Commission Resources Educational Products," for a listing of publications, videotapes, audiotapes, software, and educational programs that might be of interest to your office-based surgery practice. These resources can help with your continuous operational improvement efforts.

HM

Table 2. Whom Do I Call?

The following is a list of information resources at the Joint Commission. Contact the appropriate person by e-mail, fax, phone, or mail.

By Mail: Written correspondence should be sent to:
Joint Commission on Accreditation of Healthcare Organizations
One Renaissance Boulevard
Oakbrook Terrace, IL 60181
ATTN: ___________________
[Area Indicated (such as Account Representative or Accreditation Operations)]

By Fax: The Joint Commission's main fax number is **630/792-5005**. If you experience difficulties in transmission, please call 630/792-5541.

By Phone: The Joint Commission's **main** telephone number is **630/792-5000**. The Joint Commission's business hours are 8:30 A.M. to 5:00 P.M. Central Standard Time, Monday through Friday. The **Customer Service** telephone number is **630/792-5800**. Joint Commission customer service representatives are available from 8:00 A.M. to 5:00 P.M. Central Standard Time, Monday through Friday.

By E-mail: The Joint Commission's Web site address is http://www.jcaho.org. For an extensive e-mail or telephone list of contacts, click on **Contact Us** located near the top of the Joint Commission's home page. Throughout the online directory you will see e-mail addresses listed in parentheses. In general, e-mail addresses consist of the first letter of the person's first name and the entire last name @jcaho.org. In most cases, to reach the appropriate person and department by telephone, dial 630/792- and the extension listed.

Call Joint Commission's **Customer Service** at **630/792-5800** for questions about the following:

- General information on Joint Commission services, mission, or history
- How to apply for a survey for the first time
- Ernest A. Codman Award program and for applications
- Your practice's accreditation status or history
- Obtaining a list of accredited organizations
- Checking the current accreditation status of an organization
- Quality reports
- Help in accessing information on Joint Commission's Web site

Call the **Standards Interpretation Group** at **630/792-5900** for information and questions about:

- Interpretation of office-based surgery standards
- How to comply with office-based surgery standards
- Credentialing

Organizations seeking accreditation and wanting to learn more about the process should call **Business Development** at the following numbers:

Ambulatory Care	x5286 or x5290
Assisted Living	x5722 or x5720
Behavioral Health Care	x5771 or x5790
Critical Access Hospitals	x5822 or x5810
Disease-Specific Care	x5291 or x5256
Health Care Networks, including Managed Care Organizations, Preferred Provider Organizations, and Integrated Delivery Systems	x5291 or x5293
Home Care or Hospice	x5771 or x5742

continued on next page

HM

Table 2. Whom Do I Call? *(continued)*

Hospital	x5810 or x5811
Laboratory	x5286 or x5287
Long Term Care	x5286 or x5722
Office-Based Surgery	x5286 or x5259

Joint Commission Resources **main** telephone number is **630/268-7400**. Joint Commission Resources' business hours are 8:30 A.M. to 5:00 P.M. Central Standard Time, Monday through Friday. Visit the Web site at http://www.jcrinc.com for information, questions, or to order the following:

- Continuous service readiness
- Custom education
- Domestic consulting services
- Educational seminars
- International accreditation services
- Publications

Joint Commission Resources' **Customer Service** telephone number for publications orders and education program registrations is **877/223-6866**. Customer service representatives are available from 8:00 A.M. to 8:00 P.M. Central Standard Time, Monday through Friday. Call Customer Service for the following:

- Obtaining a free catalog for Joint Commission Resources publications or education.
- Orders for Joint Commission Resources publications and registration for education seminars.
- Multimedia education products
- Publications or education related to specific programs (such as Disease Management).
- Call **630/792-5429** with requests for permission to reprint any Joint Commission Resources publication.

Call Joint Commission **Satellite Network (JCSN)** at **800/711-6549** for information and questions about how to sign up for the series of education programs broadcast across the United States.

The New Joint Commission Accreditation Process

Overview

The Joint Commission's new accreditation process focuses on systems critical to the safety and the quality of care, treatment, and services. It represents a shift from a focus on survey preparation to a focus on continuous operational improvement by encouraging practices to incorporate the standards as a guide for routine operations.

Under this new accreditation process, the survey is the on-site evaluation piece of a continuous process. The new accreditation process encourages practices to continuously use the standards to achieve and maintain excellent operational systems. Initiatives like the sharing of Priority Focus Process (PFP) information (discussed on page ACC-4) will facilitate this.

This chapter explains the following:

- Implementation and timeline
- Revised standards and scoring format
- Priority Focus Process
- Priority focus areas
- Clinical/service groups
- Tracer methodology and changes in the on-site survey process
- Evidence of Standards Compliance and measures of success
- Accreditation decision process and decision rules

Implementation and Timeline

The time line in Figure 1 on page ACC-2 shows how components of the new accreditation process play out across a time continuum. The graphic displays the three-year accreditation cycle in terms of how it is experienced by a practice from full on-site survey in July 2002 to its next full on-site survey in July 2005.*

Key Milestones in the Time Line†

- Approximately 15 months after your last on-site survey, the Joint Commission will electronically send the output of the PFP (*see* page ACC-4 for more information) and instructions to your practice on how to proceed.
- Nine months before your next triennial on-site survey, your practice will complete an electronic application (e-App) for accreditation.
- Two weeks before your survey, the Joint Commission will provide the most current output of the PFP for your practice. (For more information on this process, please see the PFP component on page ACC-4.) The surveyor(s) scheduled to conduct your survey will also receive the PFP output for your practice This information will help the surveyor(s) develop a survey process that focuses on issues that are unique to your practice.
- The triennial on-site survey occurs. The surveyor(s) will visit various areas or services using tracer methodology. (For more information on this process, please see the Tracer Methodology component on pages ACC-11–ACC-12.)
- After evaluating your practice's performance, the survey team will review the results of its individual findings. Before the closing conference, the survey team will enter its findings into laptop computers, thus producing a report of survey findings. After the report has been rendered, the team leader will meet with your practice's chief executive officer (CEO) to provide him or her

† The Joint Commission will be transitioning to a completely unannounced survey process in 2006. These key milestones will all still be a part of the accreditation process, and their timelines will be adjusted to fit into an unannounced survey model.

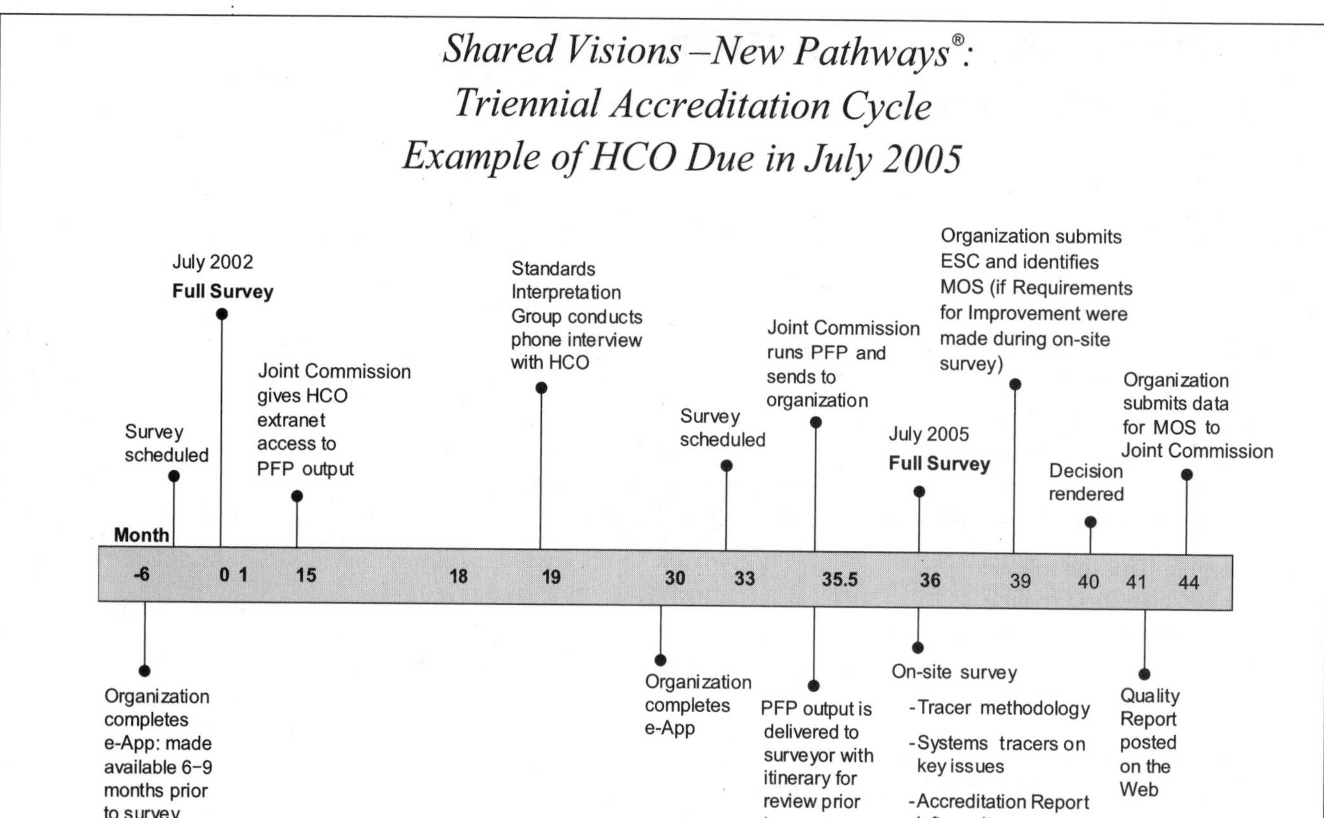

Figure 1. *This timeline depicts the events experienced by an organization through a three-year accreditation cycle from 6 months before one survey (–6) to 39 months later, or 3 months after its next full survey. Joint Commission events appear above the timeline and health care organization (HCO) events appear below the timeline.**

with a copy of the report. It is up to the CEO to decide whether the report will be distributed at the exit conference; however, the survey team will use the contents of the report during its exit conference. (For more information on this process, please *see* the "Accreditation Policies and Procedures" chapter on page APP-1.)

- Approximately 48 hours after your survey has taken place, the Joint Commission will post your report of survey findings on a secure automated area of the extranet site that is password protected for each practice. If the surveyor(s) finds requirements for improvement in your practice, you have 90 days (45 days beginning July 1, 2005) following the posting of your practice's Accreditation Report on the Jayco extranet to submit an Evidence of Standards Compliance report (ESC report). During the 90-day/45-day period, your practice's prior accreditation decision will remain in effect.
- If, at the end of the 90-day/45-day period, your practice successfully addresses its requirements for improvement, it will be moved to an accreditation decision of Accredited. After the 90-day/45-day time frame, either the ESC report is received and approved or your practice is moved to an accreditation decision of Provisional Accreditation. Your Quality Report will be made available to the public on Joint Commission's Quality Check®.

* In 2004, the Joint Commission continues to conduct voluntary unannounced surveys on a limited basis, opening the option to all types of accredited organizations, and then transitioning to a completely unannounced survey process in 2006. *See* page APP-28 of the "Accreditation Policies and Procedures" chapter for more information on random unannounced surveys.

Revised Standards and Scoring Format

As part of the Shared Visions–New Pathways® initiative, the Joint Commission conducted a major review of the standards. During this process, all standards were reviewed and subsequently streamlined to enhance the focus on key quality and safety issues. The revisions achieve the following:

- Reduce redundancy
- Improve the clarity of standards language
- Reduce the associated paperwork and documentation of compliance burden

The standards chapters have been reformatted significantly. Please refer to the section "Understanding the Parts of This Chapter" at the beginning of each functional chapter and to pages HM-3 through HM-5 in the "How To Use This Manual" chapter for a detailed explanation.

For a complete crosswalk of standards from the previous edition of the *Accreditation Manual for Office-Based Surgery Practices (AMOBS)* to the new *AMOBS*, please *see* pages CX-1–CX-19.

Scoring was also revised. The revised framework provides for the scoring of the standards as compliant or not compliant. The accreditation decision will be based on a simple count of the standards that are judged not compliant. The EPs for each standard will be scored on the following scale:

0 Insufficient compliance
1 Partial compliance
2 Satisfactory compliance
NA Not applicable

The determination as to whether a practice is compliant with a given standard is based on the scoring of that standard's EPs. An EP is a specific performance expectation related to a standard that details the specific structures or processes that must be in place for a practice to provide quality care, treatment, and services.

Two components are scored for each EP: (1) compliance with the requirement itself **and** (2) compliance with the track record* for that requirement. Scoring has been simplified from past editions of the manual, and track record achievements (which have always been part of the scoring) have been appropriately modified.

To determine your compliance with an EP, first look at the EP scoring category listed immediately preceding the scoring scale in the margin next to the EP. There are three scoring categories: A, B, and C. For more information on these scoring categories, please refer to the "Understanding the Parts of This Chapter" at the beginning of each standards chapter as well as in the "How to Use This Manual" chapter.

In addition to the requirements specifically stated in the EPs, EPs are also scored in accordance with the following track record achievements:

Score	Initial Survey†	Full Survey
2	4 months or more	12 months or more
1	2 to 3 months	6 to 11 months
0	Fewer than 2 months	Fewer than 6 months

If during an on-site survey, your practice has been found not compliant with one or more standards, you must submit an ESC report‡ for each standard that is not compliant. The ESC report must

* **Track record** The amount of time that an organization has been in compliance with a standard, EP, or other requirement.

† **Initial survey** An accreditation survey of a health care organization not previously accredited by the Joint Commission, or an accreditation survey of an organization performed without reference to any prior survey findings.

‡ **Evidence of Standards Compliance (ESC)** A report submitted by a surveyed organization within 45 days (90 days between January 1, 2004 and June 30, 2005) of its survey, which details the action(s) that it took to bring itself into compliance with a standard or clarifies why the organization believes that was in compliance with the standard for which it received a requirement for improvement. An ESC must address compliance at the EP level and include an MOS (*see* definition) for all appropriate EP corrections.

address compliance at the EP level; when an EP within a not compliant standard requires an MOS,* your practice must demonstrate achievement with the MOS when completing the ESC report.†

See the "How to Use This Manual" chapter for detailed information on sample sizes. *See* pages ACC-18–ACC-19 in this chapter for more information on the MOS decision rules.

After you have evaluated and scored each EP for a particular standard, use these simple rules to determine your compliance with the standard itself:

- Your practice is not compliant with the standard if any EP is scored 0.
- Otherwise, your practice is compliant with a standard if more than 65% of its EPs are scored 2.

Revised Accreditation Process

Presurvey Activities

Priority Focus Process

An important component of the Joint Commission's accreditation process is the PFP, which guides surveyors in planning and conducting your on-site survey. The PFP uses an automated tool, which takes available data from a variety of sources—including e-Apps, previous survey findings, complaint data—and integrates them to identify CSGs and PFAs for your practice. The PFP converts this data into information that focuses survey activities, increases consistency in the accreditation process, and customizes the accreditation process to make it specific to your practice.

Surveyors receive enhanced information and insight about a practice before the on-site survey. The PFP integrates various presurvey data (following) on each practice and recommends the PFAs and CSGs for the on-site survey. This information guides tracer activities. (*see* pages ACC-11–ACC-12 for more information on the tracer methodology.) However, the PFP does not preclude any area from being surveyed.

From these sources, the PFP identifies PFAs for each practice on which surveyors focus during the initial part of the on-site survey. Surveyors use the PFP in the following ways:

- Two weeks before the triennial survey, the surveyor(s) assigned to your practice will have access to your practice's PFP information via the surveyor extranet.
- Surveyors review the PFP information for practice-specific PFAs as well as for practice-specific CSGs
- As part of the planning process, surveyors begin to assess and plan their tracer activities.
- During the on-site survey, the surveyors use the practice's active patient list to select tracer patients.

The PFP is also used for a practice undergoing its initial survey. The only difference with this type of practice (versus a practice that has already gone through a survey) is in the available data inputs that feed the PFP. Practices undergoing initial survey do not have previous requirements for improvement (referred to as "type 1 recommendations" before January 1, 2004) available to feed into the PFP. For initial surveys, the Joint Commission is only able to feed e-App data, external data (as applicable), and Office of Quality Monitoring (OQM) data into the PFP.

---

* **Measure of success (MOS)** A numerical or quantifiable measure usually related to an audit that determines if an action was effective and sustained due four months after ESC (*see* definition) approval.

†**Note:** *Not every EP requires an MOS. EPs that do require an MOS are clearly marked in the standards chapters in this manual. Organizations are required to demonstrate achievement with an MOS* only *for EPs within a not compliant standard that require an MOS. Organizations* do not *need to demonstrate achievement with an MOS for any EP within a compliant standard.*

After these data are transformed to become the PFP information, the process for initial surveys is no different from any other type of survey. The data is aggregated in the same manner to determine the PFAs and CSGs for the practice.

Priority Focus Areas

Priority focus areas are processes, systems, or structures in a health care practice that significantly impact safety and/or the quality of care provided. The list of PFAs was developed from information provided by the Joint Commission Office of Quality Monitoring, expert literature, and expert opinions. Joint Commission categorized the different processes, systems, and structures leading to improved health care in 14 PFAs. The PFAs evolved from this process of identifying common patterns useful toward building positive health care outcomes and safe, quality health care.

The PFAs provide a consistent, yet customized approach to providing an initial focus for the on-site survey process.

The PFAs are the following:

- Assessment and Care/Services
- Communication
- Credentialed Practitioners
- Equipment Use
- Infection Control
- Information Management
- Medication Management
- Organization Structure
- Orientation & Training
- Rights & Ethics
- Physical Environment
- Quality Improvement Expertise/Activities
- Patient Safety
- Staffing

PFAs guide the surveyor throughout a portion of the survey—namely, the tracer portion. Outside of formal conferences/interviews, much of the survey consists of reviewing systems issues in the form of tracer methodology. (For more information, please *see* the "Tracer Methodology" section on pages ACC-11–ACC-12). The CSGs affect tracer selection more than the PFAs do. After a patient is selected for a tracer activity, the surveyor puts more focus on the prioritized list of PFAs for your practice.

Definitions for each PFA follow.

Assessment and Care/Services Assessment and Care/Services for patients comprise the execution of a series of processes including, as relevant: assessment; planning care, treatment, and/or services; provision of care; ongoing reassessment of care; and discharge planning, referral for continuing care, or discontinuation of services. Assessment and Care/Services are fluid in nature to accommodate a patient's needs while in a care setting. While some elements of Assessment and Care/Services may occur only once, other aspects may be repeated or revisited as the patient's needs or care delivery priorities change. Successful implementation of improvements in Assessment and Care/Services rely on the full support of leadership.

Sub-processes of Assessment and Care/Services include:

- Assessment
- Reassessment
- Planning care, treatment and/or services
- Provision of care, treatment and services
- Discharge planning or discontinuation of services

Communication Communication is the process by which information is exchanged between individuals, departments, or organizations. Effective Communication successfully permeates every aspect of a health care organization, from the provision of care to performance improvement, resulting in a marked improvement in the quality of care delivery and functioning.

Sub-processes of Communication include:
- Provider and/or staff-patient communication
- Patient and family education
- Staff communication and collaboration
- Information dissemination
- Multidisciplinary teamwork

Credentialed Practitioners Credentialed Practitioners are health care professionals whose qualifications to provide patient care services have been verified and assessed, resulting in the granting of clinical privileges. They typically are not employed staff at the health care organization. The category varies from organization to organization and from state to state. It includes licensed independent practitioners and, in some settings, nurse practitioners, advanced practice registered nurses, and physician assistants who are permitted to provide patient care services under the direction of a sponsoring physician. Licensed independent practitioners are permitted by law and the health care organization to provide care and services without clinical supervision or direction within the scope of their license and consistent with individually granted clinical privileges.

Equipment Use Equipment Use incorporates the selection, delivery, setup, and maintenance of equipment and supplies to meet patient and staff needs. It generally includes movable equipment, as well as management of supplies that staff members use (e.g., gloves, syringes). (Equipment Use does not include fixed equipment such as built-in oxygen and gas lines and central air conditioning systems; this is included in the Physical Environment focus area.) Equipment Use includes planning and selecting; maintaining, testing, and inspecting; educating and providing instructions; delivery and setup; and risk prevention related to equipment and/or supplies.

Sub-processes of Equipment Use include:
- Selection
- Maintenance strategies
- Periodic evaluation
- Orientation and training

Infection Control Infection Control includes the surveillance/identification, prevention, and control of infections among patients, employees, physicians, and other licensed independent practitioners, contract service workers, volunteers, students, and visitors. This is a system-wide, integrated process that is applied to all programs, services, and settings.

Sub-processes of Infection Control include:
- Surveillance/identification
- Prevention and control
- Reporting
- Measurement

Information Management Information Management is the interdisciplinary field concerning the timely and accurate creation, collection, storage, retrieval, transmission, analysis, control, dissemination, and use of data or information, both within a practice and externally, as allowed by law and regulation. In addition to written and verbal information, supporting information technology and information services are also included in Information Management.

Sub-processes of Information Management include:
- Planning
- Procurement
- Implementation
- Collection

- Recording
- Protection
- Aggregation
- Interpretation
- Storage and retrieval
- Data integrity
- Information dissemination

Medication Management Medication Management encompasses the systems and processes a practice uses to provide medication to individuals served by the practice. This is usually a multidisciplinary, coordinated effort of health care staff, implementing, evaluating, and constantly improving the processes of selecting, procuring, storing, ordering, transcribing, preparing, dispensing, administering (including self-administering), and monitoring the effects of medications throughout the patients' continuum of care. In addition, Medication Management involves educating patients and, as appropriate, their families, about the medication, its administration and use, and potential side effects.

Sub-processes of Medication Management include:

- Selection
- Procurement
- Storage
- Prescribing or ordering
- Preparing
- Dispensing
- Administration
- Monitoring

Organizational Structure The Organizational Structure is the framework for an organization to carry out its vision and mission. The implementation is accomplished through corporate bylaws and governing body polices, practice management, compliance, planning, integration and coordination, and performance improvement. Included are the practice's governance; business ethics, contracted organizations, and management requirements.

Sub-processes of Organizational Structure include:

- Management requirements
- Corporate by-laws and governing body plans
- Practice's management
- Compliance
- Planning
- Business ethics
- Contracted services

Orientation & Training Orientation is the process of educating newly hired staff in health care organizations to organization-wide, departmental, and job-specific competencies before they provide patient care services. "Newly hired staff" includes, but is not limited to, regular staff employees, contracted staff, agency (temporary) staff, float staff, volunteer staff, students, housekeeping, and maintenance staff.Training refers to the development and implementation of programs that foster staff development and continued learning, address skill deficiencies, and thereby help to ensure staff retention. More specifically, it entails providing opportunities for staff to develop enhanced skills related to revised processes that may have been addressed during orientation, new patient care techniques, or expanded job responsibilities. Whereas Orientation is a one-time process, Training is a continuous one.

Sub-processes of Orientation & Training include:

- Organization-wide orientation
- Departmental orientation
- Job-specific orientation
- Training and continuing or ongoing education

Patient Safety Effective patient safety entails proactively identifying the potential and actual risks to safety, identifying the underlying cause(s) of the potential, and making the necessary improvements so that risk is reduced. It also entails establishing processes to respond to sentinel events, identifying cause through root cause analysis, and making necessary improvements. This involves a systems-based approach that examines all activities within a practice that contribute to the maintenance and improvement of patient safety (such as performance improvement and risk management) to ensure the activities work together, not independently, to improve care and safety. The systems-based approach is driven by practice leadership; anchored in the practice's mission, vision, and strategic plan; endorsed and actively supported by medical staff and nursing leadership; implemented by directors; integrated and coordinated throughout the practice's staff; and continuously re-engineered using proven, proactive performance improvement modalities. In addition, effective reduction of errors and other factors that contribute to unintended adverse outcomes in a practice requires an environment in which patients/clients/residents, their families, and practice staff and leaders can identify and manage actual and potential risks to safety.

Sub-processes of patient safety include:
- Planning and designing services
- Directing services
- Integrating and coordinating services
- Error reduction and prevention
- The use of Sentinel Event Alerts
- The Joint Commission's National Patient Safety Goals
- Clinical practice guidelines
- Active patient involvement in their care

Physical Environment The Physical Environment refers to safe, accessible, functional, supportive, and effective Physical Environment for patients, staff members, workers, and other individuals, by managing physical design; construction and redesign; maintenance and testing; planning and improvement; and risk prevention, defined in terms of utilities, fire protection, security, privacy, storage, and hazardous materials and waste. The Physical Environment may include the home in the case of home care and foster care.

Sub-processes of the physical environment include:
- Physical design
- Construction and redesign
- Maintenance and testing
- Planning and improvement
- Risk prevention

Quality Improvement Expertise/Activities Quality Improvement identifies the collaborative and interdisciplinary approach to the continuous study and improvement of the processes of providing health care services to meet the needs of consumers and others. Quality Improvement depends on understanding and revising processes on the basis of data and knowledge about the processes themselves. Quality Improvement involves identifying, measuring, implementing, monitoring, analyzing, planning, and maintaining processes to ensure they function effectively. Examples of Quality Improvement Activities include designing a new service, flowcharting a clinical process, collecting and analyzing data about performance measures or patient outcomes, comparing the practice's performance to that of other practices, selecting areas for priority attention, and experimenting with new ways of carrying out a function.

Sub-processes of quality improvement expertise/activities include:
- Identifying issues and establishing priorities
- Developing measures
- Collecting data to evaluate status on outcomes, processes, or structures
- Analyzing and interpreting data
- Making and implementing recommendations
- Monitoring and sustaining performance improvement

Rights and Ethics Rights and Ethics include patient rights and organizational ethics as they pertain to patient care. Rights and Ethics address issues such as patient privacy, confidentiality and protection of health information, advance directives (as appropriate), organ procurement, use of restraints, informed consent for various procedures, and the right to participate in care decisions.

Sub-processes of Rights and Ethics include:
- Patient rights
- Organizational ethics pertaining to patient care
- Organizational responsibility
- Consideration of patient
- Care sensitivity
- Informing patients and/or family

Staffing Effective staffing entails providing the optimal number of competent personnel with the appropriate skill mix to meet the needs of a health care practice's patients based on that practice's mission, values, and vision. As such, it involves defining competencies and expectations for all staff (the competency of licensed independent practitioners are addressed in the Credentialed Practitioners priority focus area for all accreditation programs); Staffing includes assessing those defined competencies and allocating the human resources necessary for patient safety and improved patient outcomes.

Sub-processes of Staffing include:
- Competency
- Skill mix
- Number of staff

Clinical/Service Groups

Clinical/service groups (CSGs) categorize patients and/or services into distinct populations for which data can be collected. The Joint Commission created the list of CSGs based on data gathered from e-Apps from each accreditation program and on publicly available data from external sources. The list then underwent a thorough review to make sure that all categories were actually representative of populations served or services provided by the practices surveyed by the individual accreditation programs. Joint Commission surveyors use a practice's CSGs combined with other practice-specific data to get a better understanding of the practice's systems and the patients it serves. Tracer patients are selected according to CSGs.

Clinical/Service Groups for Office-Based Surgery

- Cardiac catheterization
- Endoscopy
- Gastroenterology procedures
- General surgery
- Invitro fertilization
- Ophthalmology
- Oral maxillofacial surgery
- Orthopedic surgery
- Plastic surgery
- Podiatric surgery
- Trigger point injections (pain management)
- Urologic procedures

On-Site Survey Activities

Survey Agenda

The on-site survey process shifts the focus from survey preparation and scores to continuous operational improvement in support of safe, high-quality care, treatment, and services.

The survey agenda will include the following elements (in no particular order):*

- *Opening Conference and Orientation to the Organization.* The opening session will be an opportunity for introductions and for an orientation to the structure and content of the survey. At this time, your practice will briefly explain its structures, mission, vision, and relationship with the community.
- *Surveyor Planning Session.* During this session, the surveyor(s) reviews data and information about the practice, including plans of action generated from the PPR, and plans the survey agenda. The surveyor(s) will also select initial tracer patients.
- *Leadership Session.* Surveyors discuss the following with leaders:
  - Information gathering and baseline assessment of leadership-level, system issues—system standards, management oversight and direction, and other leadership responsibilities
  - Leadership's methods used to address areas needing improvement
  - Ongoing initiatives to improve delivery of health care
  - Safety program and National Patient Safety Goals
  - Oversight by trustees or board
- *Individual Tracer Activity.* During the tracer activity, the surveyor will do the following:
  - Follow the course of a type of care, treatment, and service provided to the patient by the practice
  - Assess the interrelationships among disciplines and departments (where applicable) and the important functions in the care, treatment, and services provided
  - Evaluate the performance of processes relevant to the care, treatment, and service needs of the patient, with particular focus on the integration and coordination of distinct but related processes
  - Identify vulnerabilities in the care processes
- *Competence Assessment Process.* This process will help the practice and the surveyor to do the following:
  - Identify the competence-assessment, process-related strengths and vulnerabilities of staff and, as applicable, licensed independent practitioners
  - Begin the assessment or determine the degree of compliance with relevant standards
  - Identify human resources issues requiring further exploration
- *Environment of Care Session.* This session will help the practice and the surveyor do the following:
  - Identify vulnerabilities and strengths in their processes
  - Begin to identify or determine the action(s) necessary to address any identified vulnerabilities
  - Begin the assessment or determine the practice's actual degree of compliance with relevant standards
  - Identify EC processes requiring further evaluation of implementation
  - Identify issues requiring further exploration
- *System Tracer Sessions.* System tracers are interactive sessions with surveyors and practice staff that explore the performance of important patient-related functions that cross the practice. Surveyors and practice staff will address critical risk points and provide education during the system tracer sessions. The following are the system tracers:
  - Medication Management
  - Infection Control
  - Data Use
- Life Safety Code® (LSC)† *Building Tour.* This session will help the practice and surveyor do the following:
  - Identify areas of concern in the practice's processes for designing buildings to *LSC* requirements
  - Identify areas of concern in the practice's processes for maintaining buildings to *LSC* requirements
  - Identify areas of concern in the practice's processes for identifying and resolving *LSC* problems
  - Determine the practice's degree of compliance with relevant *LSC* requirements
  - Identify or determine the action(s) necessary to address any identified *LSC* problems

---

* Please *see* the *Survey Activity Guide,* available by calling your account representative, for more detailed information on the survey process.

† *Life Safety Code®* is a registered trademark of the National Fire Protection Association, Quincy, MA.

- *Surveyor Report Preparation.* The surveyor(s) will use this time to compile, analyze, and organize the data he or she has collected throughout the survey into a report reflecting the practice's compliance with standards.
- *CEO Exit Briefing and Organization Exit Conference.* During this conference, the surveyor(s) will do the following:
  - Report the outcome of the survey and present the Accreditation Report if desired by the CEO or administrator
  - Review the issues of standards compliance that have been identified during the survey
  - Allow the practice a final on-site opportunity to question the survey findings or provide additional material regarding standards compliance
  - Gain agreement between the surveyor(s) and the practice regarding the survey findings, when possible
  - Review required follow-up actions, as applicable

Tracer Methodology

Individual Tracer Activity

The tracer methodology is the cornerstone of the new survey process. The individual tracer activity is an evaluation method conducted during an on-site survey designed to trace the care experiences that a patient has while at the practice. The tracer methodology is a way to analyze a practice's systems of providing care, treatment, and services using actual care recipients as the framework for assessing standards compliance. Surveyors use the following general criteria to select initial individual tracers:

- Patients in top CSGs and PFAs for that practice
- Patients related to system tracer topics (see the section "System Tracers" below), such as infection control or medication management
- Patients receiving complex services.

The typical patients selected for initial tracer activity will be those identified in the practice's PFP information as listed in the CSGs. Based on identified PFAs and CSGs, the surveyor will identify patient tracers and follows specific patients through the practice's processes. A surveyor will not only examine the individual components of a system but will also evaluate how the components of a system interact with each other. In other words, a surveyor will look at the care, treatment, and services provided by each unit and service, as well as how units and services work together. Surveyors may start where the patient is currently located. They then can move to where the patient first entered the practice's systems, an area of care provided to the patient that might be a priority for that practice, or to any areas in which the patient received care, treatment, or services. The order will vary. Along the way, surveyors will speak with health care staff members who actually provided the care to that tracer patient—or, if that staff member is not available, will speak with another staff member who provides the same type of care.

Based on the surveyor's findings, he or she may select similar patients to trace. The tracer methodology permits surveyors to "pull the threads" if there is a reason to believe that an issue needs further exploration.

System Tracer Activity

System tracers differ from individual tracers in that during individual tracers, the surveyor follows a specific patient through his or her course of care, evaluating all aspects of care. System tracers follow the flow of one specific system or process across the practice. During the system tracer sessions, surveyors evaluate the system/process, including the integration of related processes, and the coordination and communication among disciplines and departments in those processes.

A system tracer includes an interactive session (involving a surveyor and relevant staff members). Points of discussion in the interactive session include the following:

- The flow of the process across the practice, including identification and management of risk points, integration of key activities, and communication among staff/units involved in the process

- Strengths in the process and possible actions to be taken in areas needing improvement
- Issues requiring further exploration in other survey activities
- A baseline assessment of standards compliance
- Education by the surveyor, as appropriate

The three topics evaluated with system tracers are data use, infection control, and medication management, although the number of system tracers varies based on survey length.

Data Use. The data use system tracer focuses on how the practice collects, analyzes, interprets, and uses data to improve patient safety and care.

The Role of Staff in Tracer Methodology

To help the surveyor or survey team in the tracer methodology, staff will be instructed to provide the surveyor or survey team with a list of active patients including the patients' names, current locations in the practice, and diagnoses, as appropriate. Surveyors may request assistance from practice staff for selection of appropriate tracer patients. As surveyors move around a practice, they will ask to speak with the staff members who have been involved in the tracer patient's care, treatment, and services. If those staff members are not available, they will ask to speak to another staff member who would perform the same function(s) as the member who has cared for or is caring for the tracer patient. Although it is preferable to speak with the direct caregiver, it is not mandatory because the questions that are asked are questions that any caregiver should be able to answer in providing care to the patient being traced.

The Accreditation Decision Process

The goal of the new accreditation decision and reporting approach is to move practices away from focusing on achieving high scores to achieving and maintaining safe, high-quality systems of care, treatment, and services. During the decision process, there will be no numerical scores, and thus no scores will be disclosed to the practices or to the public. The lack of scores will facilitate shifting the focus from passing the exam to continuous operational improvement. For more information on the practice accreditation decision rules, see pages ACC-14–ACC-20.

Changes to the new accreditation decision process include the following:

- Scoring of EPs will be on the following scale: satisfactory compliance (2), partial compliance (1), insufficient compliance (0), not applicable (NA).
- Standards will be identified as compliant or not compliant.
- Type I recommendations are replaced with "Requirements for Improvement."
- The surveyor will leave an Accreditation Report of findings on site
- The Accreditation Report will be posted on the practice's secure, password-protected extranet Web site space approximately 48 hours after survey.
- If the surveyor(s) finds requirements for improvement, there is a 90-day window to submit an ESC report. Beginning July 1, 2005, the ESC will be due within 45 calendar days of the Accreditation Report being posted on the Jayco® extranet.

For more information on the new scoring process, see pages HM-6–HM-9 in the "How to Use This Manual" chapter. Information is also available in the "Understanding the Parts of This Chapter" section at the beginning of each functional chapter in this manual.

New Accreditation Decision Categories

The accreditation decision categories—effective January 2005—are as follows:

- **Accredited**—The organization is in compliance with all standards at the time of the on-site survey or has successfully addressed all requirements for improvement in an ESC within 90 days (45 days beginning July 1, 2005) following the survey.
- **Provisional Accreditation**—The organization fails to successfully address all requirements for improvement in an ESC report within 90 days (45 days beginning July 1, 2005) following the survey.
- **Conditional Accreditation**—The organization is not in substantial compliance with the standards, as usually evidenced by a count of the number of standards identified as not compliant at

the time of survey, which is between two and three standard deviations above the mean number of noncompliant standards for organizations in that accreditation program. The organization must remedy identified problem areas through preparation and submission of ESC and subsequently undergo an on-site, follow-up survey.

- **Preliminary Denial of Accreditation**—There is justification to deny accreditation to the organization as usually evidenced by a count of the number of noncompliant standards at the time of survey, which is at least three standard deviations above the mean number of standards identified as not compliant for organizations in that accreditation program. The decision is subject to appeal prior to the determination to deny accreditation; the appeal process may also result in a decision other than Denial of Accreditation.
- **Denial of Accreditation**—The organization has been denied accreditation. All review and appeal opportunities have been exhausted.
- **Preliminary Accreditation**—The organization demonstrates compliance with selected standards in the first of two surveys conducted under the Early Survey Policy Option 1.

Components of the New Decision Process

This section provides an overview of the Joint Commission's accreditation decision process.

The survey team will leave the accreditation decision report with the practice. The survey findings will be organized by the following:

- Primary PFAs
- Standard number
- Standard text
- Applicable program
- Surveyor findings
- EP text
- Secondary PFA (as applicable)

After the on-site survey, the survey team transmits the results described to the Joint Commission Central Office.

Reports that contain flagged items or the adverse decisions of Preliminary Denial of Accreditation or Conditional Accreditation will be processed by Central Office staff within 30 days of survey. At the time of survey, an item can be flagged for Central Office review by the surveyor if there is a question about interpreting or scoring a standard. When that review is completed, the results of the survey are then posted to the pratice's secure "Jayco"extranet site.

If a practice is in compliance with all standards at the time of the on-site survey, it is Accredited at that time. The official Accreditation Decision Categories for 2005 are listed in the preceding section. If the practice is not compliant with one or more standards at the time of survey, it is required to submit an ESC report within 90 days of the Accreditation Report being posted on the Jayco extranet (starting July 1, 2005, within 45 days). As part of its ESC submission, the practice is required to demonstrate "correction" of not compliant standards (that is, detail the action(s) that it has taken—not just planned—to come into compliance with a standard) or "clarification" (explanation as to why the practice believes that it was compliant with a standard judged to be not compliant at the time of survey). The practice's ESC must address compliance at the EP level and include an MOS, if applicable for each EP found to be partially (1) or insufficiently (0) compliant.

The practice's ESC submission is evaluated by Central Office staff using the same scoring guidelines used by the surveyors at the time of survey. The ESC will be considered acceptable when the practice has demonstrated resolution of all requirements for improvement. If the practice's first ESC submission is determined to be acceptable, its decision will be Accredited, and it will be required to submit the data for applicable MOS, if required, for each EP four months later.

If it is determined that a practice's ESC submission is unacceptable, its accreditation decision will be Provisional Accreditation, and it will be required to submit an acceptable ESC within 30 days. If the second ESC is determined to be acceptable, the practice's accreditation decision will remains Provisional Accreditation until it has submitted acceptable results of the corresponding MOS four months later. If the second ESC is determined to be unacceptable, a recommendation for Conditional Accreditation will be presented to the Accreditation Committee.

Central Office staff will evaluate the MOS results, when required. If it is determined that the MOS results are acceptable, no further action will be required of the practice, and if the practice had a Provisional Accreditation decision, its accreditation status will be changed to Accredited. If it is determined that a practice's MOS submission is unacceptable and its accreditation decision is not currently Provisional Accreditation, its accreditation status will be changed to Provisional Accreditation; the practice will be required to submit a second set of MOS results in another four months. If a practice whose accreditation decision is Provisional Accreditation because of an unacceptable first ESC submission, submits an unacceptable first measure of success submission, a recommendation for Conditional Accreditation will be presented to the Accreditation Committee.

If the practice's second MOS submission is determined to be acceptable, its accreditation decision will be changed to Accredited, and no further action will be required of the practice. If the second MOS submission is determined to be unacceptable, a recommendation for Conditional Accreditation will be presented to the Accreditation Committee. *See* Figures 2 and 3, page ACC-15, for a timeline of ESC and MOS submissions.

Sustained implementation of the practice's ESC, including the MOS, are subject to review in random unannounced surveys.

A final decision letter will be posted to the practice's secure, password-protected Web site when its ESC has been reviewed and an accreditation decision has been rendered. A Quality Report will then be posted on Quality Check® on the Joint Commission Web site.

2005 Accreditation Decision Rules for Office-Based Surgery Practices

The Joint Commission makes accreditation decisions by applying decision rules to the scored standards. Decision rules determine an accreditation decision that appropriately represents a practice's overall performance as measured by evidence of compliance with the applicable standards.

Since January 2001, "weighted" decision rules have been in place to limit the impact that the performance of small or secondary components of a complex organization may have on the practice's overall accreditation decision. These rules were established based on the rationale that the poor performance of a small component of a large complex organization, as determined by standards noncompliance, should not determine the accreditation decision of the entire practice. As such, the performance factors contributing to the overall accreditation decision for a complex organization were "weighted" to account for a proportional impact on overall care. The current "weighted" decision rules can be found on page APP-24 in the "Accreditation Policies and Procedures" chapter.

The decision rules for office-based surgery practices follow.

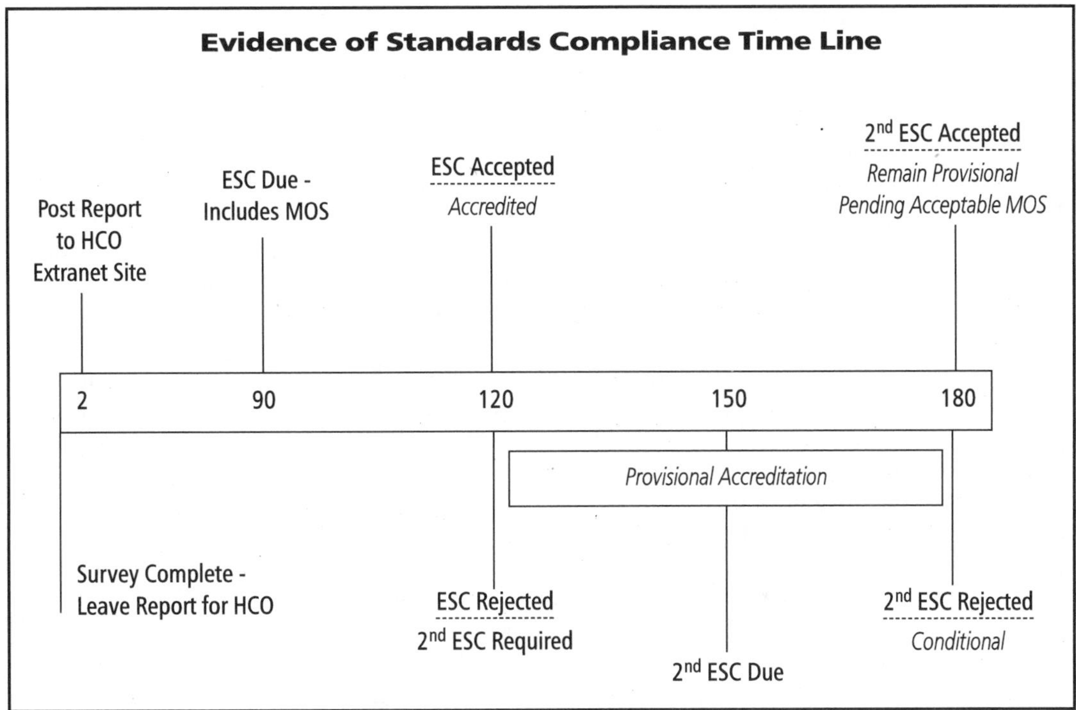

Figure 2. *This figure shows the ESC timeline.*

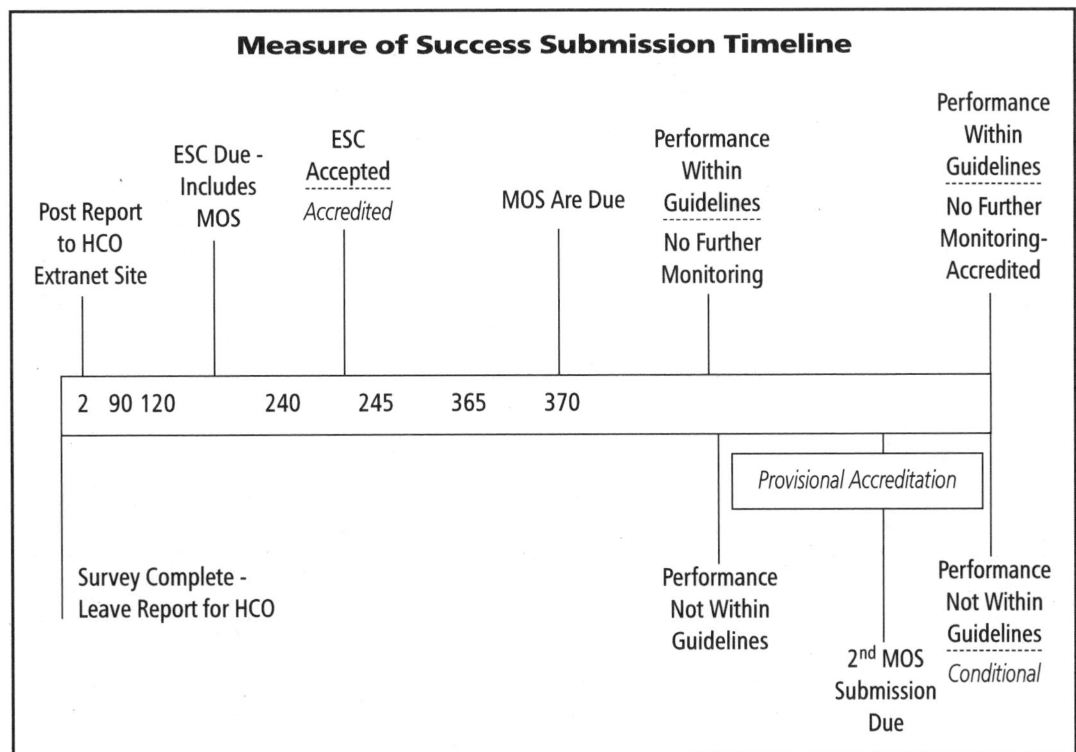

Figure 3. *This figure shows the MOS timeline.*

Preliminary Denial of Accreditation

Preliminary Denial of Accreditation is recommended when one or more of the following conditions are met:

PDA01 An immediate threat to patient/public health or safety exists within the practice.

PDA02 An individual who does not possess a license, registration, or certification is providing or has provided health care services in the practice that would, under applicable law or regulation, require such a license, registration, or certification and which placed the practice's patients at risk for a serious adverse outcome. (HR.1.20, HR.4.10)

PDA03 The Joint Commission is reasonably persuaded that the practice submitted falsified documents or misrepresented information in seeking to achieve or retain accreditation. Information provided by a practice and used by the Joint Commission for accreditation purposes must be accurate and truthful and may:

- Be provided verbally or in writing.
- Be obtained through direct observation or interview by Joint Commission surveyors.
- Be derived from documents supplied by the practice to the Joint Commission, including, but not limited to, a practice's root cause analysis in response to a sentinel event, or a practice's request for survey.
- Involve data or documents transmitted electronically to the Joint Commission, including, but not limited to, data or documents provided as part of the PPR process or the e-App process; or involve an attestation that a practice has not knowingly used Joint Commission full-time, part-time, or intermittent surveyors to provide any accreditation-related consulting services.

If accreditation is denied following implementation of this rule, the practice shall be prohibited from participating in the accreditation process for a period of one year unless the president of the Joint Commission, for good cause, waives all or a portion of this waiting period. (Accreditation Participation Requirement 10)

PDA04 The practice does not permit the performance of any survey by the Joint Commission. (Accreditation Participation Requirement 3)

PDA05 The practice has been conditionally accredited twice in a six-year period.

PDA06 The number of not compliant standards at the time of survey is three or more standard deviations above the mean.

PDA07 The practice does not possess a license(s) certificate(s), and/or permit(s), as, or when, required by applicable law and regulation, to provide the health care services for which the practice is seeking accreditation. (LD.1.30)

PDA08 The practice with a decision of Conditional Accreditation, as the result of a survey event, has failed to clear not compliant standards after two opportunities to do so (as the result of two failed ESC submissions, two failed MOS submissions, or a combination of one failed ESC submission and one failed MOS submission).

Note: *The opportunity is considered failed when the practice has not demonstrated resolution of all not compliant standards and continues to meet any of the decision rules requiring additional monitoring in the form of on-site follow-up, an ESC submission, or an MOS.*

PDA09 The result of a conditional follow-up survey is unacceptable.

Note: *The result of the conditional follow-up survey is considered unacceptable if the practice continues to meet any of the rules or an exception to the rules that caused a recommendation of Conditional Accreditation or Preliminary Denial of Accreditation.*

PDA10 A practice placed on Accreditation Watch fails to respond to a serious adverse event (sentinel event) within the defined time frame in a manner acceptable to the Joint Commission as specified in the Sentinel Event Policy.

Conditional Accreditation

Conditional Accreditation will be recommended when any one of the following conditions are met:

CON01 The number of not compliant standards at the time of survey is between two and three standard deviations above the mean.

CON02 An individual who does not possess a license, registration, or certification is providing or has provided health care services that would, under applicable law or regulation, require such a license, registration, or certification. (HR.1.20, HR.4.10)

Note: *Except as provided under rule PDA02.*

CON03 The practice has failed to clear not compliant standards after two opportunities to do so (as the result of two failed ESC submissions, two failed MOS submissions, or a combination of one failed ESC submission and one failed MOS submission).

Note: *The opportunity is considered failed* ***when the practice has not demonstrated resolution of all not compliant standards and*** *continues to* ***meet any of the decision rules*** *requiring additional monitoring in the form of on-site follow-up, an ESC Compliance submission, or an MOS submission.*

CON04 The practice has failed to implement or make sufficient progress toward the corrective actions described in an approved Statement of Conditions™ (SOC), Part 4, Plan for Improvement or has failed to implement or enforce applicable interim life safety measures.

Conditional Accreditation Follow-Up

CONF01 A conditional follow-up survey will be scheduled for practices with a Conditional Accreditation decision. The date of the survey will be established at the time the final Conditional Accreditation decision is awarded. (Conditional follow-up surveys typically occur at approximately six months from the date when the practice is notified of its official Conditional Accreditation decision.)

CONF02 A conditional accreditation follow-up survey will be scheduled for practices that have failed to clear not compliant standard(s) after two opportunities to do so (as the result of two failed ESC submissions, two failed MOS submissions, or a combination of one failed ESC submission and one failed MOS submission) and have received a Conditional Accreditation decision. The date of the survey will be established at the time the final Conditional Accreditation decision is awarded. (This survey will typically occur at approximately two to six months from the date when the practice is notified of its official Conditional Accreditation decision.)

Provisional Accreditation

Provisional Accreditation will be recommended when the following rules are met.

PROV01 The practice has failed to demonstrate resolution of all requirements for improvement at the time of its first ESC or first MOS submission. This accreditation decision results when at least one standard is scored not compliant and none of the rules for Preliminary Denial of Accreditation or Conditional Accreditation have been met.

Note 1: *Not compliant standards must be resolved within stipulated time frames (through an on-site MOS, submission of ESC, or submission of an MOS by the practice) to maintain accreditation.*

Note 2: *When a practice is placed in Provisional Accreditation as the result of a failed first ESC or failed first MOS submission, it remains in Provisional Accreditation until an MOS submission has been determined to be acceptable.*

One-Month Survey

A one-month survey will be scheduled when either of the following rules is met:

FOC01 A one-month survey will be conducted if the practice has failed to notify the Joint Commission of a request for a Public Information Interview (PII) that was submitted prior to a full accreditation survey. This one-month survey will include a PII with the individual(s) who had made the request and, as appropriate, will include an evaluation of any allegations that have implications for compliance with Joint Commission standards. (Accreditation Participation Requirement 9)

FOC02 A full laboratory survey will be conducted when a practice providing laboratory services cannot demonstrate to the Joint Commission that their laboratory accreditation decision is in good standing with a Joint Commission–recognized accreditor (such as CAP or COLA), or the accreditation is more than 30 months old.

Evidence of Standards Compliance (ESC)

An ESC report submitted by a surveyed practice within 45 days (90 days for the first 18 months of Shared Vision–New Pathways) of its survey, which details the action(s) that it took to bring itself into compliance with a standard or clarifies why the practice believes that it was in compliance with the standard for which it received a recommendation. An ESC report must address compliance at the EP level and include an MOS for all applicable EP corrections.

An ESC will be required when one or more of the following conditions exist:

ESC01 A practice has one or more standards scored not compliant at the time of a survey event.

ESC02 Failure to demonstrate continued compliance with all not compliant standards in the first ESC submission will result in Provisional Accreditation. The practice will be required to submit a second ESC within 30 days of the official notification that the first ESC was unacceptable.

Measure of Success (MOS)

MOS is a numerical or quantifiable measure, usually related to an audit that determines whether an action was effective and sustained, due four months after ESC approval.

An MOS will be required when one or more of the following conditions exist:

MOS01 A practice has submitted a successful ESC.

MOS02 Failure to demonstrate continued compliance with all not compliant standards in the first MOS submission will require the submission of a second MOS four months after official notification of the failure of the first MOS.

Note: *If the practice determines that the corrective action documented in its first ESC submission was not effective, the practice can elect to submit a second ESC that identifies new corrective action, rather than submitting a second MOS. In this case, the first MOS submission is considered failed. If this second ESC or the second MOS fails, the practice's decision is changed to Conditional or Preliminary Denial of Accreditation as appropriate.*

Four-month On-Site MOS Survey

A four-month on-site MOS survey is scheduled when the following condition is met:

MOS03 If a determination is made that on-site evaluation is required to assess compliance with the relevant standards, the assigned follow-up activity may be in the form of an on-site MOS survey rather than a MOS submission.

Preliminary Accreditation

PA01 Preliminary Accreditation will be recommended when a practice has demonstrated compliance with the selected standards used in the first of two surveys conducted under Early Survey Policy Option 1.

Note: *The first survey is conducted using a defined subset of applicable standards. The second survey is a full survey conducted approximately six months later to allow the practice sufficient time to demonstrate a track record of performance. Preliminary accreditation remains until the practice completes the second—that is initial—survey.*

Accreditation

A01 A practice's accreditation decision will be changed to Accredited when it is in compliance with all standards at the time of the on-site survey or has successfully addressed all requirements for improvement, in its first ESC submission.

Note: *Practices that are in Provisional Accreditation will have their accreditation decision changed to Accredited when their MOS submission has been determined to be acceptable.*

Administrative Rules

Changing the Time Frames for demonstrating compliance with not compliant standards:

ADM01 The follow-up time frames and nature of follow-up activity for demonstrating compliance with all not compliant standards can be changed from that stated in these decision rules when the severity of the issue requires a more timely response.

Note: *A senior member of Accreditation Operations management must approve changes to the follow-up time frames and/or nature of follow-up activity.*

Sentinel Event Policy Follow-Up

SE01 A practice that has experienced a sentinel event subject to review under the Sentinel Event Policy is required to complete a thorough and credible root cause analysis and action plan and submit them to the Joint Commission, or otherwise provide evidence of an acceptable response to the sentinel event, in a manner and time frame acceptable to the Joint Commission as specified in the Sentinel Event Policy.

SE02 Accreditation Watch will be assigned when a sentinel event subject to review by the Joint Commission has occurred, and the Joint Commission has reason to believe the practice has not completed a thorough and credible root cause analysis and action plan (or otherwise provide evidence of an acceptable response to the sentinel event) in a manner and time frame acceptable to the Joint Commission as specified in the Sentinel Event Policy.

SE03 A practice placed on Accreditation Watch is required to complete a thorough and credible root cause analysis and action plan and submit them to the Joint Commission (or otherwise provide evidence of an acceptable response to the sentinel event) in a manner and time frame acceptable to the Joint Commission as specified in the Sentinel Event Policy.

SE04 Follow-up will be scheduled, per the Sentinel Event Policy, when a sentinel event, subject to review under the Sentinel Event Policy, has occurred and the Joint Commission has determined that the practice has completed a thorough and credible root cause analysis and action plan. The purpose of the follow-up activity is to assess the implementation and effectiveness of the practice's action plan.

Accreditation Policies and Procedures

Overview

This chapter provides information on the Joint Commission's accreditation policies and procedures relevant to all health care organizations interested in Joint Commission accreditation, whether they are applying for the first time or on a renewal basis. These policies and procedures apply to all organizations either currently accredited by, or seeking accreditation by, the Joint Commission.

This chapter includes information about the continuous accreditation process and specific components that occur at various stages, including information office-based surgery practices need to know about the on-site survey and the Evidence of Standards Compliance (ESC) process. The timeline on page ACC-2 of the "The New Joint Commission Accreditation Process" chapter identifies all the stages of the continuous accreditation process and their timing in that process.

The chapter is organized into major sections reflecting the elements of the accreditation process. You will be able to locate the policies and procedures applicable to your practice according to where your practice is in the accreditation process or cycle. A practice must follow the policies and procedures described in this chapter to participate and continue to participate in the accreditation process. Failure to follow the policies and procedures described in this chapter can result in denial or withdrawal of accreditation.

Note: *The "Accreditation Participation Requirements" chapter includes specific requirements for accreditation participation. The requirements are existing policies within this "Accreditation Policies and Procedures" chapter and are currently effective for accreditation purposes. Cross-references to the Accreditation Participation Requirements (APRs) can be found in the applicable sections of this chapter.*

General Information

This section provides information relevant to a practice either applying for initial Joint Commission accreditation or seeking continued accreditation. Because this material is revised on a regular basis, all organizations are encouraged to review it.

Organizations Eligible for Accreditation

General Eligibility Requirements

Any health care organization may apply for Joint Commission accreditation under the standards in this manual* if all the following requirements are met:

- The practice is in the United States or its territories or, if outside the United States, is operated by the U.S. government, under a charter of the U.S. Congress, meeting the following criteria:
  - The nature of the health care practices in the applicant practice is compatible with that of Joint Commission standards and their elements of performance (EPs).
  - With the use of interpreters provided by the practice, as necessary, the surveyor(s) can effectively communicate with substantially all the practice's management and clinical personnel and at least half of the practice's patients, and can understand medical records and documents that relate to the practice's performance.
  - United States citizens make up at least 10% of the practice's patient population.
    or
  - A United States government agency contracts with the practice to provide services to United States citizens.
    or
  - United States citizens preferentially use the practice in that country.

* The Joint Commission will work with the organization to determine which standards from other accreditation manuals are applicable.

- The practice assesses and improves the quality of its services. This process includes a review of care by clinicians, when appropriate.
- The practice identifies the services it provides, indicating which services it provides directly, under contract, or through some other arrangement.
- The practice provides services addressed by the Joint Commission's standards.

Specific Eligibility Requirements for Survey Under the Office-Based Surgery Standards

Accreditation under the office-based surgery standards is intended for providers performing operative or invasive procedures in an office setting. Organizations seeking Medicare certification through Joint Commission accreditation must be surveyed under the *Comprehensive Accreditation Manual for Ambulatory Care* (*CAMAC*). Organizations that might recover more than one patient overnight at a time must be surveyed under the *CAMAC.* Hospital-based organizations are surveyed under the *Comprehensive Accreditation Manual for Hospitals* (*CAMH*).

Practices must meet all the following criteria to be eligible for accreditation under the office-based surgery standards:

- The organization or practice is composed of four or fewer surgeons* (physician, dentist, or podiatrist) performing operative or invasive procedures.† Multi-site office-based surgery (OBS) practices are still limited to four or fewer licensed independent practitioners.
- The organization or practice must be surgeon owned or operated, for example, a professional services corporation, private physician office, or small group practice.
- Invasive procedures are provided to patients. Practices only providing procedures such as excisions of skin lesions, moles, and warts and abscess drainage limited to the skin and subcutaneous tissue are not typically surveyed under office-based surgery standards.
- Local anesthesia, minimal sedation, conscious sedation, or general anesthesia are administered. (However, laser eye surgery using topical anesthesia does qualify.)

Office-based surgery practices that render four or more patients incapable of self-preservation at the same time are required to meet the provisions of the *Life Safety Code*® (*LSC*)‡.Practices may work with the Joint Commission to identify equivalencies to meet these requirements.

Scope of Accreditation Surveys

General Survey Categories

The Joint Commission surveys and accredits health care organizations using standards from one or more of the following manuals:

- *Accreditation Manual for Assisted Living*
- *Accreditation Manual for Critical Access Hospitals*
- *Accreditation Manual for Office-Based Surgery Practices*
- *Accreditation Manual for Preferred Provider Organizations*
- *Comprehensive Accreditation Manual for Ambulatory Care*
- *Comprehensive Accreditation Manual for Behavioral Health Care*
- *Comprehensive Accreditation Manual for Home Care* (includes standards for home health, personal/support care, hospice, home medical equipment, and pharmacies)
- *Comprehensive Accreditation Manual for Hospitals: The Official Handbook*
- *Comprehensive Accreditation Manual for Integrated Delivery Systems*
- *Comprehensive Accreditation Manual for Long Term Care* (includes standards for subacute care programs)
- *Comprehensive Accreditation Manual for Laboratory and Point-of-Care Testing*
- *Comprehensive Accreditation Manual for Managed Care Organizations*

---

* **Surgeon** Physician, dentist, or podiatrist who meets the definition of a licensed independent practitioner. A licensed independent practitioner, as defined by Joint Commission, is an individual permitted by law and by the organization to provide care, treatment, and services without direction or supervision, within the scope of the individual's license.

† **Invasive procedure** A procedure involving puncture or incision of the skin or insertion of an instrument or foreign material into the body (other than venipuncture and IV therapy). This includes laser surgery and other evolving technologies.

‡ *Life Safety Code*® is a registered trademark of the National Fire Protection Association, Quincy, MA.

In addition to standards, the Joint Commission also surveys office-based surgery practices using the standards' EPs, performance measurement data (when applicable), and APRs, including the Joint Commission National Patient Safety Goals (*see* the "Accreditation Participation Requirements" chapter). Used in conjunction with the standards, these items help assess an office-based surgery practice's performance.

Tailored Survey Policy

The Joint Commission survey, assuming satisfactory compliance, provides one accreditation award for all the office-based surgery practice's services, programs, and related organizations. Another service, program, or related entity (that is, component), whether providing services or through a contractual arrangement, is included in the survey of the applicant practice under the following circumstances:

- There are Joint Commission standards applicable to the component.
- The component is overseen and managed by the applicant practice through organizational and functional integration.

Note: *Any service, program, or related entity that is a component of an accreditation-eligible practice may independently seek accreditation if it can meet Joint Commission survey-eligibility requirements.*

Organizational and functional integration refers to the degree to which the component is overseen and managed by the applicant practice. An applicant practice refers both to a practice seeking accreditation and to a practice that is currently accredited. A component is a service, program, or related entity that delivers care or services and is eligible for survey under one of the Joint Commission's accreditation programs. These include the following:

- General, psychiatric, pediatric, critical access, surgical specialty, and rehabilitation hospitals
- Home care organizations, including those that provide home health services, personal care and support services, home infusion and other pharmacy services, long term care pharmacies and infusion centers, durable medical equipment services, and hospice services
- Nursing homes and other long term care facilities, including subacute care programs and dementia programs
- Assisted living residences that provide or coordinate personal services, 24-hour supervision and assistance (scheduled and unscheduled) activities, and health-related services
- Behavioral health care organizations, including those that provide mental health services, substance abuse treatment services, foster care services, and services for persons with developmental disabilities for individuals of various ages in various organized service settings
- Ambulatory care providers, including outpatient surgery facilities and office-based surgery, rehabilitation centers, sleep labs, imaging centers, group practices, and others
- Clinical laboratories

Organizational integration exists when the applicant practice's governing body, either directly or ultimately, controls budgetary and resource allocation decisions for the component or, where individual corporate entities are involved, there is greater than 50% common governing board membership for the applicant practice and on the board of the component.

Functional integration exists when the entity meets at least three of the following eight criteria:

1. The applicant practice and the component do the following:
   - Use the same process for determining membership of licensed independent practitioners in practitioner panels or medical or professional staff
     and/or
   - Have a common organized medical or professional staff for the applicant practice and the component
2. The applicant practice's human resources function hires and assigns staff at the component and has the authority to do the following:
   - Terminate staff at the component
   - Transfer or rotate staff between the applicant practice and the component
   - Conduct performance appraisals of the staff who work in the component

3. The applicant practice's policies and procedures are applicable to the component with few or no exceptions.
4. The applicant practice manages significant operations of the component; that is, the component has little or no management authority or autonomy independent of the applicant practice.
5. The component's patient records are integrated in the applicant practice's patient record system.
6. The applicant practice applies its performance improvement program to the component and has authority to implement actions intended to improve performance at the component.
7. The applicant practice bills for services provided by the component under the name of the applicant practice.
8. The applicant practice and/or the component portrays to the public that the component is part of the practice through the use of common names or logos; references on letterheads, brochures, telephone-book listings, or Web sites; or representations in other published materials.

The Joint Commission evaluates all health care services provided by the practice for which the Joint Commission has standards and makes one accreditation decision and survey report. A practice must be prepared to provide evidence of its compliance with each applicable standard. To gain accreditation, a practice must demonstrate overall compliance with the standards and their EPs.

Complex Organization Survey Process

The complex organization survey process is applied to organizations that are governed by the Tailored Survey Policy (*see* pages APP-3–APP-4). The Joint Commission conducts a complex organization survey based on the services provided by the organization, as reported in its application for accreditation. Because a complex organization survey process involves standards in more than one of the manuals listed in this chapter, the Joint Commission provides the organization with a copy of each of the manuals to be used in the survey before it is conducted.

Organizations that have acquired a new component are given a 12-month grace period from the time the component is acquired before the performance of that component is factored into the organization's overall accreditation decision. The newly acquired component is usually surveyed within six months of its acquisition as an extension survey; however, the accreditation decision rendered from the extension survey is in effect for the component *only* for 12 months following the acquisition before impacting the organization's overall accreditation decision.

Contracted Services

The Joint Commission evaluates the practice's assessment of the quality of services provided under contractual arrangements. The Joint Commission reserves the right to evaluate, as part of its survey, services provided by another practice or provider. It may survey performance issues between the contracted practice and the applicant practice, regardless of the accreditation decision of the contracted practice. The Joint Commission also surveys services provided on-site under contract.

Unannounced Surveys

Historically, Joint Commission regular, triennial surveys have been conducted in an announced fashion. Beginning in 2004 and through 2005, the Joint Commission will conduct unannounced triennial surveys on an optional and limited basis. The Joint Commission plans to transition to all unannounced surveys by 2006.

For practices that elect to undergo an unannounced survey in 2004 or 2005, the following policies are applicable:

- The survey can be scheduled anywhere between January and December in the year that the practice is due for survey.
- The practice will be invoiced immediately after the survey.
- The practice will be removed from the pool of practices eligible for a random unannounced survey throughout its accreditation cycle.
- Because the date of a practice's survey cannot be announced and, therefore, a public information interview will most often not be able to be scheduled during the practice's survey, the PII

policy no longer applies. In place of the PII policy, the practice is required to fulfill the new APR for continuous public involvement. This APR is effective in 2006 for all programs and immediately for the practices that voluntarily undergo unannounced surveys. Through this APR, the practice is required to demonstrate how it communicates with its public to provide information on how an individual can contact the Joint Commission with any patient safety or quality-of-care concerns.

All other policies and procedures in this chapter apply to practices undergoing an unannounced regular survey.

Early Survey Policy

The sidebar on page APP-6 highlights Early Survey Policy Options 1 and 2 described in the following sections. A practice wishing to be accredited for the first time by the Joint Commission may choose one of two Early Survey Policy Options described here. Under both Option 1 and Option 2, practices are required to undergo two surveys. However, the nature of the surveys and potential outcomes differ. The first survey under Option 1 is a more limited survey, while the first survey under Option 2 is a full accreditation survey. The Public Information Policy (pages APP-9–APP-12) applies to both Option 1 and Option 2.

Early Survey Policy Option 1 (Preliminary Accreditation)

A. Eligibility. This option is available to any practice that is currently not accredited except a practice that has been denied accreditation. Practices must declare during the application process that they wish to be surveyed under this option.

B. The First Survey. When a practice chooses Option 1, the Joint Commission conducts two on-site surveys. The Joint Commission can conduct the first survey as early as two months before the practice begins operating, provided the practice meets the following criteria:

- It is licensed or has a provisional license, according to applicable law and regulation.
- The building in which the services will be offered or from which the services will be coordinated is identified, constructed, and equipped to support such services.
- It has identified its chief executive officer or administrator, its director of clinical or medical services, and its nurse executive, if applicable.
- It has identified the date it will begin operations.

Generally, the first survey uses a limited set of standards and assesses only the practice's physical facilities, policies and procedures, plans, and related structural considerations. For this reason, the Early Survey Policy Option 1 has not been recognized by the Centers for Medicare & Medicaid Services (CMS) to meet the requirements for Medicare certification.

C. Preliminary Accreditation. The Joint Commission grants Preliminary Accreditation to a practice in satisfactory compliance with a subset of the standards and their EPs assessed in the first survey under Option 1. A practice not in satisfactory compliance must reapply and begin the accreditation process again. A practice that meets the decision rules for Conditional Accreditation will also be granted a Preliminary Accreditation decision.

The Preliminary Accreditation decision will include assignment of an additional survey against the full set of applicable standards within six months of the first survey. The survey will assess evidence of compliance with the standards for at least four months.

For a practice operating when the survey is conducted, the effective date for its Preliminary Accreditation decision is the day after the survey is conducted. For a practice not in operation, the effective date is the day after it begins operating. If the practice is not in operation at the time of survey, the practice must confirm in writing the date it begins operating.

A Preliminary Accreditation decision remains until the practice has completed a second, full survey or until the Joint Commission has withdrawn the Preliminary Accreditation. The Joint Commission may withdraw Preliminary Accreditation in the following situations:

- When a practice that was not providing services at the time of the first survey does not begin services when expected

APP

Early Survey Policy Options

Early Survey Policy Option 1

First Survey

- Conducted up to two months before opening
  - Licensed
  - Building identified, constructed, and equipped
  - CEO or administrator, director of clinical or medical services (medical director) identified
  - Identified opening date
- Limited set of standards (physical plant, policies and procedures)
- Outcome: Preliminary Accreditation

Second Survey

- Six months after first survey.
- Full survey.
- Outcome: Change in Preliminary Accreditation decision to Accredited, Provisional Accreditation, Conditional Accreditation, or Preliminary Denial of Accreditation. The effective date of the accreditation decision is the day after the *second* survey.

Early Survey Policy Option 2

First Survey

- Conducted when an organization:
  - Has been in operation (licensed) at least one month
  - Has cared for at least 10 patients
  - Has 1 patient in active treatment at time of survey
- Full survey; no track record
- Outcome: Accredited, Conditional Accreditation, or Preliminary Denial of Accreditation

Second Survey

- A full, follow-up survey four months after first survey.
- Addresses track record and standards compliance issues.
- Outcome: Accredited, Provisional Accreditation, Conditional Accreditation, or Preliminary Denial of Accreditation. The effective date of the accreditation decision is the day after the *first* survey.

Note: For all surveys, the organization incurs a fee. Contact the Department of Planning and Financial Affairs at 630/792-5115 for more information.

- If a practice does not meet the survey eligibility criteria (*see* pages APP-1–APP-2) or
- If a practice fails to accept the date of the second survey
- If a practice is found not in satisfactory compliance with the applicable standards and their EPs

In these cases, the practice must begin the accreditation process again.

D. The Second Survey. The second survey is a full accreditation survey. The Joint Commission conducts this survey at the following times:

- Approximately six months after the first survey
- At least four months after the practice has begun operating

The practice's accreditation status, based on survey results, changes to one of the following:

- Accredited
- Provisional Accreditation
- Conditional Accreditation
- Preliminary Denial of Accreditation
- Denial of Accreditation

The effective date of the accreditation decision is the day after the second survey. The practice's three-year accreditation cycle begins the day after the second survey is conducted, unless the Joint Commission reaches a decision to deny accreditation. Submission of ESC may be required based on the survey findings of the second survey under this option.

Early Survey Policy Option 2

A. Eligibility. Option 2 is available only to a practice that has the following:

- Never been surveyed by the Joint Commission or has been unaccredited by the Joint Commission for the previous two years
- Been in actual operation for at least one month
- Cared for at least 10 patients by the time of the first survey with at least 1 patient in active treatment at the time of survey
- Not been denied participation in the Medicare program as a result of a survey conducted by or action taken by CMS or the state on behalf of CMS

B. The First Survey. When a practice chooses Early Survey Policy Option 2, the Joint Commission will conduct an initial full accreditation survey. If the practice demonstrates satisfactory compliance with standards and their EPs in the first survey, it is granted an Accredited decision,* including a requirement for a second survey to assess for sufficient track record of compliance. This accreditation decision reflects the preliminary nature of the assessed performance. The effective date of the accreditation decision is the day after the first survey.

C. The Second Survey. The practice will undergo a full follow-up survey in four months to address track record achievements that could not be assessed during the first survey due to the limited time of operation. The full scope of applicable standards will be reviewed with particular attention being paid to the issue of sustained performance since the first survey. Practices surveyed under the Early Survey Policy are also required to complete an ESC after the first and second surveys, as appropriate.

Initial Surveys

Practices that are seeking Joint Commission accreditation for the first time or have been unaccredited by the Joint Commission during the previous two years are eligible for an initial survey. The full scope of applicable standards will be reviewed during the survey. The scoring of the standards will be based on a 4-month track record of compliance (prior to survey), rather than the 12-month track record of compliance required for triennial surveys.

Information Accuracy and Truthfulness Policy

The accuracy and veracity of relevant information, whether actually used in the accreditation process or not, are essential to the integrity of the Joint Commission's accreditation process. Information provided at any time by the practice must be accurate and truthful.† Such information may do the following:

- Be provided verbally or in writing.
- Be obtained through direct observation or interview by Joint Commission surveyors.
- Be derived from documents supplied by the practice to the Joint Commission including, but not limited to, a practice's root cause analysis in response to a sentinel event, a practice's request for accreditation, or a plan of correction submitted as part of the Conditional Accreditation process.
- Involve data or documents transmitted electronically to the Joint Commission, including, but not limited to, data or documents provided as part of the electronic application process.
  or
- Involve an attestation that a practice has not knowingly used Joint Commission full-time, part-time, or intermittent surveyors to provide any accreditation-related consulting services after January 1, 2004. Examples of such services include, but are not limited to, the following:
  - Helping a practice to meet Joint Commission standards
  - Conducting mock surveys for a practice
    or
  - Providing consultation to a practice to address Priority Focus Process (PFP) information

* Effective immediately.

† *See* APR 10 on page APR-4 in the "Accreditation Participation Requirements" chapter.

Falsification, as the term is used in this policy, applies to both commissions and omissions in sharing information with the Joint Commission.

Policy Requirements

The Joint Commission's Information Accuracy and Truthfulness Policy includes the following:

1. A practice must never provide the Joint Commission with falsified information relevant to the accreditation process. The Joint Commission construes any efforts to do so as a violation of the practice's obligation to engage in the accreditation process in good faith.
2. Falsification is defined for this policy as the fabrication, in whole or in part, and through commission or omission, of any information provided by an applicant or accredited practice to the Joint Commission. This includes, but is not limited to, any redrafting, reformatting, or content deletion of documents.
3. The practice may submit additional material that summarizes or otherwise explains original information submitted to the Joint Commission. These materials must be properly identified, dated, and accompanied by the original documents.
4. The Joint Commission conducts an evaluation when it has cause to believe that an accredited practice might have provided falsified information to the Joint Commission relevant to the accreditation process. Except as otherwise authorized by the president of the Joint Commission, the evaluation includes an unannounced on-site survey. This survey uses special protocols designed to address the alleged information falsification. It assesses the degree of actual practice compliance with the standards and their EPs that are the subject of the allegation, if appropriate.
5. The Joint Commission immediately takes action to deny accreditation or remove the accreditation award from an accredited practice whenever the Joint Commission is reasonably persuaded that the practice has provided falsified information. If nonmanagerial employees or contractors have undertaken the falsification and the practice's leadership takes no immediate action upon becoming aware of the falsification, or at least one individual in a supervisory or managerial position directs or participates in the falsification, the Joint Commission will act to declare Preliminary Denial of Accreditation or to remove the accreditation award from an accredited practice.
6. The Joint Commission notifies responsible federal and state government agencies of any practice subject to such action.
7. If a practice is denied accreditation because it provided falsified information, the Joint Commission prohibits it from participating in the accreditation process for a period of one year. The president of the Joint Commission, for good cause only, may waive all or a portion of this waiting period.

Good Faith Participation in Accreditation

The Joint Commission requires each practice seeking accreditation or reaccreditation to engage in the accreditation process in good faith. The Joint Commission may deny accreditation to any practice failing to participate in good faith in the accreditation process.

Certain categories of issues interfering with good faith participation can be described as follows:

- Deceiving the Joint Commission. Compliance with the Information Accuracy and Truthfulness Policy requires a commitment on the part of the accredited practice not to deceive the Joint Commission in any aspect of the accreditation process. The Joint Commission believes that appropriate preparation for an accreditation survey is a fully acceptable and positive practice, which helps improve the quality and safety of individual care. It is rare that such preparation would overstep the bounds of good faith activity to reach the level of deception. For example, to hire additional caregiving staff shortly before a survey for the express purpose of their presence during the survey, with the intent to terminate the employment of such caregivers promptly after survey, is an act of such deception.
- Deceiving the Public. Accredited practices are not acting in good faith if they mislead the public about the meaning and limitations of accreditation. Also, accredited practices must not inaccurately suggest to the public that their accreditation award applies to any unaccredited affiliated or otherwise related activities.

- Reprisals. The Joint Commission invites open communication from any accredited practice's staff and recipients of care, treatment, and services about any standards compliance or other issues relating to the accreditation process. A practice's good faith participation in the accreditation process would be questioned if the practice does the following:
  - Attempts to discourage such communication, for example, by taking disciplinary steps against an employee solely because that employee provides information to the Joint Commission
  - Threatens those who communicate with the Joint Commission with a defamation lawsuit based solely on what was said to the Joint Commission

    or
  - Allows the treatment or access to services of any individual or staff to be adversely impacted by his or her or a family member's communication with the Joint Commission
- Standards Compliance. If a practice's conduct reflects a lack of commitment to standards compliance, issues of good faith may be raised. For example, an intentional refusal to attempt to comply with a standard could suggest a cavalier view of the accreditation process.

The Good Faith Participation requirement applies continuously throughout the accreditation cycle.

Public Information Policy*

The Joint Commission is committed to making relevant and accurate information about surveyed health care organizations available to interested parties. Information regarding a health care organization's quality and safety of care helps organizations improve their services. This information can also help educate consumers and health care purchasers in making informed choices about health care. At the same time, it is important that confidentiality be maintained for certain information to encourage candor in the accreditation process.

Quality Reports

The Quality Report provides summary information about the provision of quality and safety at an accredited practice. Quality Reports are created at the practice level and are designed to provide national and state information that can be compared against other accredited practices and nonaccredited practices.

Joint Commission Quality Reports for each accredited practice include the following information:

- The date of the most recent triennial survey
- The accreditation decision based on the most recent triennial survey
- A practice's current accreditation decision
- The current decision of any component or program whose accreditation decision is different from that of the practice as a whole
- The date of the most recent evaluation activity for the practice, if any
- Standards areas with requirements for improvement
- Subsequent satisfaction of requirements for improvement and the date(s) of resolution for specific standards areas
- Subsequent new requirements for improvement and the date(s) assigned
- Services included in the accreditation survey
- Joint Commission policies or rules that lead to Preliminary Denial of Accreditation or Denial of Accreditation
- Disease-specific care certification(s) and the effective date of each certification
- The receipt of Special Quality Recognition Awards, as recognized by the Joint Commission's Board of Commissioners (for example, the Ernest A. Codman Awards, Magnet Status)
- Achievement of National Patient Safety Goals

Each accredited practice is afforded the opportunity to prepare a commentary of up to two pages regarding its Quality Report. The commentary accompanies any practice Quality Reports distributed by the Joint Commission, whether via hard copy or the Joint Commission's Web site.

* This policy meets the requirements of the Health Insurance Portability and Accountability Act of 1996 (HIPAA).

Each Quality Report released by the Joint Commission also includes appropriate background information.

The Joint Commission may also make information contained in Quality Reports available to other third-party providers of information. A practice's Quality Report may be obtained via the Customer Service Department or through Quality Check®, a directory on the Joint Commission's Web site (http://www.jcaho.org).

Performance measurement data will be included in Quality Reports when all the following conditions are met:

- Accredited practices are reporting data on standardized core measures.
- Performance measurement data have been integrated into the accreditation process.
- Sufficient data to assure statistical significance are available.
- Appropriate reporting formats have been developed and approved by the Board of Commissioners.

In addition, released data must satisfy the following requirements:

- The data are accompanied by an explanation of the following:
  - Source or derivation
  - Accuracy, reliability, and validity
  - Appropriate uses
  - Limitations and potential misuses

Information That Is Publicly Disclosed on Request

In addition to information provided in Quality Reports, the following information may be obtained by writing or calling the Joint Commission:

- A practice's accreditation history
- Survey fees paid by an accredited practice
- A practice's scheduled survey date(s) after the practice has been notified of the dates
- Applicable standards used for an accreditation survey
- For a complex survey, the organizational component(s) contributing to a Conditional Accreditation or Denial of Accreditation decision
- Requirements for improvements for which the Joint Commission had no or insufficient evidence of resolution when a practice withdrew from accreditation
- The standards areas for which the Joint Commission had no or insufficient evidence of resolution of requirements for improvement when a practice withdrew from accreditation
- As applicable, confirmation of the occurrence of a sentinel event at an accredited practice and the Joint Commission's intent to apply its Sentinel Event Policy to this occurrence

Release of Complaint-Related Information on Request

The Joint Commission addresses all complaints that pertain to patient safety or quality-of-care issues within the scope of Joint Commission standards. Complaints may be forwarded by CMS or other federal or state agencies having oversight responsibilities for health care organizations, or may be received directly from consumers, payers, or health care professionals.

The Joint Commission has a toll-free hotline to provide patients, their families, caregivers, and others with an opportunity to share concerns regarding quality-of-care issues at accredited health care organizations. The toll-free number is 800/994-6610 and is available 24 hours a day, seven days a week; however, staff members are available weekdays between 8:30 A.M. and 5:00 P.M. Central Standard Time to answer calls.

Upon request from any party, the Joint Commission releases the following aggregate information relating to complaints about an accredited practice for the three-year period prior to receipt of the request:

- The number of standards-related written complaints filed against an accredited practice that have met criteria for review
- The applicable standards areas involved in a specific complaint review

- The standards areas in which requirements for improvement were issued as a result of complaint evaluation activities
- When an unannounced or unscheduled survey is based on information derived from a complaint or public sources, the standards areas related to the complaint

The Joint Commission also provides the following information as appropriate to complainants regarding their complaints:

- Any determination that the complaint is not related to Joint Commission standards
- If the complaint is related to standards, the course of action to be taken regarding the complaint
- Whether the Joint Commission has decided to take action regarding a practice's accreditation decision following completion of the complaint investigation
- Any change in a practice's accreditation decision following completion of the complaint investigation

Release of Aggregate Performance Data

The Joint Commission reserves the right to publish or release aggregate performance data.

Data Release to Government Agencies*

The Joint Commission makes available to federal, state, local, or other government certification or licensing agencies specific accreditation-related information under the following circumstances:

- When the Joint Commission identifies a serious situation in a practice that might jeopardize the health or safety of patients or the public and immediately takes action to deny accreditation
- Upon request, when the request involves otherwise publicly available information

Additional information is made available when a practice is certified for participation in a federal or state program or licensed to operate by a state agency on the basis of its accreditation. The Joint Commission so advises the practice's chief executive officer and provides timely notice to local, state, and federal authorities having jurisdiction. The information available to government agencies includes the following:

- The official accreditation decision and any subsequent change in this decision or any designation, such as Accreditation Watch
- Complaint information requested by CMS or state agencies in accordance with deemed status or other recognition requirements, including the following:
  - Action taken on the complaint
  - The standards area(s) in which a requirement for improvement was issued as a result of the complaint evaluation
  - The status of the case
- Specific information when a practice is assigned a Conditional Accreditation, Preliminary Denial of Accreditation, or Denial of Accreditation decision, which includes the following:
  - All final requirements for improvement
  - A statement, if any, from the practice regarding its views on the validity of the Joint Commission survey findings
  - A copy of the approved plan of correction and the results of the plan of correction follow-up survey
- Notification of upcoming triennial or focused surveys and retrospective dates of other surveys conducted, such as random unannounced, other announced, or unannounced for-cause surveys

---

* Section 92, PL 96-499, the Omnibus Budget Reconciliation Act of 1980, requires that Medicare providers include, in all their contracts for services costing $10,000 or more in any 12-month period, a clause allowing the Secretary of the U.S. Department of Health and Human Services (DHHS), the U.S. Comptroller General, or their representatives to examine the contract and the contractor's books and records. The Joint Commission herein stipulates that if its charges to any such provider amount to $10,000 or more in any 12-month period, the contract or any agreement on which such charges are based and any of the Joint Commission's books, documents, and records that might be necessary to verify the extent and nature of Joint Commission costs will be available to the Secretary of DHHS, the Comptroller General, or any of their duly authorized representatives for four years after the survey. The same conditions apply to any related subcontracts the Joint Commission has if the payments under such subcontracts amount to $10,000 or more in any 12-month period.

- A copy of the Accreditation Report is included for the following:
  - CMS upon request respecting deemed status determinations
  - State agencies that have entered into specific information-sharing agreements that permit provider-authorized release of such reports to the state agency

Joint Commission Right to Clarify

The Joint Commission reserves the right to clarify information, even if the information involved would otherwise be considered confidential, when a practice disseminates inaccurate information regarding its accreditation.

Confidential Information

The Joint Commission keeps confidential the following information received or developed during the accreditation process:

- The Accreditation Report unless its submission is required by a government agency (*see* "Data Release to Government Agencies" on page APP-11)
- Information learned from the practice before, during, or following the accreditation survey, which is used to determine compliance with specific accreditation standards
- A practice's root cause analysis and related action plan prepared in response to a sentinel event or in response to other circumstances specified by the Joint Commission
- All other materials that might contribute to the accreditation decision
- Written staff analyses and Accreditation Committee minutes and agenda materials
- The algorithms used in the PFP
- The PFP information used in a practice's survey

This policy applies to all practices with an accreditation history, subject to any requirements of any applicable laws.

Survey Fees

The Joint Commission determines survey fees annually as needed to meet the cost of its operations. Surveyed practices are charged for all surveys with the exception of random unannounced surveys. The Joint Commission bases a practice's survey fees on several factors, including the volume and type of services provided, and the sites to be included in the practice's accreditation. Contact the Pricing Unit at the Joint Commission at 630/792-5115 for a fee schedule or more information on survey fees.

The survey fee is not finalized until the Joint Commission has received and reviewed the practice's application. The Joint Commission sends an invoice when it schedules a practice for survey. It asks the practice to pay the fees according to specified terms. The Joint Commission charges a practice the fee rate in effect at the time of survey. For an initial survey, a practice must send a nonrefundable processing fee with the e-App. The Joint Commission credits this payment toward the practice's total fee.

The Joint Commission offers practices two payment options. A practice can do one of the following:

- Pay the full survey fee upon receipt of the invoice, which is sent approximately 30 calendar days before the survey is scheduled
- Pay 50% of the fee upon receipt of the invoice and the remaining 50% within 60 calendar days after completion of the survey

A practice that did not pay its survey fee in full prior to issuance of the accreditation decision and report must remit the outstanding balance within 60 calendar days from receipt of the report. Failure to provide timely payment may result in the loss of accreditation. The Joint Commission notifies a practice with significant standards compliance problems of either a Conditional Accreditation or a Preliminary Denial of Accreditation decision as soon as possible, whether or not payment has been received.

Practices participating in optional, voluntary unannounced triennial surveys in 2004 and 2005 will be invoiced after their survey takes place.

Before the Survey

This section provides information on the steps leading to a full accreditation survey. These include the application process, the assignment of an account representative, the PFP, survey scheduling, the assignment of a survey team, policies regarding survey scheduling, postponements and delays, the notification of the public about a forthcoming Joint Commission survey, and the conduct of a PII. The accreditation timeline included on page ACC-2 is also a good reference for viewing the accreditation process as a whole. In accordance with the requirements of the Health Insurance Portability and Accountability Act of 1996 (HIPAA), a health care organization and the Joint Commission must have a signed Business Associate agreement before the practice's survey can begin.

A Practice's Extranet Site

A key feature of the Shared Visions–New Pathways initiative is increased use of technology in the accreditation process. The use of technology better enables the Joint Commission and accredited practices to communicate accreditation-related information in a more efficient and timely manner.

To fully use technology in the accreditation process, each practice will have a secured Web site on the Joint Commission's extranet—access to the site can only be accomplished through the use of the practice's password. This site will permit practices to complete their application electronically. In addition, approximately 48 hours following a practice's survey, the practice's Accreditation Report and its ESC report will be posted on the practice's Web site. Only the accredited practice will have access to this site when it is ready for the practice to complete.

Application for Accreditation

A practice begins the accreditation process by completing an application. An electronic version of the application for accreditation can be completed via the practice's extranet site. When a practice is due to complete its application, the Joint Commission electronically notifies the practice about how to access its application electronically. Likewise, when a practice notifies the Joint Commission that it wishes to become accredited, the Joint Commission provides the practice with information explaining how to access and complete its application on the extranet site.

Practices using this e-App will type data directly in the application and, when complete, will submit the application to the Joint Commission electronically. The application provides essential information about a practice, including ownership, demographics, and types and volume of services provided.

The application does the following:

- Describes the practice seeking accreditation
- Requires the practice to provide the Joint Commission with all official records and reports of public or publicly recognized licensing (for example, a state license), examining, reviewing, or planning bodies*
- Authorizes the Joint Commission to obtain any records and reports not possessed by the practice
- When accepted, establishes the terms of the relationship between the practice and the Joint Commission

For a practice that chooses not to complete its application via the extranet site, the practice may request a print copy of the application by contacting its account representative. If you do not know who your account representative is, please call 630/792-3007.

Except for unannounced surveys, the Joint Commission will notify the practice of the scheduled survey at least four weeks before the survey date. For information on receiving applications for resurvey, see "Continuing Accreditation" on page APP-26.

---

* *See* APR 1 on page APR-2 in the "Accreditation Participation Requirements" chapter.

Accuracy of the Application Information

The Joint Commission schedules surveys based on information provided in the practice's e-App. With the information provided, the Joint Commission determines the number of days required for a survey and the composition of the survey team.

Inaccurate or incomplete information in the e-App might necessitate an additional survey, which could delay the Joint Commission's survey report and accreditation decision. The practice might also incur additional survey charges.

Handling Changes Affecting the Application Information*

At any time during the accreditation process, if a practice undergoes a change that modifies the information reported in its e-App, the practice must notify the Joint Commission in writing within 30 calendar days after such change is made. Information that must be reported includes the following:

- A change in ownership
- A change in location
- A significant increase or decrease in the volume of services
- The addition of a new type of health service or site of care
- The acquisition of a new component
- The deletion of an existing health service or site of care or
- The deletion of an existing component

The Joint Commission may schedule an additional survey for a later date if its surveyor or survey team arrives at the practice and discovers that a change was not reported. The Joint Commission may also survey any unreported services and sites addressed by its standards. The Joint Commission makes the final accreditation decision for the practice only after surveying all or an appropriate sample of all services and sites provided by the practice for which the Joint Commission has standards. Information reported in the e-App is subject to the Joint Commission's Information Accuracy and Truthfulness (see pages APP-7–APP-9).

Role of the Account Representative

The Joint Commission assigns an account representative to each practice after receipt of the e-App. This person serves as the primary contact between the practice and the Joint Commission. He or she coordinates survey planning and covers policies, procedures, accreditation issues or services, and inquiries throughout the accreditation process. If your practice does not know who your account representative is, please call 630/792-3007.

Survey Scheduling and Postponements

Note: *This section is not applicable to practices that choose to have their survey conducted unannounced.*

Schedules for Surveys

The Joint Commission schedules surveys systematically and efficiently to keep survey fees to a minimum. Resurveys are scheduled within 45 calendar days before or after the practice's triennial due date. A practice's first full accreditation survey, an initial survey, must be scheduled within six months from the time the Joint Commission receives the practice's application.

Survey Postponement Policy

A postponement is a practice's request to alter an already scheduled survey date. A practice should direct a request for a postponement to its account representative. A request to postpone a survey may be granted if one or more of the following criteria are met:

- A natural disaster or other major unforeseen event has occurred that has totally or substantially disrupted operations.

* *See* APR 2 on page APR-2 in the "Accreditation Participation Requirements" chapter.

- The practice is involved in a major strike, has ceased admitting patients, and is transferring patients to other facilities or practices.
- Patients and/or the practice is being moved to a new building on the day or days of the survey.
- The Joint Commission has provided fewer than four weeks' advance notice to the practice (by telephone or in writing) of the survey date(s).

Note: *If a survey postponement is requested because of a natural disaster, strike, or movement to a new building, an on-site extension survey may be required if the practice is continuing to provide patient care services.*

A practice undergoing its first Joint Commission survey will be asked to specify on its application the month in which it wishes to be surveyed. Following the scheduling of the survey, the practice will be permitted to postpone its survey only if it meets the preceding criteria.

Fees for Postponements

In rare circumstances, the Joint Commission may, at its discretion, approve a request to postpone a survey for a practice not meeting any of the criteria described above. In such cases, the practice may be charged a fee to defray costs and may be required to undergo an extension survey. Please contact your account representative or the Pricing Unit at 630/792-5115.

Timeliness of Application and Deposits

The Joint Commission requires a practice to submit a new e-App if the practice does not accept a scheduled survey within six months. This ensures that the practice's information is current.

A nonrefundable, nontransferable survey deposit is required for initial surveys only. The Joint Commission applies the deposit to the practice's survey fee if a survey is conducted.

Forfeiture of Survey Deposit

A practice scheduled for an initial survey will forfeit its survey deposit if its survey is not conducted within six months of submission of its application. The practice must then reapply and submit a new survey deposit to begin the accreditation process again.

The Survey Agenda

The Joint Commission's account representative works with the practice to develop a tentative survey agenda based on survey task assignments required as part of the survey. A generic agenda template will be sent to all practices with a similar number of required survey days and similar survey teams. The draft of the tentative agenda is reviewed and revisions made, as appropriate.

Notifying the Public About a Joint Commission Survey

The Joint Commission evaluates all relevant information about a practice's compliance with applicable standards and intent statements. It therefore requires a practice to inform the public of a scheduled full survey and invite them to provide the surveyor or survey team with relevant information.* The practice must provide an opportunity for members of the public to participate in a PII during a full survey, including the second survey under Early Survey Policy Option 1 and both surveys under Early Survey Policy Option 2 (see pages APP-5–APP-7). A full survey refers to the survey of all components of a practice under all applicable standards and intent statements. The public includes, but is not limited to, the following:

- Patients and their families
- Patient advocates and advocacy groups
- Members of the community for whom services are provided
- Staff

Public Posting

* *See* APR 8 on pages APR-3–APR-4 in the "Accreditation Participation Requirements" chapter.

PUBLIC NOTICE

The Joint Commission on Accreditation of Healthcare Organizations will conduct an accreditation survey of

______________________________ on ______________________________

(Insert the name of your organization) *(Insert your survey dates)*

The purpose of the survey will be to evaluate the organization's compliance with nationally established Joint Commission standards. The survey results will be used to determine whether, and the conditions under which, accreditation should be awarded the organization.

Joint Commission standards deal with organization quality and safety-of-care issues and the safety of the environment in which care is provided. Anyone believing that he or she has pertinent and valid information about such matters may request a Public Information Interview with the Joint Commission's field representatives at the time of the survey. Information presented at the interview will be carefully evaluated for relevance to the accreditation process. Requests for a public information interview must be made in writing and should be sent to the Joint Commission no later than five working days before the survey begins. The request must also indicate the nature of the information to be provided at the interview. Such requests should be addressed to

Division of Accreditation Operations
Office of Quality Monitoring
Joint Commission on Accreditation of Healthcare Organizations
One Renaissance Boulevard
Oakbrook Terrace, IL 60181

Or
Faxed to 630/792-5636

Or
E-mailed to complaint@jcaho.org

The Joint Commission's Office of Quality Monitoring will acknowledge in writing or by telephone requests received 10 days before the survey begins. An Account Representative will contact the individual requesting the public information interview prior to survey, indicating the location, date, and time of the interview and the name of the surveyor who will conduct the interview.

This notice is posted in accordance with the Joint Commission's requirements and may not be removed before the survey is complete.

Date Posted:______________________

Figure 1. *This is a sample Public Notice form.*

The practice is responsible for making the PII process widely known and effective as a source of compliance information in the accreditation process. The Joint Commission requires a practice scheduled for full survey to post or make announcements of the following:

- The survey date
- The opportunity for a PII
- How to request an interview

In the event that all practice components are not surveyed at the same time, the requirement to announce the upcoming full survey applies at the time the primary program is surveyed.

To maximize participation, postings or announcements must be made throughout the practice, including components being surveyed at a different time, in a form consistent with one provided by the Joint Commission. See Figure 1, on this page, for an example of a Public Notice form. This example may be used by the practice, or the practice may design its own Public Notice form that conveys the same information as this example. A practice should post notices in staff eating areas, break rooms, on bulletin boards near major entrances, and in treatment areas. In addition, the practice must provide each staff person with a written announcement of the survey if such postings are not likely to be seen by all staff.

Advance Notice

The Joint Commission requires a practice scheduled for survey to post public notices at least 30 calendar days before the scheduled date. A practice receiving the scheduled date fewer than 30 calendar days before the survey date should post public notices promptly. Notices must remain posted until the survey is complete.

Informing the Public to Notify the Joint Commission Regarding Safety and Quality of Care Concerns

The practice must take reasonable steps to inform its community of the opportunity for PII during the full survey at least 30 calendar days before the survey. Steps include the following:

- Informing all advocacy groups (such as organized patient groups and unions) that have substantively communicated with the practice in the previous 12 months
- Reaching other members of the community through means such as a public service announcement on radio or television, a classified advertisement in a local newspaper, postings on the practice's Web site, or a notice in a community newsletter or other publication*
- Informing individuals who inquire about the survey of the survey date(s) and opportunity to participate

A practice opting to have its survey conducted on an unannounced basis is not required to comply with the requirements of this policy. Rather, the practice is required, by a new APR, to demonstrate how it informs its public(s) that they should notify the Joint Commission if they have issues concerning safety and quality of care in that practice on a continuous basis. The practice can demonstrate its compliance with this APR, by distributing information about the Joint Commission through including contact information in published materials such as admission brochures and/or posting this information on the practice's Web site.

Compliance with the Public Information Interview Policy

The surveyor(s) reviews the practice's compliance with the policy outlined in the preceding section. The team indicates at the exit conference whether it believes the practice has complied with the policy and reports on this to the Joint Commission. Failure to comply with the PII Policy ordinarily results in a recommendation, which needs to be addressed as part of the ESC process (see "Accreditation Decisions" on page APP-23). As a result, the Joint Commission may also conduct a postsurvey PII at the practice's expense, if requested.

In addition, the surveyor(s) conducting a postsurvey PII also conducts whatever follow-up survey he or she believes appropriate in view of the information obtained during the public information interview. A practice's subsequent failure to comply with the Joint Commission's PII Policy may result in loss or denial of its accreditation.

Conduct of the Public Information Interview

Handling Requests†

Individuals requesting a PII are to forward their requests and the nature of the information they will provide in writing to the Joint Commission. The practice must explain this process in its communications. To ensure participation, individuals are encouraged to forward written requests as soon as possible, and no later than five calendar days before the scheduled survey.

Sometimes an individual might make a written request for a PII directly to the practice. When this occurs, the practice must promptly forward it to the Office of Quality Monitoring at the Joint Commission. A practice receiving oral requests should instruct individuals to make the requests in writ-

* This type of notification must be published or broadcast at least once.

† *See* APR 9 on page APR-4 in the "Accreditation Participation Requirements" chapter.

ing and mail them to the Joint Commission. The practice should provide individuals needing assistance in doing this with the necessary support.

Scheduling Interviews

The practice must provide potential PII participants with sufficient advance notice. The Joint Commission acknowledges all PII requests to the individual participants. Prior to the survey, the Joint Commission schedules a time-limited PII to be conducted during the survey. The Joint Commission is responsible for notifying the individuals requesting PIIs of the interview's exact date, time, and place. The practice must try to alleviate any potential concerns about reprisals to individuals who participate in the interview process.

Interview Eligibility

Individuals whose written requests arrive late or who simply appear at the stated time, requesting the opportunity to be heard without a prior written request, are heard by a Joint Commission surveyor if time permits. Otherwise, the surveyor informs them that it is not possible to honor their requests and then offers them the opportunity to provide a subsequent written statement.

Individuals contacting the Joint Commission and stating an interest in supplying information anonymously are informed that they may provide written complaints through the Joint Commission's Office of Quality Monitoring at 800/994-6610. The Joint Commission will maintain confidentiality, as requested.

The Interview Process

The Joint Commission's survey team conducts the PII. A representative of the practice may attend, unless the individual requesting the PII asks that no representative from the practice be present. The Joint Commission will honor such requests. The interview will be conducted on the practice's premises, whether a representative from the practice is present or not.

The practice is expected to provide reasonable accommodations for all PIIs.

An interview consists of the orderly receipt of information, orally or in writing, within a set time limit. The interview is not a debate between an organization's representative and an interviewee. Surveyors may, however, ask clarifying questions.

In addition, surveyors will not debate with or convey conclusions to any interviewee. Rather, the Joint Commission considers the information gathered in the interview by the surveyor along with the surveyor's findings and recommendations during the survey process.

The On-Site Survey

This section includes information relevant to a practice that has applied for an accreditation survey and is ready for the survey process. It provides an overview of the survey process, including use of the PFP.

Priority Focus Process

The PFP guides the overall survey process, including planning and the on-site survey, by providing enhanced insight into and information about each practice before its survey. This focuses survey activities on practice-specific issues that are most relevant to safety and quality of care (referred to as priority focus areas [PFAs]). The PFP can be considered a process for standardizing the PFAs for review during survey.

As part of the PFP, an automated tool called the Priority Focus Tool (PFT) takes data gathered before the survey about a practice and, through the use of algorithms or sets of rules, transforms the data into information that guides the survey process. Examples of sources for the data may include, but are not limited to, the following:

- Data from a practice's application
- Complaint and sentinel event information
- A practice's previous survey results

For additional information on the PFP process, see "The New Joint Commission Accreditation Process" chapter.

The Survey Process in Brief

Overview

During an accreditation survey, the Joint Commission evaluates a practice's performance of functions and processes aimed at continuously improving patient outcomes. The survey process focuses on assessing performance of important patient-centered and practice functions that support the safety and quality of patient care and may include the conduct of a PII. This assessment is accomplished through evaluating a practice's compliance with the applicable standards in this manual based on the following:

- Tracing the care delivered to patients
- Verbal and written information provided to the Joint Commission
- On-site observations and interviews by Joint Commission surveyors
- Documents provided by the practice

The Joint Commission's accreditation process seeks to help practices identify and correct problems and improve the safety and quality of the, treatment, care, and services provided. In addition to evaluating continuous compliance with standards and their EPs, significant time is spent on education.

Beginning in 2006, all accreditation resurveys will be unannounced. Initial surveys will remain announced.

Surveys are designed to be individualized to each practice, to be consistent, and to support the practice's efforts to improve performance. The length of the survey is determined by the Joint Commission based on information supplied in the application describing practice size and scope of services.

Survey Agenda

The survey agenda will contain the following elements:

Opening Conference and Orientation to the Practice. The opening session of the survey process will be an opportunity for practice leaders and key staff to meet with the surveyor(s) and make any last-minute adjustments to the survey schedule or elements.

Leadership Conference. During the conference, surveyors will discuss with leaders (including nursing, performance improvement, and safety leadership) their roles in performance improvement and other key issues of practice operations, such as patient safety, review of National Patient Safety Goals, and PFP output related to clinical/service groups (CSGs) and clinical focus areas. Some practices may experience two Leadership Conferences, as necessary.

Visits to Care, Treatment, and Service Areas Guided by the PFP Using the Tracer Methodology. These two elements of the Joint Commission's survey process, PFP and tracer, allow surveyors to analyze the functioning of practice systems.

Tracer Methodology. One element driving this revised accreditation process is analysis of the practice's systems of providing care, treatment, and services using actual patients as the framework for assessing compliance with selected standards. This process, called tracer methodology, works with PFP to trace patients, using PFAs as a starting point, within the health care practice's systems. For more information on tracer methodology, *see* "The New Joint Commission Accreditation Process" chapter.

Systems Tracer Session. During this session, high-priority safety and quality of care issues on a systemwide basis are evaluated throughout the practice.

Closing Conference. The closing or exit conference will be devoted to a discussion of the surveyor's findings. At the completion of the survey, the surveyors will provide the practice's Accreditation Report before leaving the practice.

Scoring Compliance and Track Record Achievements

Accredited practices are expected to remain in continuous compliance with the standards and their EPs throughout their accreditation cycle. Standards will be judged "compliant" or "not compliant." EPs will be scored on the following scale:

0 Insufficient compliance
1 Partial compliance
2 Satisfactory compliance
NA Not applicable

For a complete discussion on the scoring methodology, *see* "The New Joint Commission Accreditation Process" chapter.

For practical purposes in conducting the survey, surveyors will ordinarily limit their evaluation of the practice's track record of compliance, which is 12 months for a triennial survey and 4 months prior to an initial survey.

Surveyors may evaluate compliance over a shorter or longer time frame depending on circumstances encountered during the survey. For example, the required time frame for full compliance with applicable standards and EPs for new services will not exceed the time the service has been in operation. In another example, certain activities that are conducted infrequently, such as biennial credentialing, may require evaluation over a longer interval to ensure an adequate sample size for valid assessment. For a triennial survey, a practice's track record will generally impact the scoring of standards according to the following:

Score 0 Fewer than 6 consecutive months before survey
Score 1 6 to 11 consecutive months before survey
Score 2 12 consecutive months or more before survey

During initial surveys, a practice's track record will generally impact the scoring of standards according to the following:

Score 0 Fewer than 2 consecutive months before survey
Score 1 2 to 3 consecutive months before survey
Score 2 4 consecutive months or more before survey

Feedback Sessions

Final scores about compliance are not reached until all required patient care settings have been visited and all survey activities have been conducted. However, surveyors will communicate their observations at the daily briefing, as requested by the practice. If the practice has additional information that would demonstrate compliance with a standard that the surveyor has indicated may be a recommendation, the practice should supply that information to the surveyor(s) as soon as possible.

Final On-Site Survey Activities

At the leadership closing conference, the survey team will present survey findings and a written Accreditation Report.

Immediate Threat to Life

The Joint Commission may consider for accreditation purposes a surveyor's finding that some aspect of a practice's operation is having or might potentially have a serious, adverse effect on patient health or safety, and that immediate action must be taken.

In these cases, surveyors will notify the practice's chief executive officer and Joint Commission's headquarters staff immediately if they identify any condition they believe poses a serious threat to public or patient health and safety. The president of the Joint Commission, or if the president is unavailable his or her designee, can then issue an expedited Preliminary Denial of Accreditation decision based on such notification. He or she will promptly inform the practice's chief executive officer and appropriate governmental authorities of this decision and the findings that led to this action. The Accreditation Committee of the Board of Commissioners will confirm or reverse the decision at its next meeting. The Accreditation Committee may take into consideration a practice's corrective actions or responses to a serious threat situation. The practice can provide information to demonstrate that the serious threat-to-life situation has been corrected prior to the Accreditation Committee's consideration of the Preliminary Denial of Accreditation decision.

In these situations, the corrective action will be considered when a single issue leads to the adverse finding and the practice demonstrates that it did the following:

- Took immediate action to completely remedy the situation
- Prepared a thorough and credible root cause analysis
- Adopted systems changes to prevent a future recurrence of the problem

Accreditation Reports

Following evaluation of the practice's performance of functions and processes, the survey team reviews the results of integrated individual findings. Then, with the use of laptop-based decision support software, the team produces the practice's Accreditation Report. The team leader meets with the practice's chief executive officer prior to the closing conference and provides him or her with a copy of the report. The CEO determines whether or not the preliminary report is distributed at the closing conference. The survey team uses the report contents in making its closing conference presentations.

Within approximately 48 hours of a survey, the practice's report of survey findings will be posted on the practice's secured extranet site. The report includes, as appropriate, a practice's strengths, requirements for improvement, and supplemental findings.

If a practice does not receive any recommendations, then the practice's accreditation decision will be rendered at the same time that the practice's Accreditation Report is available and will be effective the day after the completion of the survey. If a practice receives requirements for improvement, then the practice's accreditation decision will be rendered following the submission of an ESC report. The ESC report is due within 90 calendar days following the survey; however, the practice's accreditation decision will be retroactive to the day after the last day of the survey.* For practices that receive a notification that they will be recommended for either Conditional Accreditation or Preliminary Denial of Accreditation, their accreditation decisions will be rendered by the Joint Commission's Accreditation Committee. (*See* ACC-18.)

After the Survey

This section includes information relevant to a practice that recently has participated in an accreditation survey. Material includes information on the ESC process, the MOS process, the types of accreditation decisions, how to request review of Preliminary Denial of Accreditation decisions, how to appeal Denial of Accreditation decisions, and how to use and display an accreditation award.

Evidence of Standards Compliance Process

For every requirement for improvement cited in a practice's Accreditation Report, the practice must submit an ESC. The ESC report will be available for completion on the practice's extranet site at the same time the practice's Accreditation Report is posted, which is approximately 48 hours after the practice's survey.

The ESC report must detail the action(s) that the practice took to bring itself into compliance with a standard or clarify why the practice believes that it is in compliance with the standard in which it

* Beginning July 1, 2005, the ESC will be due within 45 days of survey.

Table 1. Types of Joint Commission Accreditation Decisions

The Joint Commission has six accreditation decision categories. Each decision and the conditions that lead to it are described below.

Accreditation Decision Category	Conditions That Lead to This Type of Decision
Accredited	The organization is in compliance with all standards at the time of the on-site survey or has successfully addressed all requirements for improvement in an Evidence of Standards Compliance within 90 days following the survey (45 days beginning July 1, 2005)
Provisional Accreditation	The organization fails to successfully address all requirements for improvement in an Evidence of Standards Compliance within 90 days following the survey (45 days beginning July 1, 2005)
Conditional Accreditation	The organization is not in substantial compliance with the standards, as usually evidenced by a count of the number of standards identified as not compliant at the time of survey which is between two and three standard deviations above the mean number of noncompliant standards for organizations in that accreditation program. The organization must remedy identified problem areas through preparation and submission of an ESC and subsequently undergo an on-site, follow-up survey.
Preliminary Denial of Accreditation	There is justification to deny accreditation to the organization as usually evidenced by a count of the number of noncompliant standards at the time of survey which is at least three standard deviations above the mean number of standards identified as not compliant for organizations in that accreditation program. The decision is subject to appeal prior to the determination to deny accreditation; the appeal process may also result in a decision other than Denial of Accreditation.
Denial of Accreditation	The organization has been denied accreditation. All review and appeal opportunities have been exhausted.
Preliminary Accreditation	The organization demonstrates compliance with selected standards in the first of two surveys conducted under Early Survey Policy Option 1.

received a requirement for improvement. An ESC must address compliance at the EP level and include an MOS, if applicable. An MOS is a numerical or quantifiable measure usually related to an audit that determines whether if an action is effective and sustained. (*See* Measure(s) of Success Report on APP-23.)

The ESC report is due within 90 calendar days* after a practice's survey. Following submission of the report, a practice will receive an accreditation decision. If a practice implements actions to address its requirements for improvement, the practice's accreditation decision will be Accredited. If a practice's ESC report does not address its requirements for improvement, then the practice's accreditation decision will be Provisional Accreditation.

Conditional Accreditation, Preliminary Denial of Accreditation, and the ESC Report

If a practice is notified that a recommendation will be made to the Joint Commission's Accreditation Committee for either Conditional Accreditation or Preliminary Denial of Accreditation, the practice will have an opportunity to provide information to clarify any of the recommendations cited in its Accreditation Report through its ESC report. This information will be provided to the Accreditation Committee.

Measure(s) of Success Report

A practice will be required to submit an MOS report within four months of submitting an acceptable ESC report. The MOS report demonstrates whether each MOS identified in the practice's ESC report was reached.

Accreditation Decisions

A practice's accreditation decision becomes official following submission of its ESC report, which is retroactive to the day after the last day of the survey, or, in the case of Conditional Accreditation or Preliminary Denial of Accreditation, on the date the Accreditation Committee makes a decision. When a practice's accreditation decision becomes official, it is publicly disclosable. There are six possible accreditation decisions, as follows:

1. Accredited
2. Provisional Accreditation
3. Conditional Accreditation
4. Preliminary Denial of Accreditation
5. Denial of Accreditation
6. Preliminary Accreditation

A practice's request to withdraw from the accreditation process after undergoing survey and before a final decision has been made does not terminate the decision-making process. The Joint Commission will issue a final accreditation decision.

Table 1 (page APP-22) provides a description of each category and the condition that lead to it.

Review and Appeal of Preliminary Denial of Accreditation or Denial of Accreditation Decisions

The appeal procedures are set forth in the "Review and Appeal Procedures" section of this chapter on pages APP-28–APP-35. Two additional procedures specific to Preliminary Denial of Accreditation and Denial of Accreditation decisions are listed here.

When a practice receives written notice from the Joint Commission that a recommendation of Preliminary Denial of Accreditation is proposed for submission to the Accreditation Committee, the practice has 10 calendar days from receipt of that notification to submit to the Joint Commission an ESC report, clarifying information that demonstrates that it was in fact in compliance with one or more standards in question at the time of survey. If after Joint Commission review of any submitted materials, the Preliminary Denial of Accreditation recommendation will still be made, the practice will have five business days from receipt of notification to submit a written response directly to the Accreditation Committee.

* Forty-five days beginning July 1, 2005.

Weighted Decision Rules

Recently, the Joint Commission has reevaluated how a complex organization's overall accreditation decision should be impacted by a component's decision involving threats to patient safety, instances in which inaccurate information is provided to the Joint Commission, or violation of other APRs.

As such, the Joint Commission has revised the weighted decision rules so that, when a secondary component of a complex organization meets rules of Conditional Accreditation or Preliminary Denial of Accreditation as a consequence of invoking the Immediate Threat to Life Policy or not complying with the Information Accuracy and Truthfulness Policy or APRs, that accreditation decision applies equally to the component and the complex organization of which the component is a part. See Table 2 on page APP-25 for more information on the weighted decision rules.

Award Display and Use

The Joint Commission provides each accredited practice with one certificate of accreditation per site. There is no charge for the initial certificate(s). Additional certificates may be purchased. Such requests should be sent to the Certificate Coordinator, Division of Accreditation Operations at the Joint Commission.

The certificate and all copies remain the Joint Commission's property. They must be returned if either of the following situations occur:

- The practice is issued a new certificate reflecting a name change.
  or
- The practice's accreditation status is changed, withdrawn, or denied, for any reason.

A practice accredited by the Joint Commission must be accurate in describing to the public the nature and meaning of its accreditation and its award.* When a practice receives an accreditation award, the Joint Commission sends the practice guidelines for characterizing the accreditation award.

Accreditation award certificates include language about educating patients and their families on how to contact the Joint Commission.

A practice may not engage in any false or misleading advertising of the accreditation award. Any such advertising may be grounds to deny accreditation. For example, a practice may not represent its accreditation as being awarded by any of the Joint Commission's corporate members. These include the American College of Physicians, the American College of Surgeons, the American Dental Association, the American Hospital Association, and the American Medical Association. The Joint Commission has permission to reprint the seals of its corporate members on the certificates of accreditation. However, these seals must not be reproduced or displayed separately from the certificate.

Any practice that materially misleads the public about any matter relating to its accreditation must undertake corrective advertising of a degree acceptable to the Joint Commission in the same medium in which the misrepresentation occurred. If a practice fails to undertake the required corrective advertising following the communication of false or misleading advertising about its accreditation status, the practice may be subject to loss of accreditation.

The Joint Commission's logo is a registered trademark. An accredited practice may use the logo if it follows the following guidelines:

- The logo must remain in the same proportional relationship as provided and should not be displayed any larger than a practice's own logo.
- The logo's format cannot be changed, the name may not be separated from the symbol, and it must be printed in the original color.
- Graphic devices such as seals, other words, or slogans cannot be added to the logo except for the words "Accredited by."

* *See* APR 11 on page APR-5 in the "Accreditation Participation Requirements" chapter.

Table 2. Weighted Decision Rules	
Primary Program	**Secondary Programs**
One program in a complex organization is to be identified as "primary" (this is not a change from the previous rule). If the primary program meets a rule for Provisional Accreditation, Conditional Accreditation, or Preliminary Denial of Accreditation, the overall decision for the organization will be Provisional Accreditation, Conditional Accreditation, or Preliminary Denial of Accreditation, respectively.	If one of the secondary programs meets a rule for Preliminary Denial of Accreditation, the overall decision for the organization will be Conditional Accreditation. If one of the secondary programs meets a rule for Conditional Accreditation, the overall decision for the organization will be Provisional Accreditation. If two or more of the secondary programs meet rules for Preliminary Denial of Accreditation, the overall decision for the organization will be Preliminary Denial of Accreditation. If two or more of the secondary programs meet rules for Conditional Accreditation, the overall decision for the organization will be Conditional Accreditation. If the primary or any secondary program meets a rule for Provisional Accreditation, the overall decision for the organization will be Provisional Accreditation.

These guidelines apply to logo use on all print materials, Internet Web pages, and promotional items, such as coffee mugs, T-shirts, and notepads. Contact the Department of Communications at the Joint Commission at 630/792-5631 for questions about using the Joint Commission logo.

Before the Next Survey

This section provides information relevant to practices between Joint Commission surveys. Material includes the duration of an accreditation award; the process for continuing accreditation; how to notify the Joint Commission in the event of organizational changes, including the opening or closing of a unit or services, addition or deletion of components, leadership changes, mergers, consolidations, and acquisitions; and unscheduled and unannounced for-cause surveys.

Re-entering the Accreditation Process

For a previously accredited practice to be designated as "new" and be subject to only a four-month track record period for demonstrating standards compliance, it must not have participated in the accreditation process during the previous 6 months. If a practice is re-entering the accreditation process before 6 months have passed, it must demonstrate a continuing 12-month track record of compliance with the standards.

Duration of Accreditation Award

An accreditation award is continuous until the practice has its next full survey, which is usually around three years unless revoked for cause or as otherwise outlined in this chapter. Accreditation is effective on the first day after the Joint Commission completes the practice's survey. A practice may request a full accreditation survey more frequently than once every three years. The Joint Commission will, at its discretion and in accordance with its mission, determine whether to honor the request. Such requests should be sent to the practice's account representative.

Continuous Compliance

The Joint Commission expects an accredited practice to be in continuous compliance with all applicable standards and EPs. It may ask a practice to supply, in writing, information about compliance with standards. It may also survey a practice at any time with or without notice in response to complaints, media coverage, or other information that raises questions about the adequacy of patient health and safety protections (see "Unscheduled and Unannounced For-Cause Surveys" on page APP-27). The Joint Commission might also conduct a survey if a practice fails to respond to a request for more information.

A practice's failure to permit a survey can be viewed by the Joint Commission as the practice no longer wanting to participate in the accreditation process. Therefore, the Joint Commission will begin proceedings to deny accreditation to the practice.*

Continuing Accreditation

The Joint Commission does not automatically renew a practice's accreditation. A practice seeking to continue its accreditation must reapply for accreditation, undergo a full accreditation survey, and be found in compliance with the standards and intent statements.

Accreditation Renewal Process

The Joint Commission will notify a practice approximately six to nine months before the practice's triennial accreditation due date that it needs to complete an application for a resurvey and provide information about how the application can be accessed, completed, and transmitted to the Joint Commission electronically via the practice's extranet site. The practice should call 630/792-5800 if it has not received such a notification four months before its accreditation due date.

Note: *Effective January 1, 2006, all triennial surveys will be conducted on an unannounced basis. As such, the accreditation renewal process will change. Please consult future issues of* Perspectives *or the next edition of this manual for more information on the anticipated changes.*

Generally, the Joint Commission conducts a triennial survey in the time period between 45 calendar days before the practice's three-year survey due date and 45 calendar days after the due date. The Joint Commission notifies the practice of the survey date at least four weeks before the survey. If there are any specific dates within the 45 calendar days before and after the due date range that would conflict with other practice activities, the practice should identify those dates in the application as dates to avoid.

Accreditation Decision During Triennial Survey

A practice's previous accreditation decision remains in effect until a decision is made either to accredit or to preliminarily deny accreditation to the practice.

Notification of Changes Made Between Surveys

Accreditation is neither automatically transferred nor continued if significant changes occur within the practice. When significant changes occur, the practice must notify the Joint Commission in writing not more than 30 calendar days after such change is made. The practice must also notify the Joint Commission in writing if it opens or closes any units or services.

Failure to provide timely notification to the Joint Commission of these changes may result in the loss of accreditation.

Mergers, Consolidations, and Acquisitions

In the case of a merger, consolidation, or acquisition, the Joint Commission may decide that the practice responsible for services must have a survey. Barring exceptional circumstances, the Joint Commission continues the accreditation of the practice undergoing the kind of changes described previously until it determines whether an extension survey is necessary.

Note: *When an accredited practice acquires another practice and an extension survey is conducted, the survey findings resulting from the extension survey would be maintained separately from, and would not be reflected in, the accreditation decision of the acquiring practice for 12 months following*

* *See* APR 3 on pages APR-2–APR-3 in the "Accreditation Participation Requirements" chapter.

the acquisition. After the 12-month period, any outstanding standards compliance problems in the acquired component(s) would be reflected in the accreditation decision of the acquiring practice.

Extension Surveys

An extension survey is conducted at an accredited practice or at a site that is owned and operated by the practice if the accredited practice's current accreditation is not due to expire for at least nine months and when at least one of the preceding conditions is met. The results of an extension survey may affect the practice's accreditation decision. An extension survey of the practice may be necessary if the practice has the following:

- Instituted a new service or program for which the Joint Commission has standards
- Changed ownership and there are a significant number of changes in the management and clinical staff or operating policies and procedures
- Offered at least 25% of its services at a new location or in a significantly altered physical plant
- Expanded its capacity to provide services by 25% or more as measured by patient volume, pieces of equipment, or other relevant measures
- Provided a more intensive level of service

  or
- Merged with, consolidated with, or acquired an unaccredited site, service, or program for which there are applicable Joint Commission standards and EPs

An extension survey may also occur with the following situations:

- The Joint Commission grants a practice's request to continue its current accreditation beyond the conclusion of the three-year cycle.*

  or
- A practice has merged, consolidated, or acquired an accredited practice whose accreditation expiration date is within three months of the merger, consolidation, or acquisition, while its own accreditation expiration date is at least nine months away.

Unscheduled and Unannounced "For-Cause" Surveys

The Joint Commission may perform either an unscheduled survey or an unannounced survey when it becomes aware of potentially serious standards compliance or patient care or safety issues, or it has other valid reasons for surveying in an accredited practice.†

Note: *The "for-cause" unscheduled or unannounced surveys should not be confused with "random unannounced" surveys, as described on page APP-28.*

Either type of survey can take place at any point in a practice's three-year accreditation cycle. The Joint Commission usually provides the practice with 24 to 48 hours' advance notice of an unscheduled survey. No preliminary report is generated after an unscheduled survey whether announced or unannounced.

Note: *Practices are charged for these surveys, regardless of the outcome. The cost of the survey can be obtained by calling the Pricing Unit at 630/792-5115. However, practices are not charged for random unannounced surveys. (For additional information on random unannounced surveys, see page APP-28).*

No advance notice is provided for unannounced surveys. Reasons for unannounced surveys include occurrence of any event or series of events in an accredited practice that creates the following significant situations:

- Concern that a continuing threat might exist to the safety or care of patients

  or
- Indication that the practice is not or has not been in compliance with the Joint Commission's Information Accuracy and Truthfulness Policy

---

* Such requests are granted only for unusual or compelling reasons.

† *See* APR 3 on pages APR-2–APR-3 in the "Accreditation Participation Requirements" chapter.

Such a survey can either include all the practice's services or only those areas where a serious concern exists.

Results of any unannounced or unscheduled surveys may generate follow-up activities and can affect a practice's current accreditation decision. The Joint Commission may deny accreditation if the practice does not allow the Joint Commission to conduct unscheduled or unannounced surveys.

Random Unannounced Surveys

The Joint Commission also conducts unannounced surveys on a 5% random sample of accredited practices. The survey is generally conducted 9–30 months following the accreditation date (that is, the date after the last day of the full survey). A practice receives no advance notice of the random unannounced survey. One surveyor conducts each such survey for one day. Practices are not charged for random unannounced surveys.

Note: *As part of the move toward all accreditation surveys be conducted on an unannounced basis in 2006, the Joint Commission will no longer conduct random unannounced surveys after January 1, 2006.*

During the random unannounced survey, the surveyor assesses both fixed and variable components, or performance areas. Fixed components are identified each year for practices based on the highest PFAs and selected National Patient Safety Goals. Fixed components are identified based on the degree of actual or perceived risk to the care of patients posed by noncompliance with standards related to these elements. Fixed components for each accreditation program are published in *Perspectives* and are listed on the Joint Commission Web site. Variable components are identified through the PFP. Presurvey information run through PFP identifies prioritized practice-specific PFAs to be evaluated. (*See* the "Priority Focus Process" section of this chapter on pages APP-18–APP-19 for more on presurvey information.) The surveyor may also expand the scope of the random unannounced survey based on findings at the time of the survey.

No random unannounced surveys will be conducted at a practice undergoing an unannounced triennial survey.

Review and Appeal Procedures

After any Preliminary Denial of Accreditation decision, a practice has the right to make a detailed presentation before a Review Hearing Panel. The Accreditation Committee will then review the findings of the Review Hearing Panel and either deny accreditation to the practice or select an appropriate alternative accreditation decision. The practice may appeal any decision of the Accreditation Committee to deny accreditation before the decision becomes the final decision of the Joint Commission.

The following outline details review and appeal procedures.

I. Evaluation by the Joint Commission Staff

A. Review and Determination by Joint Commission Staff. Following a triennial or other survey activity, the Joint Commission staff shall review survey findings, survey documents, and any other relevant materials or information received from any source. Except as provided in paragraphs I.B, I.C, and I.D, Joint Commission staff shall, in accordance with decision rules approved by the Accreditation Committee of the Board of Commissioners, do the following:

1. Determine or recommend to the Accreditation Committee that the practice be accredited, as described in paragraph VII of these procedures.
   or
2. Recommend to the Accreditation Committee that the practice be conditionally accredited.
   or
3. Determine that the practice be conditionally accredited if the practice does not submit ESC in accordance with paragraph I.B.I.a or I.B.I.b
   or

4. Recommend to the Accreditation Committee that the practice be preliminarily denied accreditation.
   or
5. Defer consideration while additional information regarding the practice's compliance status is reviewed by the Joint Commission staff.
   or
6. Determine or recommend to the Accreditation Committee that the practice be preliminarily accredited in accordance with the Early Survey Policy set forth on pages APP-5–APP-7.
   or
7. Recommend to the Accreditation Committee that the practice be initially denied Preliminary Accreditation in accordance with the Early Survey Policy set forth on pages APP-5–APP-7.

B. Determination to Recommend Conditional Accreditation Based on Full Triennial Surveys.

1. Notification to Practice of Areas of Noncompliance with Standards. In the case of full triennial surveys, if the Joint Commission staff, based on survey findings, survey documents, and any other relevant materials or information received from any source, determines to recommend that the practice be conditionally accredited, it will outline its findings and determination. The practice may do the following:
   a. Accept the findings and determination of the staff through submission of the ESC
      or
   b. Submit to the Joint Commission, through ESC, any clarification of its compliance with Joint Commission standards at the time of the survey that is not reflected in the Accreditation Report, along with an explanation of why such documentation was not available for review at the time of the survey.
2. Consideration of the Practice's Response. Joint Commission staff shall review the practice's submission of any additional information and shall, in accordance with decision rules approved by the Accreditation Committee, do the following:
   a. Recommend to the Accreditation Committee that the practice be conditionally accredited.
      or
   b. Recommend to the Accreditation Committee that the practice be preliminarily denied accreditation.
      or
   c. Recommend to the Accreditation Committee that the practice be accredited, as described in paragraph VII of these procedures.

C. Determination to Recommend That Accreditation Be Preliminarily Denied Based on Full Triennial or Other Survey Activity.

1. Notification to Practice of Areas of Noncompliance with Standards. In the case of full triennial surveys, if the Joint Commission staff, based on survey findings, survey documents, and any other relevant materials or information received from any source, determines, in accordance with decision rules approved by the Accreditation Committee, to recommend to the Accreditation Committee that the practice be preliminarily denied accreditation, it will outline its findings and determination. The practice may do the following:
   a. Accept the findings and determination of the staff through submission of the ESC
      or
   b. Submit to the Joint Commission, through the ESC, any clarification of its compliance with Joint Commission standards at the time of the survey that is not reflected in the Accreditation Report, along with an explanation of why such information was not available for review at the time of the survey.

2. Consideration of the Practice's Response. Joint Commission staff members shall review the practice's submission of any additional information and shall, in accordance with decision rules approved by the Accreditation Committee, do the following:
   a. Recommend to the Accreditation Committee that the practice be conditionally accredited.
   or
   b. Recommend to the Accreditation Committee that the practice be preliminarily denied accreditation.
   or
   c. Recommend to the Accreditation Committee that the practice be accredited, as described in paragraph VII of these procedures.

D. Decisions by the President of the Joint Commission. Notwithstanding anything outlined in paragraphs I.A—I.C.1 of these procedures to the contrary, if the findings of any survey identify any condition that poses a threat to public or resident safety, the president of the Joint Commission, or if the president is not available, a vice president of the Joint Commission designated by the president to do so, may promptly decide that the practice be immediately placed in Preliminary Denial of Accreditation. This action and the findings that led to this action shall be reported by telephone and in writing to the practice's chief executive officer and in writing to the authorities having jurisdiction. The president's or his or her designee's decision shall be promptly reviewed by the Accreditation Committee in accordance with paragraph II of these procedures.

II. Review by the Accreditation Committee

A. Scope of Review. The Accreditation Committee shall consider the Joint Commission president's, or the president's designee's, decision and the Joint Commission staff's report and recommendation and may review the survey findings, survey documents, any other relevant materials or information received from any source, including any additional information supplied by the practice in response to this information or, in the case of a Preliminary Denial of Accreditation decision by the president or his or her designee, information supplied by the practice regarding corrective actions taken in response to the identification of a serious threat to resident or public health or safety.

B. Decision. Following such consideration, the Accreditation Committee shall do the following:

1. Accredit the practice, as described in paragraph VII of these procedures.
2. Or conditionally accredit the practice.
3. Or preliminarily deny accreditation to the practice or confirm a decision by the president or his or her designee to preliminarily deny accreditation.
4. Or defer consideration while additional information regarding the practice's compliance status is gathered and reviewed by Joint Commission staff.
5. Or order a resurvey or partial resurvey of the practice and an evaluation of the results, to the extent appropriate, by the Joint Commission staff. Thereafter, Joint Commission staff shall transmit the report and recommendation to the Accreditation Committee for action, as provided in paragraph II.C of these procedures.
6. Or preliminarily accredit the practice.
7. Or initially deny Preliminary Accreditation to those practices that apply for Early Survey Policy Option 1.

C. Deferred Consideration. When the Accreditation Committee defers consideration pursuant to paragraph II.B.4 or II.B.5 of these procedures, Joint Commission staff shall review and report to the Accreditation Committee concerning the practice's compliance decision. The Accreditation Committee may order any resurvey or partial resurvey necessary to determine such a decision.

Following such consideration and review, the Accreditation Committee shall do the following:

1. Accredit the practice, as described in paragraph VII of these procedures.

2. Or conditionally accredit the practice.
3. Or preliminarily deny accreditation or confirm a decision of the president or his or her designee to preliminarily deny accreditation to the practice.
4. Or defer consideration while additional information regarding the practice's compliance status is gathered and reviewed by the Joint Commission staff.
5. Or order an additional resurvey or partial resurvey of the practice and an evaluation of the results, to the extent appropriate, by the Joint Commission staff. Thereafter, Joint Commission staff shall transmit the report and recommendations to the Accreditation Committee for action, as provided in paragraph II.C of these procedures.
6. Or preliminarily accredit the practice.
7. Or preliminarily deny Preliminary Accreditation to those practices applying under Early Survey Policy Option 1.

III. Conditional Accreditation

A. Survey to Determine Implementation of Evidence of Standards Compliance (ESC). Within approximately six months from the date the practice is notified of its Conditional Accreditation decision, the Joint Commission shall conduct a survey of the practice to determine the degree to which deficiencies have been corrected or improvements implemented, although the Joint Commission upon occasion may shorten that time period, as appropriate.

B. Review and Determination by Joint Commission Staff. Joint Commission staff shall review the survey findings, survey documents, and any other relevant materials or information received from any source. In accordance with decision rules approved by the Accreditation Committee, the Joint Commission staff shall do the following:

1. Determine or recommend to the Accreditation Committee that the practice be accredited, as described in paragraph VII of these procedures.
2. or recommend to the Accreditation Committee that the practice be preliminarily denied accreditation.
3. Or defer consideration while additional information regarding the practice's compliance status is gathered and reviewed by the Joint Commission staff. At the conclusion of this review, one of the recommendations outlined in paragraph III.D of these procedures shall be made to the Accreditation Committee.

C. Action by the Accreditation Committee. Following review of the recommendations of the Joint Commission staff, the Accreditation Committee shall do the following:

1. Accredit the practice, as described in paragraph VII of these procedures.
2. Or preliminarily deny accreditation to the practice.
3. Or defer consideration while additional information regarding the practice's compliance status is gathered and reviewed by the Joint Commission staff.
4. Or order a resurvey or partial resurvey of the practice and an evaluation of the results, to the extent appropriate, by the Joint Commission staff. Thereafter, Joint Commission staff shall transmit the report and recommendation to the Accreditation Committee for action, as provided in paragraph III.C of these procedures.

D. Charges to the Practice. The full costs of the Conditional Accreditation process shall be paid by the practice that receives Conditional Accreditation.

IV. Review Hearing Panels

A. Right to a Hearing Before a Review Hearing Panel. A practice that has been preliminarily denied accreditation* or Preliminary Accreditation pursuant to paragraph II.B.3, II.B.7, II.C.3, II.C.7, or III.C.2 of these procedures is entitled to a hearing in which to make a detailed presentation before a Review Hearing Panel if the Joint Commission receives the

* The Preliminary Denial of Accreditation decision, if subsequently changed to other than Denial of Accreditation, following review and action by the Accreditation Committee, is no longer disclosable as part of the organization's accreditation decision history.

practice's written request for the hearing within five business days after the practice receives the written notice of the Accreditation Committee's decision, including confirmation of a decision by the president, or his or her designee, to preliminarily deny accreditation, as provided in paragraph I.D of these procedures. A Review Hearing Panel shall be composed of two health care professionals who are not on the Accreditation Committee and one member of the Accreditation Committee who is familiar with the practice's decision.

B. Notice of the Time and Place of the Presentation Before a Review Hearing Panel. The presentation before the Review Hearing Panel shall be held at the Joint Commission's headquarters except when the president of the Joint Commission, or his or her designee, determines otherwise for good cause shown. At least 30 calendar days before the presentation, the Joint Commission shall send the practice written notice of the time and place of the hearing and copies of any supplemental materials or information received from any source that the practice does not already have and that may affect any accreditation decision. The notice shall advise the practice of the agenda to be followed and, if feasible, of the identity and professional qualifications of the panel members. At least 10 calendar days before the scheduled hearing date, the practice must submit to the Joint Commission any materials it wishes to be considered by the Review Hearing Panel.

C. Procedure for the Conduct of a Hearing. A Review Hearing Panel may proceed with only two of the three panel members present, provided one of them is the member of the Accreditation Committee. Representatives of the practice may make oral and written presentations and may be accompanied by legal counsel. Presentations or information concerning actions taken by the practice subsequent to the survey upon which the Preliminary Denial of Accreditation decision was based are not considered relevant to the validity of the decision. A Joint Commission surveyor who participated in the survey will ordinarily appear at the hearing.

D. Report of Review Hearing Panel. After a hearing has been completed, the Review Hearing Panel shall review the facts regarding the original Preliminary Denial of Accreditation decision. The panel will submit a written report of its findings on factual matters for consideration by the Accreditation Committee.

E. Charges to the Practice. The practice is charged a nominal fee for the conduct of a Review Hearing Panel.

V. Second Consideration by the Accreditation Committee

A. Scope of Review. The report of the Review Hearing Panel shall be considered by the Accreditation Committee.

B. Decision. Following such consideration, the Accreditation Committee shall do the following:

1. Accredit or preliminarily accredit the practice, as described in paragraph VII of these procedures.
   or
2. Conditionally accredit the practice.
   or
3. Deny accreditation to the practice.
   or
4. Defer consideration while additional information regarding the practice's compliance status is gathered and reviewed by Joint Commission staff.
   or
5. Order a resurvey or partial resurvey of the practice and an evaluation of the results, to the extent appropriate, by the Joint Commission staff.

VI. Review by the Board Appeal Review Committee

A. Review Request. A practice that has been denied accreditation or Preliminary Accreditation pursuant to paragraph V.B.3 of these procedures is entitled to request a review of the decision by the Board Appeal Review Committee if the Joint Commission receives the practice's request for review within five business days after the practice receives the written notice of the Accreditation Committee's decision. The Board Appeal Review Committee is composed of four members of the Board of Commissioners who are not members of the Accreditation Committee.

B. Notice of Time and Procedure for Review. The Joint Commission shall send the practice a copy of the report of the Review Hearing Panel at least 20 business days before the meeting of the Board Appeal Review Committee at which the practice's request for review will be considered. Two members of the Board Appeal Review Committee will constitute a quorum. This meeting will generally held by telephone conference, except when it is held in conjunction with meetings of the Board of Commissioners or other committee(s) of the Board of Commissioners. The practice must submit any materials that it wishes the Board Appeal Review Committee to consider at least 10 calendar days before the scheduled meeting date. The Board Appeal Review Committee shall review the decision of the Accreditation Committee, which considered the report of the Review Hearing Panel, and any written materials submitted by the practice, and shall do one of the following:

1. Deny accreditation or Preliminary Accreditation to the practice, after finding that there is substantial evidence to support the Accreditation Committee's decision.
   or
2. Make an independent evaluation of the Accreditation Committee's decision and then decide to conditionally accredit, preliminarily accredit, or accredit the practice, as described in paragraph VII of these procedures.
   The action taken by the Board Appeal Review Committee shall constitute the final accreditation decision of the Joint Commission.

C. Participation. No member of the Accreditation Committee or of the Review Hearing Panel who participated in an accreditation decision or review of findings on factual matters concerning an organization shall participate in any deliberations or vote of the Board Appeal Review Committee in its review of that accreditation decision or report of findings on factual matters. This provision shall not preclude any commissioner who participated in a review hearing as a member of the Review Hearing Panel from presenting and responding to questions about the report of that Review Hearing Panel to the Board Appeal Review Committee.

VII. Procedure Relating to Not Compliant Standards and Determination of Corrected Not Compliant Standards

A. A decision of the Joint Commission staff pursuant to paragraph I.A.1, I.B.2.c, or I.C.2.c of these procedures, of the Accreditation Committee pursuant to paragraph II.B.1, II.C.1, or III.C.1 of these procedures, or of a Board Appeal Review Committee, as provided in paragraph VI.B of these procedures, to accredit a practice may be made contingent upon satisfactory correction of not compliant standards or, when appropriate, upon compliance with interim life safety measures. The practice may be conditionally accredited or its accreditation may be withdrawn if it does not correct or document the correction of the specified not compliant standards within the time specified in the notice of the decision to the practice, or, when applicable, fails to demonstrate compliance with the interim life safety measures. Joint Commission staff, through the use of surveys or partial surveys or through other means, such as ESC and MOS, shall determine whether the practice has corrected the not compliant standards within the time provided or, when applicable, has demonstrated compliance with interim life safety measures, and shall report its findings to the practice. If the Joint Commission staff determines that the practice has not corrected the not compliant standards within the time provided or, when applicable, has not demonstrated compliance with interim life safety measures, the practice's status will change to Provisional Accreditation. The Joint Commission shall report its findings to the practice, and, after reviewing any comments of the practice, as appropriate and in accordance with decision rules approved by the Accreditation Committee, do the following:

1. Provide another opportunity to the practice to correct or document the correction of not compliant standards, as provided in any applicable decision rules approved by the Accreditation Committee.
   or
2. Determine or recommend that the practice be placed in Conditional Accreditation status with a conditional follow-up survey in approximately four months or other time as appropriate.
   or
3. Recommend to the Accreditation Committee that the practice be preliminarily denied accreditation, if certain not compliant standards, specified in decision rules approved by the Accreditation Committee, have not been corrected or the correction of which has not been documented after the specified number of opportunities given to the practice to do so, and, when applicable and as specified in decision rules approved by the Accreditation Committee, the practice has failed to demonstrate compliance with interim life safety measures.

B. If the Joint Commission staff determines to recommend to the Accreditation Committee that the practice be preliminarily denied accreditation in accordance with paragraph VII.A.3, or be conditionally accredited in accordance with VII.A.2, the staff shall submit its recommendation and any comments of the practice to the Accreditation Committee for action, as provided in paragraphs II.B.1 through II.B.7.

VIII. Final Accreditation Decision

A. The action taken by the Joint Commission staff shall constitute the final decision of the Joint Commission to do the following:

1. Accredit the practice, when taken pursuant to paragraph I.A.1, I.B.2.c, or I.C.2.c of these procedures.
   or
2. Conditionally accredit the practice, when taken pursuant to paragraph I.A.3 or VII.A.2 of these procedures.
   or
3. Preliminarily accredit the practice, when taken pursuant to paragraph I.A.6 of these procedures.

B. The action taken by the Accreditation Committee shall constitute the final decision of the Joint Commission to do the following:

1. Accredit the practice, when taken pursuant to paragraph II.B.1, II.C.1, or III.C.1 of these procedures.
   or
2. Conditionally accredit the practice, when taken pursuant to paragraph II.B.2 or II.C.2 of these procedures.
   or
3. Deny accreditation to the practice, when taken pursuant to paragraph II.B.3, II.C.3, III.C.2, or VII.B of these procedures, and the practice does not request the opportunity to make a presentation before a Review Hearing Panel pursuant to paragraph IV.A of these procedures.
   or
4. Preliminarily accredit the practice, when taken pursuant to paragraph II.B.6 of these procedures.
   or

5. Deny Preliminary Accreditation to the practice, when taken pursuant to paragraph II.B.7 of these procedures, and the practice applying for Early Survey Policy Option 1 or 2 does not request the opportunity to make a presentation before a Review Hearing Panel pursuant to paragraph IV.A of these procedures.

C. The action taken by the Board Appeal Review Committee shall constitute the final decision of the Joint Commission to do the following:

1. Accredit the practice, conditionally accredit the practice, or deny accreditation, when taken pursuant to paragraph VI.B of these procedures.

IX. Status of the Practice Pending a Final Decision and Effective Date of a Final Decision

A. The accreditation status of an accredited practice shall continue in effect pending any final accreditation decision.

B. A final decision to accredit, preliminarily accredit, or conditionally accredit a practice that follows an initial Accreditation Committee decision of Preliminary Denial of Accreditation pursuant to paragraph II.B shall be considered effective as of the first day after completion of the practice's survey from which the decision results.

C. A final decision to deny accreditation or Provisional Accreditation to a practice shall become effective as follows:

1. As of the date of the decision made by the Board Appeal Review Committee pursuant to paragraph VI.B of these procedures.
   or
2. At the expiration of the time during which a practice may, but does not, request a review by the Board Appeal Review Committee, pursuant to paragraph VI.A of these procedures.
   or
3. At the expiration of the time during which a practice may, but does not, request the opportunity to make a presentation before a Review Hearing Panel pursuant to paragraph IV.A of these procedures.
   or
4. On receipt by the Joint Commission, before a final decision, of notification from the practice that it withdraws its request for review of a Preliminary Denial of Accreditation decision before a Review Hearing Panel or its request for appeal of a Denial of Accreditation decision before the Board Appeal Review Committee.

X. Notice

Any notice required by these accreditation procedures to be given to a practice shall be addressed to the practice at its post office address as shown in Joint Commission records and shall be sent to the practice by certified letter as forwarded by a recognized package delivery service. Any notice required to be given to the Joint Commission by the practice shall be sent by the practice in the same manner and shall be addressed to the Office of the Executive Vice President for Accreditation Operations, Joint Commission on Accreditation of Health care Practices, One Renaissance Boulevard, Oakbrook Terrace, IL 60181.

Sentinel Events

I. Sentinel Events

In support of its mission to continuously improve the safety and quality of health care provided to the public, the Joint Commission reviews practices' activities in response to sentinel events in its accreditation process, including all full accreditation surveys and random unannounced surveys.

- A sentinel event is an unexpected occurrence involving death or serious physical or psychological injury, or the risk thereof. Serious injury specifically includes loss of limb or function. The phrase "or the risk thereof" includes any process variation for which a recurrence would carry a significant chance of a serious adverse outcome.
- Such events are called "sentinel" because they signal the need for immediate investigation and response.
- The terms "sentinel event" and "medical error" are not synonymous; not all sentinel events occur because of an error, and not all errors result in sentinel events.

SE

II. Goals of the Sentinel Event Policy

The policy has four goals:

1. To have a positive impact in improving patient care, treatment, and services and preventing sentinel events
2. To focus the attention of a practice that has experienced a sentinel event on understanding the causes that underlie the event, and on changing the practice's systems and processes to reduce the probability of such an event in the future
3. To increase the general knowledge about sentinel events, their causes, and strategies for prevention
4. To maintain the confidence of the public and accredited practices and practices in the accreditation process

III. Standards Relating to Sentinel Events

Standards

Each Joint Commission accreditation manual contains standards in the "Improving Practice Performance" (PI) chapter that relate specifically to the management of sentinel events. These standards are PI.1.10, PI.2.20, PI.2.30, and PI.3.10.

Practice-Specific Definition of Sentinel Event

The Improving Practice Performance standard, PI.2.30, requires each accredited practice to define "sentinel event" for its own purposes in establishing mechanisms to identify, report, and manage these events. While this definition must be consistent with the general definition of sentinel event as published by the Joint Commission, accredited practices have some latitude in setting more specific parameters to define "unexpected," "serious," and "the risk thereof." At a minimum, a practice's definition must include those events that are subject to review under the Sentinel Event Policy as defined in Section IV of this chapter.

Expectations Under the Standards for an Organization's Response to a Sentinel Event

Accredited practices are expected to identify and respond appropriately to all sentinel events (as defined by the practice in accordance with the preceding paragraph) occurring in the practice or associated with services that the practice provides, or provides for. Appropriate response includes conducting a timely, thorough, and credible root cause analysis; developing an action plan designed to implement improvements to reduce risk; implementing the improvements; and monitoring the effectiveness of those improvements.

Root Cause Analysis

Root cause analysis is a process for identifying the basic or causal factors that underlie variation in performance, including the occurrence or possible occurrence of a sentinel event. A root cause analysis focuses primarily on systems and processes, not on individual performance. It progresses from special causes* in clinical processes to common causes† in practice processes and identifies potential improvements in processes or systems that would tend to decrease the likelihood of such events in the future or determines, after analysis, that no such improvement opportunities exist.

Action Plan

The product of the root cause analysis is an action plan that identifies the strategies that the practice intends to implement to reduce the risk of similar events occurring in the future. The plan should address responsibility for implementation, oversight, pilot testing (as appropriate), timelines, and strategies for measuring the effectiveness of the actions.

Survey Process

When conducting an accreditation survey, the Joint Commission seeks to evaluate the practice's compliance with the applicable standards and to score those standards based on performance throughout the practice over time (for example, the preceding 12 months for a full accreditation survey). Surveyors are instructed not to seek out specific sentinel events beyond those already known to the Joint Commission.

If, in the course of conducting the usual survey activities, a sentinel event is identified, the surveyor will take the following steps:

- Inform the CEO that the event has been identified.
- Inform the CEO that the event will be reported to the Joint Commission for further review and follow-up under the provisions of the Sentinel Event Policy.

During the on-site survey, the surveyor(s) will assess the practice's compliance with sentinel event–related standards in the following ways:

- By reviewing the practice's process for responding to a sentinel event.
- By interviewing the practice's leaders and staff about their expectations and responsibilities for identifying, reporting, and responding to sentinel events.
- By Asking for an example of a root cause analysis that has been conducted in the past year to assess the adequacy of the practice's process for responding to a sentinel event. Additional examples may be reviewed if needed to more fully assess the practice's understanding of, and ability to conduct, root cause analyses. In selecting an example, the practice may choose a *closed case* or a near miss‡ to demonstrate its process for responding to a sentinel event.

---

* **Special cause** is a factor that intermittently and unpredictably induces variation over and above what is inherent in the system. It often appears as an extreme point (such as a point beyond the control limits on a control chart) or some specific, identifiable pattern in data.

† **Common cause** is a factor that results from variation inherent in the process or system. The risk of a common cause can be reduced by redesigning the process or system.

‡ **Near miss** Used to describe any process variation that did not affect an outcome but for which a recurrence carries a significant chance of a serious adverse outcome. Such a near miss falls within the scope of the definition of a sentinel event but outside the scope of those sentinel events that are subject to review by the Joint Commission under its Sentinel Event Policy.

SE

IV. Reviewable Sentinel Events

Definition of Occurrences That Are Subject to Review by the Joint Commission Under the Sentinel Event Policy

The definition of a reviewable sentinel event takes into account a wide array of occurrences applicable to a wide variety of health care organizations. Any or all occurrences may apply to a particular type of health care organization. Thus, not all the following occurrences may apply to your particular practice. The subset of sentinel events that is subject to review by the Joint Commission includes any occurrence that meets any of the following criteria:

- The event has resulted in an unanticipated death or major permanent loss of function, not related to the natural course of the patient's illness or underlying condition.*†
  or
- The event is one of the following (even if the outcome was not death or major permanent loss of function unrelated to the natural course of the patient's illness or underlying condition):
  - Suicide of a patient in a setting where the patient receives around-the-clock care, treatment, and services (for example, hospital, residential treatment center, crisis stabilization center)
  - Unanticipated death of a full-term infant
  - Infant abduction or discharge to the wrong family
  - Rape‡
  - Hemolytic transfusion reaction involving administration of blood or blood products having major blood group incompatibilities
  - Surgery on the wrong patient or wrong body part§

How the Joint Commission Becomes Aware of a Sentinel Event

Each practice is encouraged, but not required, to report to the Joint Commission any sentinel event meeting the preceding criteria for reviewable sentinel events. Alternatively, the Joint Commission may become aware of a sentinel event by some other means such as communication from a patient, a family member, an employee of the practice, a surveyor, or through the media.

Reasons for Reporting a Sentinel Event to the Joint Commission

Although self-reporting a sentinel event is not required and there is no difference in the expected response, time frames, or review procedures, whether the practice voluntarily reports the event or the Joint Commission becomes aware of the event by some other means, there are several advantages to the practice that self-reports a sentinel event:

---

* A distinction is made between an adverse outcome that is primarily related to the natural course of the resident's illness or underlying condition (not reviewed under the Sentinel Event Policy) and a death or major permanent loss of function that is associated with the treatment (including "recognized complications") or lack of treatment of that condition, or otherwise not clearly and primarily related to the natural course of the patient's illness or underlying condition (reviewable). In indeterminate cases, the event will be presumed reviewable and the practice's response will be reviewed under the Sentinel Event Policy according to the prescribed procedures and time frames without delay for additional information such as autopsy results.

† "Major permanent loss of function" means sensory, motor, physiologic, or intellectual impairment not present on admission requiring continued treatment or life-style change. When "major permanent loss of function" cannot be immediately determined, applicability of the policy is not established until either the patient is discharged with continued major loss of function, or two weeks have elapsed with persistent major loss of function, whichever occurs first.

‡ *Rape,* as a reviewable sentinel event, is defined as unconsented sexual contact involving a patient and another patient, staff member, or other perpetrator while being treated or on the premises of the health care organization, including oral, vaginal, or anal penetration or fondling of the patient's sex organ(s) by another individual's hand, sex organ, or object. One or more of the following must be present to determine reviewability:

- Any staff-witnessed sexual contact as described previously
- Sufficient clinical evidence obtained by the organization to support allegations of unconsented sexual contact
- Admission by the perpetrator that sexual contact, as described previously, occurred on the premises

§ All events of surgery on the wrong patient or wrong body part are reviewable under the policy, regardless of the magnitude of the procedure or the outcome.

SE

Table 1. Examples of Reviewable and Nonreviewable Sentinel Events*

Examples of Sentinel Events That Are Reviewable Under the Joint Commission's Sentinel Event Policy

Any patient death, paralysis, coma, or other major permanent loss of function associated with a medication error.

Any suicide of a patient in a setting where the patient is housed around-the-clock, including suicides following elopement from such a setting.

Any elopement, that is unauthorized departure, of a patient from an around-the-clock care setting resulting in a temporally related death (suicide or homicide) or major permanent loss of function.

Any procedure on the wrong patient, wrong side of the body, or wrong organ.

Any intrapartum (related to the birth process) maternal death.

Any perinatal death unrelated to a congenital condition in an infant having a birth weight greater than 2,500 grams.

Assault, homicide, or other crime resulting in patient death or major permanent loss of function.

A patient fall that results in death or major permanent loss of function as a direct result of the injuries sustained in the fall.

Hemolytic transfusion reaction involving major blood group incompatibilities.

> **Note:** An adverse outcome that is *directly related* to the natural course of the patient's illness or underlying condition, for example, terminal illness present at the time of presentation, is **not** reportable **except** for suicide in, or following elopement from, a 24-hour care setting (*see* above).

Examples of Sentinel Events That Are Nonreviewable Under the Joint Commission's Sentinel Event Policy

Any "near miss."

Full return of limb or bodily function to the same level as prior to the adverse event by discharge or within two weeks of the initial loss of said function.

Any sentinel event that has not affected a recipient of care (patient, client, resident).

Medication errors that do not result in death or major permanent loss of function.

Suicide other than in an around-the-clock care setting or following elopement from such a setting.

A death or loss of function following a discharge against medical advice (AMA).

Unsuccessful suicide attempts.

Unintentionally retained foreign body without major permanent loss of function.

Minor degrees of hemolysis with no clinical sequelae.

> **Note:** In the context of its performance improvement activities, an organization may choose to conduct intensive assessment, for example, root cause analysis, for some nonreportable events. Please refer to the "Improving Practice Performance" chapter of this Joint Commission accreditation manual.

* **Note:** *This list may not apply to all settings.*

- Reporting the event enables the addition of the "lessons learned" from the event to be added to the Joint Commission's Sentinel Event Database, thereby contributing to the general knowledge about sentinel events and to the reduction of risk for such events in many other practices.
- Early reporting provides an opportunity for consultation with Joint Commission staff during the development of the root cause analysis and action plan.
- The practice's message to the public that it is doing everything possible to ensure that such an event will not happen again is strengthened by its acknowledged collaboration with the Joint Commission to understand how the event happened and what can be done to reduce the risk of such an event in the future.

Required Response to a Reviewable Sentinel Event

If the Joint Commission becomes aware (either through voluntary self-reporting or otherwise) of a sentinel event that meets the preceding criteria (see page SE-3) and the event has occurred in an accredited practice, the practice is expected to do the following:

- Prepare a thorough and credible root cause analysis and action plan within 45 calendar days of the event or of becoming aware of the event.
- Submit to the Joint Commission its root cause analysis and action plan, or otherwise provide for Joint Commission evaluation of its response to the sentinel event under an approved protocol (see Section VI), within 45 calendar days of the known occurrence of the event.

The Joint Commission will then determine whether the root cause analysis and action plan are acceptable. If the determination that an event is reviewable under the Sentinel Event Policy occurs more than 45 calendar days following the known occurrence of the event, the practice is allowed 15 calendar days for its response. If the practice fails to submit an acceptable root cause analysis within the 45 calendar days (or within 15 calendar days, if the 45 calendar days have already elapsed), it will be at risk for being placed on Accreditation Watch by the Accreditation Committee. A practice that experiences a sentinel event that does not meet the criteria for review under the Sentinel Event Policy is expected to complete a root cause analysis but does not need to submit it to the Joint Commission.

Review of Root Cause Analyses and Action Plans

A root cause analysis will be considered acceptable if it has the following characteristics:

- The analysis focuses primarily on systems and processes, not on individual performance.
- The analysis progresses from special causes in clinical processes to common causes in practice processes.
- The analysis repeatedly digs deeper by asking "Why?"; then, when answered, "Why?" again, and so on.
- The analysis identifies changes that could be made in systems and processes (either through redesign or development of new systems or processes) which would reduce the risk of such events occurring in the future.
- The analysis is thorough and credible.
- To be thorough, the root cause analysis must include the following:
  - A determination of the human and other factors most directly associated with the sentinel event and the process(es) and systems related to its occurrence
  - An analysis of the underlying systems and processes through a series of "Why?" questions to determine where redesign might reduce risk
  - An inquiry into all areas appropriate to the specific type of event as described in Table 2 (see page SE-7)
  - An identification of risk points and their potential contributions to this type of event
  - A determination of potential improvement in processes or systems that would tend to decrease the likelihood of such events in the future, or a determination, after analysis, that no such improvement opportunities exist
- To be credible, the root cause analysis must do the following:
  - Include participation by the leadership of the practice and by individuals most closely involved in the processes and systems under review

- Be internally consistent (that is, not contradict itself or leave obvious questions unanswered)
- Provide an explanation for all findings of "not applicable" or "no problem"
- Include consideration of any relevant literature
- An action plan will be considered acceptable if it does the following:
  - Identifies changes that can be implemented to reduce risk or formulates a rationale for not undertaking such changes
  - Identifies, in situations where improvement actions are planned, who is responsible for implementation, when the action will be implemented (including any pilot testing), and how the effectiveness of the actions will be evaluated

All root cause analyses and action plans will be considered and treated as confidential by the Joint Commission. A detailed listing of the minimum scope of root cause analysis for specific types of sentinel events is included in Table 2.

Accreditation Watch Designation

A practice is placed on Accreditation Watch when a reviewable sentinel event has occurred and has come to the Joint Commission's attention, and a thorough and credible root cause analysis of the sentinel event and action plan has not been completed in specified time frames. Although Accreditation Watch status is not an official accreditation category, it can be publicly disclosed by the Joint Commission.

Follow-Up Activities

After the Joint Commission has determined that a practice has conducted an acceptable root cause analysis and developed an acceptable action plan, the Joint Commission will notify it that the root cause analysis and action plan are acceptable and will assign an appropriate follow-up activity, typically an MOS or follow-up survey within six months.

V. The Sentinel Event Database

To achieve the third goal of the Sentinel Event Policy, "to increase the general knowledge about sentinel events, their causes, and strategies for prevention," the Joint Commission collects and analyzes data from the review of sentinel events, root cause analyses, action plans, and follow-up activities. These data and information form the content of the Joint Commission's Sentinel Event Database.

The Joint Commission is committed to developing and maintaining this Sentinel Event Database in a fashion that will protect the confidentiality of the practice, the caregiver, and the patient. Included in this database are three major categories of data elements:

1. Sentinel event data
2. Root cause data
3. Risk reduction data

Aggregate data relating to root causes and risk-reduction strategies for sentinel events that occur with significant frequency will form the basis for future error-prevention advice to practices through *Sentinel Event Alert* and other media. The Sentinel Event Database is also a major component of the evidence base for the National Patient Safety Goals.

VI. Procedures for Implementing the Sentinel Event Policy

Voluntary Reporting of Reviewable Sentinel Events to the Joint Commission

If a practice wishes to report an occurrence in the subset of sentinel events that are subject to review by the Joint Commission, the practice will be asked to complete a form to be sent to the Joint Commission's Office of Quality Monitoring by mail or by facsimile transmission (630/792-5636). Copies of the sentinel event reporting form may be obtained by calling the Sentinel Event Hotline at 630/792-3700 or the Office of Quality Monitoring at 630/792-5642. This form may also be accessed via the Joint Commission Web site at http://www.jcaho.org.

SE

Table 2. Minimum Scope of Root Cause Analysis for Specific Types of Sentinel Events

Detailed inquiry into these areas is expected when conducting a root cause analysis for the specified type of sentinel event. Inquiry into areas not checked (or listed) should be conducted as appropriate to the specific event under review.

	Suicide (24-Hour Care)	Medication Error	Procedural Complication	Wrong-Site Surgery	Treatment Delay	Restraint Death	Elopement Death	Assault/Rape/ Homicide	Transfusion Death	Infant Abduction
Behavioral assessment process*	X					X	X	X		
Physical assessment process †	X		X	X	X	X	X			
Patient identification process		X		X					X	
Patient observation procedures	X					X	X	X	X	
Care planning process	X		X			X	X			
Continuum of care	X				X	X				
Staffing levels	X	X	X	X	X	X	X	X	X	X
Orientation and training of staff	X	X	X	X	X	X	X	X	X	X
Competency assessment/ credentialing	X	X	X		X	X	X	X	X	X
Supervision of staff ‡		X	X		X	X			X	
Communication with patient/family	X			X	X	X	X			X
Communication among staff members	X	X	X	X	X	X			X	X
Availability of information	X	X	X	X	X	X			X	
Adequacy of technological support		X	X							
Equipment maintenance/ management		X	X			X				
Physical environment§	X	X	X				X	X	X	X
Security systems and processes	X						X	X		X
Control of medications: storage/access		X							X	
Labeling of medications		X							X	

* Includes the process for assessing patient's risk to self (and to others, in cases of assault, rape, or homicide where a patient is the assailant).

† Includes search for contraband.

‡ Includes supervision of physicians in training.

§ Includes furnishings; hardware (for example, bars, hooks, rods); lighting; distractions.

Reviewable Sentinel Events That Are Not Reported by the Organization

If the Joint Commission becomes aware of a sentinel event subject to review under the Sentinel Event Policy that was not reported to the Joint Commission by the practice, the CEO of the practice is contacted, and a preliminary assessment of the sentinel event is made. An event that occurred more than one year before the date the Joint Commission became aware of the event will not, in most cases, reviewed under the Sentinel Event Policy. In such a case, a written response will be requested from the practice, including a summary of processes in place to prevent similar occurrences.

Determination That a Sentinel Event Is Reviewable Under the Sentinel Event Policy

Based on available factual information received about the event, Joint Commission staff will apply the preceding definition (page SE-3) to determine whether the event is reviewable under the Sentinel Event Policy. Challenges to a determination that an event is reviewable will be resolved through consultation with senior staff in the Division of Accreditation Operations.

Initial On-Site Review of a Sentinel Event

An initial on-site review of a sentinel event will usually not be conducted unless it is determined that there is a potential ongoing threat to patient health or safety or potentially significant noncompliance with Joint Commission standards. If an on-site ("for-cause") review is conducted, the practice will be billed an appropriate amount based on the established fee schedule to cover the costs of conducting such a survey.

Disclosable Information

If the Joint Commission receives an inquiry about the accreditation status of a practice that has experienced a reviewable sentinel event, the practice's accreditation status is reported in the usual manner without making reference to the sentinel event. If the inquirer specifically references the specific sentinel event, the Joint Commission acknowledges that it is aware of the event and currently is working or has worked with the practice through the sentinel event review process.

Initiation of Accreditation Watch

If the Joint Commission becomes aware that a practice has experienced a reviewable sentinel event, but the practice fails to submit or otherwise make available an acceptable root cause analysis and action plan, or otherwise provide for Joint Commission evaluation of its response to the sentinel event under an approved protocol, within 45 calendar days of the event, or of its becoming aware of the event, or within 15 calendar days if the determination that the event is reviewable under the Sentinel Event Policy occurs more than 45 calendar days following the known occurrence of the event, unless Joint Commission staff for good reason has agreed to a short extension of time, a recommendation will be made to the Accreditation Committee to place the practice on Accreditation Watch. If the Accreditation Committee places the practice on Accreditation Watch, the practice will then be permitted an additional 15 calendar days to submit an acceptable root cause analysis and action plan, or otherwise provide for Joint Commission evaluation of its response to the sentinel event under an approved protocol.

The practice will be offered advisory assistance in performing a root cause analysis of the event.

Accreditation Watch status is considered publicly disclosable information.

In all cases of a practice refusing to permit review of information regarding a reviewable sentinel event in accordance with the Sentinel Event Policy and its approved protocols, the initial response by the Joint Commission is assignment of Accreditation Watch. Continued refusal may result in loss of accreditation.

Submission of Root Cause Analysis and Action Plan

A practice that experiences a sentinel event subject to the Sentinel Event Policy is asked to submit two documents (in addition to the sentinel event reporting form discussed on page SE-6):

(1) the complete root cause analysis, including its findings; and (2) the resulting action plan that describes the practice's risk reduction strategies and a strategy for evaluating their effectiveness. The template, "A Framework for a Root Cause Analysis and Action Plan in Response to a Sentinel Event," is available to practices as an aid in organizing the steps in a root cause analysis and developing an action plan. This three-page form can be obtained by calling the Sentinel Event Hotline at 630/792-3700 or by accessing it on the Joint Commission Web site at http://www.jcaho.org.

The root cause analysis and action plan are not to include the patient's name or the names of caregivers involved in the sentinel event.

Alternatively, if the practice has concerns about waivers of confidentiality protections as a result of sending the root cause analysis documents to the Joint Commission, the following alternative approaches to a review of the practice's response to the sentinel event are acceptable:

1. A review of the root cause analysis and action plan documents brought to Joint Commission headquarters by practice staff, then taken back to the practice on the same day.
2. An on-site visit by a specially trained surveyor to review the root cause analysis and action plan.
3. An on-site visit by a specially trained surveyor to review the root cause analysis and findings without directly viewing the root cause analysis documents through a series of interviews and a review of relevant documentation. For purposes of this review activity, "relevant documentation" includes, at a minimum, any documentation relevant to the practice's process for responding to sentinel events, the patient's medical record, and the action plan resulting from the analysis of the subject sentinel event. The latter serves as the basis for appropriate follow-up activity.
4. When the practice affirms that it meets specified criteria respecting the risk of waiving confidentiality protections for root cause analysis information shared with the Joint Commission, an on-site visit by a specially trained surveyor to conduct the following:
   a. Interviews and review relevant documentation, including the patient's medical record, to obtain information about the following:
      - The process the practice uses in responding to sentinel events
      - The relevant policies and procedures preceding and following the practice's review of the specific event, and the implementation thereof, sufficient to permit inferences about the adequacy of the organization's response to the sentinel event
   b. A standards-based survey of the patient care, treatment, and services and the practice management functions relevant to the sentinel event under review.

Any one of the four alternatives results in a sufficient charge to the practice to cover the average direct costs of the visit. Inquiries about the fee should be directed to the Joint Commission's pricing unit at 630/792-5115.

The Joint Commission must receive a request for review of a practice's response to a sentinel event using any of these alternative approaches within at least five business days of the self-report of a reviewable event or of the initial communication by the Joint Commission to the practice that it has become aware of a reviewable sentinel event.

The Joint Commission's Response

Staff assesses the acceptability of the practice's response to the reviewable sentinel event, including the thoroughness and credibility of any root cause analysis information reviewed and the practice's action plan. If the root cause analysis and action plan are found to be thorough and credible, the response will be accepted and an appropriate follow-up activity will be assigned.

If the response is unacceptable, staff will provide consultation to the practice on the criteria that have not yet been met and will allow an additional 15 calendar days beyond the original submission period for the practice to resubmit its response. This additional time is provided only if the practice's initial submission of its root cause analysis and action plan was within the time frame as outlined previously.

If the response continues to be unacceptable, staff will recommend to the Accreditation Committee that the practice be placed on Accreditation Watch and be required to address the inadequacies and to submit, or make available for review, a new root cause analysis and action plan within

15 calendar days of notification that the Accreditation Committee has found the response to be unacceptable and has placed the practice on Accreditation Watch, or staff will provide for further Joint Commission evaluation of the practice's response to the event.

Depending on the practice's initial response to the Accreditation Watch decision, the Joint Commission will determine whether an on-site visit should be made to help the practice conduct an appropriate root cause analysis and develop an action plan.

When the practice's response (initial or revised) is found to be acceptable, the Joint Commission issues a letter that does the following:

- Reflects the Joint Commission's determination to (1) continue or modify the practice's current accreditation status and (2) terminate the Accreditation Watch if previously assigned
- Assigns an appropriate follow-up activity, typically an MOS or a follow-up visit to be conducted within six months

If on review the practice's response is still not acceptable or the practice fails to respond, staff will recommend to the Accreditation Committee that the practice be placed in Preliminary Denial of Accreditation. If approved by the Accreditation Committee, this accreditation decision would be considered publicly disclosable information and the process for resolution of Preliminary Denial of Accreditation would be initiated.

Action Plan Follow-up Activity

The follow-up activity will assess (based on applicable standards) the following:

- The practice's response to additional relevant information obtained since completion of the root cause analysis
- The implementation of system and process improvements identified in the action plan
- The means by which the practice will continue to assess the effectiveness of those efforts
- The practice's response to data collected to measure the effectiveness of the actions
- The resolution of any outstanding requirements for improvement

A decision to maintain or change the practice's accreditation status as a result of the follow-up activity or to assign additional follow-up requirements is based on existing decision rules unless otherwise determined by the Accreditation Committee.

Handling Sentinel Event–Related Documents

Handling of any submitted root cause analysis and action plan is restricted to specially trained staff in accordance with procedures designed to protect the confidentiality of the documents.

Upon completion of the Joint Commission review of any submitted root cause analysis and action plan and the abstraction of the required data elements for the Joint Commission's Sentinel Event Database, the original root cause analysis documents and any copies will be destroyed. Upon request, the original documents will be returned to the practice.

The action plan resulting from the analysis of the sentinel event will initially be retained to serve as the basis for the follow-up activity. When the action plan has been implemented to the satisfaction of the Joint Commission as determined through follow-up activities, the Joint Commission will destroy the action plan.

Oversight of the Sentinel Event Policy

The Accreditation Committee of the Joint Commission's Board of Commissioners is responsible for overseeing the implementation of this policy and procedure. In addition to reviewing and deciding individual cases involving Accreditation Watch, the Accreditation Committee periodically audits root cause analyses and action plans reviewed by staff. For the purposes of these audits, the Joint Commission temporarily retains random samples of these documents. Upon completion of the audit, these documents are also destroyed.

For more information about the Joint Commission's Sentinel Event Policy and Procedures, visit the Joint Commission's Web site at http://www.jcaho.org or call the Sentinel Event Hotline at 630/792-3700.

National Patient Safety Goals

This chapter addresses the National Patient Safety Goals and requirements. Office-based surgery practices providing care relevant to each of the goals are responsible for implementing the applicable requirements or, with Joint Commission approval, effective alternatives.

As with Joint Commission standards, accredited office-based surgery practices are evaluated for continuous compliance with the specific requirements associated with the National Patient Safety Goals. Compliance with these requirements is assessed by the Joint Commission through on-site surveys and Evidences of Standards Compliance (ESC). Practices are judged to be either compliant or not compliant with each goal. If an office-based surgery practice does not fully comply with all the requirements associated with a goal, the practice will be assigned a requirement for improvement for the goal in the same way that noncompliance with an EP for a standard generates a requirement for improvement for that standard. All requirements for improvement generate follow-up requirements, and can impact the accreditation decision, as determined by established accreditation decision rules. (*See* pages ACC-14–ACC-20 of "The New Joint Commission Accreditation Process" chapter for the current decision rules.) Failure to resolve a requirement for improvement for a goal can ultimately lead to loss of accreditation.

Note: *You might notice that some goals appear to be misnumbered or missing from the numerical sequence. This is not a typographical error. Some goals do not apply to office-based surgery programs practices and therefore have not been included in the chapter.*

Scoring Grid
0 Insufficient compliance
1 Partial compliance
2 Satisfactory compliance
NA Not applicable

NP SG

The purpose of the Joint Commission's National Patient Safety Goals is to promote specific improvements in patient safety. The goals highlight problematic areas in health care and describe evidence- and expert-based solutions to these problems. Recognizing that sound system design is intrinsic to the delivery of safe, high-quality health care, the goals focus on systemwide solutions, wherever possible.

Although the requirements associated with the National Patient Safety Goals are generally more prescriptive than Joint Commission standards requirements, organizations may request Joint Commission approval of specific alternative approaches to meeting National Patient Safety Goal requirements. The Joint Commission also provides guidance on how to achieve effective compliance with each goal's requirements. This guidance includes detailed answers to Frequently Asked Questions (FAQs).

Three of the requirements associated with the 2004 National Patient Safety Goals that related to preventing wrong site, wrong procedure, and wrong person surgery have been incorporated into the Universal Protocol for ambulatory care, critical access hospitals, hospitals, and office-based surgery, effective July 1, 2004. The 2004 goals and requirements are now replaced by the Universal Protocol for these programs, and their compliance with these three requirements are now scored at the Universal Protocol, which is also provided in this chapter on pages NPSG-4–NPSG-5.

The National Patient Safety Goals are derived primarily from informal recommendations made in the Joint Commission's safety newsletter, *Sentinel Event Alert.* The Sentinel Event Database, which contains de-identified aggregate information on sentinel events reported to the Joint Commission, is the primary, but not the sole, source of information from which the alerts, as well as the National Patient Safety Goals, are derived. A broadly representative Sentinel Event Advisory Group works with Joint Commission staff on a continuing basis to determine priorities for, and develop, goals and associated requirements. As part of this development process, candidate goals and requirements are sent to the field for review and comment. Selected existing and new goals and requirements are annually recommended by the Advisory Group to the Joint Commission's Board of Commissioners for final review and approval. The Advisory Group also assists the Joint Commission in evaluating potential alternatives to goal requirements that have been suggested by individual organizations.

❑ Compliant
❑ Not Compliant

Goal 1

Improve the accuracy of patient identification.

Requirement 1A

Use at least two patient identifiers (neither to be the patient's physical location) whenever administering medications or blood products; taking blood samples and other specimens for clinical testing, or providing any other treatments or procedures.

Note: *The preceding requirement is not scored here. It is scored at standard PC.5.10, EP 4.* See *page PC-12.*

❑ Compliant
❑ Not Compliant

Goal 2

Improve the effectiveness of communication among caregivers.

Requirement 2A

For verbal or telephone orders or for telephonic reporting of critical test results, verify the complete order or test result by having the person receiving the order or test result "read-back" the complete order or test result.

Note: *The preceding requirement is not scored here. It is scored at standard IM.6.50, EP 4.* See *page IM-11.*

Scoring Grid
0 Insufficient compliance
1 Partial compliance
2 Satisfactory compliance
NA Not applicable

Requirement 2B

Standardize a list of abbreviations, acronyms, and symbols that are not to be used throughout the practice.

A | 0 | 1 | 2 | NA

Requirement 2C

Measure, and assess and, if appropriate, take action to improve the timeliness of reporting, and the timeliness of receipt by the responsible licensed caregiver, of critical test results and values.

A | 0 | 1 | 2 | NA

Goal 3

Improve the safety of using medications.

❑ Compliant
❑ Not Compliant

Requirement 3A

Remove concentrated electrolytes (including, but not limited to, potassium chloride, potassium phosphate, sodium chloride > 0.9%) from patient care units.

Note: *The preceding requirement is not scored here. It is scored at standard MM.2.20, EP 9.* See *page MM-9.*

Requirement 3B

Standardize and limit the number of drug concentrations available in the practice.

Note: *The preceding requirement is not scored here. It is scored at standard MM.2.20, EP 8.* See *page MM-9.*

Requirement 3C

Identify and, at a minimum, annually review a list of look-alike/sound-alike drugs used in the practice, and take action to prevent errors involving the interchange of these drugs.

A | 0 | 1 | 2 | NA

Goal 5

Improve the safety of using infusion pumps.

❑ Compliant
❑ Not Compliant

Requirement 5A

Ensure free-flow protection on all general-use and PCA (patient controlled analgesia) intravenous infusion pumps used in the practice.

A | 0 | 1 | 2 | NA

Goal 7

Reduce the risk of health care–associated infections.

❑ Compliant
❑ Not Compliant

Requirement 7A

Comply with current Centers for Disease Control and Prevention (CDC) hand hygiene guidelines.*

Note: *The preceding requirement is not scored here. It is scored at standard IC.4.10, EP 2.* See *page IC-9.*

Requirement 7B

Manage as sentinel events all identified cases of unanticipated death or major permanent loss of function associated with a health care–associated infection.

A | 0 | 1 | 2 | NA

Goal 8

Accurately and completely reconcile medications across the continuum of care.

❑ Compliant
❑ Not Compliant

* Organizations are required to comply with all 1A, 1B, and 1C CDC recommendations or requirements.

Scoring Grid

0 Insufficient compliance
1 Partial compliance
2 Satisfactory compliance
NA Not applicable

A | 0 | 1 | 2 | NA |

Requirement 8A

During 2005, for full implementation by January 2006, develop a process for obtaining and documenting a complete list of the patient's current medications upon the patient's entry to the practice and with the involvement of the patient. This process provides for comparing the medications the practice provides to those on the list.

A | 0 | 1 | 2 | NA |

Requirement 8B

A complete list of the patient's medications is communicated to the next provider of service when it refers or transfers a patient to another setting, service, practitioner, or level of care within or outside the practice.

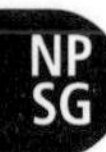

❑ Compliant
❑ Not Compliant

Goal 11

Reduce the risk of surgical fires.

A | 0 | 1 | 2 | NA |

Requirement 11A

Educate staff, including operating licensed independent practitioners and anesthesia providers, on how to control heat sources and manage fuels with enough time for patient preparation, and establish guidelines to minimize oxygen concentration under drapes.

Universal Protocol

Wrong site, wrong procedure, wrong person surgery can be prevented. This Universal Protocol is intended to achieve that goal. It is based on the consensus of experts from the relevant clinical specialties and professional disciplines and is endorsed by more than 40 professional medical associations and practices.

In developing this protocol, consensus was reached on the following principles:

- Wrong site, wrong procedure, wrong person surgery can and must be prevented.
- A robust approach—using multiple, complementary strategies—is necessary to achieve the goal of eliminating wrong site, wrong procedure, wrong person surgery.
- Active involvement and effective communication among all members of the surgical team is important for success.
- To the extent possible, the patient (or legally designated representative) should be involved in the process.
- Consistent implementation of a standardized approach using a universal, consensus-based protocol will be most effective.
- The protocol should be flexible enough to allow for implementation with appropriate adaptation when required to meet specific patient needs.
- A requirement for site marking should focus on cases involving right/left distinction, multiple structures (fingers, toes), or levels (spine).
- The Universal Protocol should be applicable or adaptable to all operative and other invasive procedures that expose patients to harm, including procedures done in settings other than the operating room.

In concert with these principles, the following steps, taken together, comprise the Universal Protocol for eliminating Wrong Site, WrongProcedure, Wrong Person Surgery™:

- Pre-operative verification process
    - Purpose: To ensure that all of the relevant documents and studies are available prior to the start of the procedure and that they have been reviewed and are consistent with each other and with the patient's expectations and with the team's understanding of the intended patient, procedure, site and, as applicable, any implants. Missing information or discrepancies must be addressed before starting the procedure.
    - Process: An ongoing process of information gathering and verification, beginning with the determination to do the procedure, continuing through all settings and interventions

Scoring Grid
0 Insufficient compliance
1 Partial compliance
2 Satisfactory compliance
NA Not applicable

involved in the preoperative preparation of the patient, up to and including the "time out" just before the start of the procedure.

- Marking the operative site
  - Purpose: To identify unambiguously the intended site of incision or insertion.
  - Process: For procedures involving right/left distinction, multiple structures (such as fingers and toes), or multiple levels (as in spinal procedures), the intended site must be marked such that the mark will be visible after the patient has been prepped and draped.
- "Time out" immediately before starting the procedure
  - Purpose: To conduct a final verification of the correct patient, procedure, site and, as applicable, implants.
  - Process: Active communication among all members of the surgical/procedure team, consistently initiated by a designated member of the team, conducted in a fail-safe mode; that is the procedure is not started until any questions or concerns are resolved.

NP SG

UP 1

The practice fulfills the expectations set forth in the Universal Protocol for Preventing Wrong site, Wrong Procedure, Wrong Person Surgery and associated implementation guidelines.

❑ Compliant
❑ Not Compliant

Requirement 1A

Conduct a pre-operative verification process as described in the Universal Protocol.

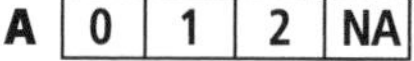
A | 0 | 1 | 2 | NA

Requirement 1B

Mark the operative site as described in the Universal Protocol.

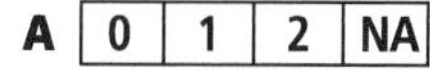
A | 0 | 1 | 2 | NA

Requirement 1C

Conduct a "time out" immediately before starting the procedure as described in the Universal Protocol.

Note: *The preceding element of performance is not scored here. It is scored at standard PC.13.20, EP 9.* *See page PC-19.*

NP SG

Accreditation Participation Requirements

This chapter includes specific requirements for participation in the accreditation process and for maintaining an accreditation award. These differ from survey eligibility criteria in that the accreditation process may be initiated even when all Accreditation Participation Requirements (APRs) have not yet been met.

For a practice seeking accreditation for the first time, compliance with the APRs is assessed during the initial survey. For the accredited practice, compliance with these requirements is assessed throughout the accreditation cycle through on-site surveys, Evidence of Standards Compliance (ESCs), and periodic updates of practice-specific data and information. Organizations are either compliant or not compliant with APRs. When a practice does not comply with an APR, the practice is assigned a requirement for improvement in the same context that noncompliance with a standard or element of performance (EP) generates a requirement for improvement. However, refusal to permit performance of an unscheduled or unannounced for-cause survey (APR 3) or falsification of information (APR 10) will immediately lead to preliminary Denial of Accreditation. All requirements for improvement can impact the accreditation decision and follow-up requirements, as determined by established accreditation decision rules. Failure to resolve a requirement for improvement can ultimately lead to loss of accreditation.

Scoring Grid
0 Insufficient compliance
1 Partial compliance
2 Satisfactory compliance
NA Not applicable

APR

Application for Accreditation

❑ Compliant
❑ Not Compliant

APR 1

When requested, the practice provides the Joint Commission with all official records and reports of public or publicly recognized licensing (for example, a state license), examining, reviewing, or planning bodies.*

Element of Performance for APR 1

A | 0 | 1 | 2 | NA

1. The practice provides the Joint Commission with all official records and reports of licensing, examining, reviewing, or planning bodies.

❑ Compliant
❑ Not Compliant

APR 2

The practice immediately reports any changes in the information provided in the application for accreditation and any changes made between surveys.†

Rationale for APR 2

A practice that experiences a significant change in ownership or control, location, capacity, or the categories of services offered must notify the Joint Commission in writing not more than 30 days after such changes. The Joint Commission may decide that the practice must be resurveyed when a significant merger or consolidation has taken place. The Joint Commission continues the practice's accreditation until it determines whether a resurvey is necessary. Failure to provide timely notification to the Joint Commission of ownership, merger or consolidation, and service changes may result in interruption or loss of accreditation.

Element of Performance for APR 2

A | 0 | 1 | 2 | NA

1. The practice notifies the Joint Commission not more than 30 days before or after a significant change in ownership or control, location, capacity, or the categories of services offered.

Acceptance of Survey

❑ Compliant
❑ Not Compliant

APR 3

A practice permits the performance of an unscheduled or unannounced for-cause survey‡ at the discretion of the Joint Commission.

Rationale for APR 3

The Joint Commission may perform either an unscheduled or unannounced for-cause survey when it becomes aware of potentially serious patient care or safety issues in a practice. Either type of survey can take place at any point in a practice's three-year accreditation cycle. An unscheduled or unannounced survey can either include all of the practice's services or address only those areas where a serious concern may exist. A practice's failure to permit an unscheduled or unannounced survey is grounds for withdrawal of accreditation.

* *See also* page APP-13 in the "Accreditation Policies and Procedures" chapter.

† *See also* pages APP-13–APR-14.

‡ *See also* pages APP-27–APR-28 for an explanation of the difference between an unscheduled and unannounced for-cause survey. In addition, *see* the last paragraph of the "Continuous Compliance" section on page APP-26.

Scoring Grid
0 Insufficient compliance
1 Partial compliance
2 Satisfactory compliance
NA Not applicable

Elements of Performance for APR 3

1. The practice permits the performance of an unscheduled for-cause survey. **A** 0 1 2 NA
2. The practice permits the performance of an unannounced for-cause survey. **A** 0 1 2 NA

Performance Measurement

APR 4 Through 7

Not applicable.

Public Information Interviews

APR 8

The practice provides notice of an upcoming full accreditation survey and of the opportunity for a Public Information Interview.*

❑ Compliant
❑ Not Compliant

Rationale for APR 8

A practice must provide an opportunity for the public to participate in a PPI during a full survey. The public includes the following:

- Patients and their families
- Patient advocates and advocacy groups
- Members of the community for whom services are provided
- Practice personnel and staff.

The practice is responsible for making the PII process widely known and effective as a source of compliance information in the accreditation process. The Joint Commission requires a practice scheduled for a full survey to post announcements of the survey date, the opportunity for a PII, and how to request an interview. To maximize participation, postings must be made throughout the practice in the form provided by the Joint Commission (*see* Public Notice Form on page APP-16). Practices should post notices in public eating areas and on bulletin boards near major entrances. In addition, if all staff members are not likely to see such postings, the practice must provide each staff member with a written announcement of the survey.

The practice must also provide potential PII participants with sufficient advance notice. The Joint Commission requires practices to post public notices at least 30 days before the scheduled survey date. Notices must remain posted until the survey is completed.

The practice should also promptly initiate community advertising or other communications as soon as it receives notice of the survey date. Appropriate steps to take in notifying the community of the opportunity for PII include the following:

- Informing all advocacy groups (such as organized patient groups and unions) that have substantively communicated with the practice in the previous 12 months
- Reaching other members of the community, for example, through a public service announcement on radio or television, a classified advertisement in a local newspaper, or notice in a community newsletter or other publication
- Informing individuals who inquire about the survey of the survey date(s) and opportunity to participate

* *See also* pages APP-17 and APP-18.

Scoring Grid
0 Insufficient compliance
1 Partial compliance
2 Satisfactory compliance
NA Not applicable

Elements of Performance for APR 8

A 0 1 2 NA
1. The practice provides notice of an upcoming full survey and of the opportunity for a PII.

❑ Compliant
❑ Not Compliant

APR 9

The practice notifies the Joint Commission of any requests for a PII.*

Rationale for APR 9

The practice must promptly forward to the Joint Commission all written requests to participate in a PII. Practices receiving an oral request should instruct the individual(s) to make the request in writing and mail it to the Joint Commission. The practice should provide the individual(s) needing assistance in doing this with the necessary support. The practice is responsible for notifying the interviewee(s) of the exact date, time, and place of the PII.

Elements of Performance for APR 9

A 0 1 2 NA
1. The practice notifies the Joint Commission of any requests for a PII.

A 0 1 2 NA
2. The practice notifies any interviewee(s) of the exact date, time, and place of a PII.

Misrepresentation of Information

❑ Compliant
❑ Not Compliant

APR 10

The practice does not misrepresent information in the accreditation process.†

Rationale for APR 10

Information provided by a practice and used by the Joint Commission for the accreditation process must be accurate and truthful. Such information may be provided in the following ways:

- Provided orally
- Obtained through direct observation by Joint Commission surveyors
- Derived from documents supplied by the practice to the Joint Commission
- Involve data submitted electronically by the practice through the performance measurement system to the Joint Commission

The Joint Commission requires each practice seeking accreditation to engage in the accreditation process in good faith. Any practice that fails to participate in good faith by falsifying information presented in the accreditation process may have its accreditation denied or removed by the Joint Commission.

For the purpose of this requirement, *falsification* is defined as the fabrication, in whole or in part, and through commission or omission, of any information provided by an applicant or accredited practice to the Joint Commission. This includes any redrafting, reformatting, or content deletion of documents. However, the practice may submit additional material that summarizes or otherwise explains the original information submitted to the Joint Commission. These additional materials must be properly identified, dated, and accompanied by the original documents.

Element of Performance for APR 10

A 0 1 2 NA
1. A practice provides accurate and truthful information throughout the accreditation process.

---

* *See also* pages APP-17 and APP-18.

† *See also* pages APP-7–APP-9.

Scoring Grid
0 Insufficient compliance
1 Partial compliance
2 Satisfactory compliance
NA Not applicable

APR 11

❑ Compliant
❑ Not Compliant

A practice does not publicly misrepresent its accreditation status or the scope of facilities and services to which the accreditation applies.*

Rationale for APR 11

Practices accredited by the Joint Commission must be accurate when describing to the public the nature and meaning of their accreditation. On request, the Joint Commission's Department of Communications will provide accredited practices with appropriate guidelines for characterizing the accreditation award. A practice may not engage in any false or misleading advertising with respect to the accreditation award. Any such advertising may be grounds for denying or revoking accreditation.

Elements of Performance for APR 11

1. The practice accurately represents its accreditation status as to the scope of facilities and services to which the accreditation applies. A | 0 | 1 | 2 | NA |
2. The practice does not engage in any false or misleading advertising with respect to the accreditation award. A | 0 | 1 | 2 | NA |

APR 12

❑ Compliant
❑ Not Compliant

Accredited practices or practices seeking accreditation are not permitted to use Joint Commission full-time, part-time, or intermittent surveyors to provide any accreditation-related consulting services.

Rationale for APR 12

Consulting services include, but are not limited to, the following:
- Helping a practice to meet Joint Commission standards
- Conducting mock surveys for a practice
- Providing consultation to a practice to address Priority Focus Process (PFP) information

Element of Performance for APR 12

1. The practice does not use Joint Commission full-time, part-time, or intermittent surveyors to provide any accreditation-related consulting services. A | 0 | 1 | 2 | NA |

Survey Observers

APR 13

❑ Compliant
❑ Not Compliant

A practice that applies for survey is obligated to accept Joint Commission on Accreditation of Healthcare Organizations' surveyor management staff and/or a member of the Board of Commissioners to observe a survey under two specific circumstances:
- Observation and mentoring of surveyors as part of surveyor management and development
- Preceptorship of new surveyors

The observer will not participate in the on-site survey process in any fashion, including the scoring of standards compliance. The presence of an observer will not result in any additional charge to the practice nor will it be accepted as de facto grounds for score revisions or decision appeal.

Element of Performance for APR 13

1. The practice accepts Joint Commission on Accreditation of Healthcare Organizations' surveyor management staff and/or a member of the Board of Commissioners to observe a survey under either of the two specific circumstances. A | 0 | 1 | 2 | NA |

---

* *See also* pages APP-24–APP-25.

APR

Practice Ethics, and Patient Rights and Responsibilities

Overview

The **goal** of patient rights and practice ethics in an office-based surgery practice is to help improve patient outcomes by respecting each patient's rights and conducting business relationships with patients and the public ethically. Patients have a fundamental right to considerate care that safeguards their personal dignity and respects their psychological, cultural, and spiritual values. Understanding these values guides the practitioner in meeting patients' care needs and preferences. A practice's behavior toward its patients and its business practices significantly affect the patient's experience of and response to care.

RI

Glossary Terms

These key terms have specific Joint Commission definitions. Please access the Glossary found near the end of your manual for the Joint Commission definition and appropriate use.

abuse
- mental abuse
- physical abuse
- sexual abuse

advance directive
confidentiality
exploitation
family
guardian
neglect
surrogate decision maker

Standards

The following is a list of all standards for this function. They are presented here for your convenience without footnotes or other explanatory text. If you have a question about a term used here, please check the Glossary.

Note: *A revised standard numbering system is being used with the reformatted standards. This revised numbering system allows for more flexibility to add standards while maintaining the current label for each standard.*

RI

Practice Ethics

RI.1.10 The practice follows ethical behavior in its business practices.

RI.1.20 The practice addresses conflicts of interest.

RI.1.30 The integrity of decisions is based on identified care, treatment, and service needs of the patients.

RI.1.40 Not applicable

Individual Rights

RI.2.10 The practice respects the rights of patients.

RI.2.20 Not applicable

RI.2.30 Patients are involved in decisions about care, treatment, and services provided.

RI.2.40 Informed consent is obtained.

RI.2.50 Not Applicable

RI.2.60 Patients receive adequate information about the person(s) responsible for the delivery of their care, treatment, and services.

RI.2.70 Patients have the right to refuse care, treatment, and services in accordance with law and regulation.

RI.2.80 Not applicable

RI.2.90 Patients and, when appropriate, their families are informed about the outcomes of care, including unanticipated outcomes.

RI.2.100 The practice respects the patient's right to and need for effective communication.

RI.2.110 Not applicable

RI.2.120 The practice addresses the resolution of complaints from patients and their families.

RI.2.130 The practice respects the needs of patients for confidentiality, privacy, and security.

RI.2.140 Through RI.2.170 Not applicable

RI.2.180 The practice protects research subjects and respects their rights during research, investigation, and clinical trials involving human subjects.

Individual Responsibilities

RI.3.10 Patients are given information about their responsibilities while receiving care, treatment, and services.

Understanding the Parts of This Chapter

To help you navigate this reformatted standards chapter, it may be helpful to think of its parts this way:

- The **standard** is the "goal."
- The **rationale** explains why it's important to achieve this goal.
- The **elements of performance** identify the step(s) needed to achieve this goal.

These parts are defined as follows.

Standard A statement that defines the performance expectations and/or structures or processes that must be in place in order for a practice to provide safe, high-quality care, treatment, and services. An practice is either "compliant" or "not compliant" with a standard as reflected by the check boxes in the margin by the standard:

❑ Compliant
❑ Not Compliant

Accreditation decisions are based on simple counts of the standards that are determined to be "not compliant."

Rationale A statement that provides background, justification, or additional information about a standard. A standard's rationale is not scored. In some instances, the rationale for a standard is self-evident. Therefore, not every standard has a written rationale.

Elements of performance (EPs) The specific performance expectations and/or structures or processes that must be in place in order for a practice to provide safe, high-quality care, treatment, and services. The scoring of EP compliance determines a practice's overall compliance with a standard. EPs are evaluated on the following scale:

0 Insufficient compliance
1 Partial compliance
2 Satisfactory compliance
NA Not applicable

You will find a **measure of success** icon—Ⓜ—next to some EPs. Measures of success (MOS) need to be developed for certain EPs when a standard is judged to be out of compliance through the on-site survey. An MOS is defined as a quantifiable measure, usually related to an audit, that can be used to determine whether an action has been effective and is being sustained.*

Using the Self-Assessment Grid to Assess Your Compliance

Once you are familiar with the parts of this chapter, you can begin to assess your compliance with its requirements. A self-assessment grid (otherwise known as a scoring grid) has been provided in the margins for your convenience. If you would like to assess your practice's performance, mark your scores for the EPs on the scoring grid by following the simple steps described below. **Note:** *You are **not** required to complete this scoring grid. It is provided simply to help you assess your own performance.*

Two components are scored for each EP: (1) compliance with the requirement itself **and** (2) compliance with the track record† for that requirement. Scoring has been simplified from the past edition of the manual, and track record achievements (which have always been part of the scoring) have been appropriately modified.

* For more information about Measures of Success, *see* "The New Joint Commission Accreditation Process" chapter in this manual.

† **Track record** The amount of time that a practice has been in compliance with a standard, element of performance, or other requirement.

Note: *Some standards and EPs do not apply to a particular type of practice; these standards and EPs are marked "not applicable" and the related text is not included. Your practice is not expected to comply with standards and EPs marked "not applicable."*

In addition, some standards and EPs that do apply to practices may not apply to the specific care, treatment, and services that your individual practice provides. Although these standards and EPs are included in the manual, you are not expected to comply with them. If you are unsure about the standards or EPs that apply to your practice, please contact the Joint Commission's Standards Interpretation Group at 630/792-5900.

Step 1: Score Your Compliance with Each Element of Performance

Before you can determine your compliance with the standards, you must score your compliance with each EP. First look at the EP scoring criterion category listed immediately preceding the scoring scale in the margin next to the EP. There are three scoring criterion categories: A, B, and C (described below). Please note that for each EP scoring criterion category, your practice must meet the performance requirement itself and the track record achievements (*see* below).

Category A

These EPs relate to the presence or absence of the requirement(s) and are scored either yes (2) or no (0); however, score 1 for partial compliance is also possible based on track record achievements (*see* below).

If an A EP has multiple components designated by bullets, your practice must be compliant with all the bullets to receive a score of 2. If your practice does not meet one or more requirements in the bullets, you will receive a score of 0.

Category B

Category B EPs are scored in two steps:

1. As with category A EPs, category B EPs relate to the presence or absence of the requirement(s). If your practice *does not meet* the requirement(s), the EP is scored 0; there is no need to assess your compliance with the principles of good process design (*see* below).
2. If your practice *does meet* the requirement(s), but there is concern about the quality or comprehensiveness of the effort, then and only then should you assess the qualitative aspect of the EP. That is, review the applicable principles of good process design and ask how the principles were applied in the situation under discussion. Good process design has the following characteristics:
   - Is consistent with your practice's mission, values, and goals
   - Meets the needs of patients
   - Reflects the use of currently accepted practices (doing the right thing, using resources responsibly, using practice guidelines)
   - Incorporates current safety information and knowledge such as sentinel event data and National Patient Safety Goals
   - Incorporates relevant performance improvement results

This two-part evaluation applies to both simple and bulleted B EPs. First, the EPs are assessed to determine if the requirements are present. If the EP has multiple components designated by bullets, as with the category A EPs, your practice must meet the requirements in *all* the bulleted items to get a score of 2. If your practice meets *none* of the requirements in the bullets, it receives a score of 0. If your practice meets *at least one, but not all,* of the bulleted requirements, it will receive a score of 1 for the EPs.

Use the following rules to determine your EP score:

- Your EP score is 0 if your practice does not meet the requirement(s); you *do not* need to assess your compliance with the preceding applicable principles of good process design
- Your EP score is 1 if your practice does meet the requirement(s), but considered only *some* of the preceding applicable principles of good process design

- Your EP score is 2 if your practice does meet the requirement(s) *and* considered *all* the preceding principles of good process design

Category C

C EPs are scored 0, 1, or 2 based on the number of times your practice does not meet the EP. These EPs are frequency based and require totaling the number of occurrences (that is, results of performance or nonperformance) related to a particular EP. Each situation discovered by a surveyor(s) will be counted as a separate occurrence.

Note: *Multiple events of the same type related to a single patient and single practitioner/staff member are counted as* one occurrence only.

Use the following rules to determine your EP score:
- Your EP score is 2 if you find one or fewer occurrences of noncompliance with the EP
- Your EP score is 1 if you find two occurrences of noncompliance with the EP
- Your EP score is 0 if you find three or more occurrences of noncompliance with the EP

If an EP in the C category has multiple requirements designated by bullets, the following scoring guidelines apply:
- If there are fewer than 2 findings in all bullets, the EP is scored 2
- If there are three or more findings in all bullets, the EP is scored 0
- In all other combinations of findings, the EP is scored 1

Track Record Achievements

In addition to meeting the requirement(s) in each EP, regardless of category, your practice must also meet the following track record achievements:

Score	Initial Survey	Full Survey
2	4 months or more	12 months or more
1	2 to 3 months	6 to 11 months
0	Fewer than 2 months	Fewer than 6 months

Sample Sizes

If during an on-site survey, your practice has been found to be not compliant with one or more standards, you must demonstrate Evidence of Standards Compliance (ESC) for each standard that is not compliant. The ESC must address compliance at the EP level; when an EP within a noncompliant standard requires an MOS, your practice must demonstrate achievement with the MOS when completing the ESC.

Note: *Not every EP requires an MOS. EPs that do require an MOS are clearly marked in this chapter. Practices are required to demonstrate achievement with an MOS* only *for EPs within a noncompliant standard that require an MOS. Practices* do not *need to demonstrate achievement with an MOS for any EP within a compliant standard.*

When demonstrating achievement with an MOS during the ESC process, your practice is **required** to use the following sample sizes, which were established because of their statistical significance, their relative simplicity in application, and their sensitivity to a practice's population size:
- For a population size of fewer than 30 cases,* sample 100% of available cases
- For a population size of 30 to 100 cases, sample 30 cases
- For a population size of 101 to 500 cases, sample 50 cases
- For a population size greater than 500 cases, sample 70 cases

When demonstrating an ESC (mandatory use), use the following percentages to determine your EP score: 90% through 100% of your sample size is in compliance = score 2; 80% through 89% of your sample size is in compliance = score 1; less than 80% of your sample size is in compliance = score 0.

* "Case" refers to a single instance in which a situation related to a survey finding occurs. For example, if a survey finding was related to **pain assessment,** then a "case" would be any patient record. If a survey finding was related to **pain management,** a "case" would be any patient record for patients receiving pain management.

In addition, the following information should govern your practice's selection of samples:

- The appropriate sample size should be determined by the specific population related to the survey findings
- The sampling approach should involve either systematic random sampling (for example, your practice selects every second or third case for review) or simple random sampling (for example, your practice uses a series of random numbers generated by a computer to identify the cases to be reviewed)
- When submitting a clarifying ESC, if your practice selects records as part of its sample, the records should be from a period of no more than three months before the last date of the survey
- Assessment of MOS compliance is conducted for a four-month period following the date of ESC approval. Your practice should select records as a part of your sample following the date of ESC approval and use the required sample sizes. MOS percentage compliance rates are derived from the average of all four months.

Step 2: Use Your EP Scores to Gauge Your Compliance with the Standards

Now that you have evaluated and scored each EP for a particular standard, use these simple rules to determine your compliance with the standard itself:

- Your practice is not in compliance (that is, "not compliant") with the standard if any EP is scored 0
- Otherwise, your practice is in compliance with a standard if 65% or more of its EPs are scored 2

Standards, Rationales, Elements of Performance, and Scoring

Practice Ethics

Introduction

A practice has an ethical responsibility to the patients and community it serves. To fulfill this responsibility, ethical care, treatment, and service practices and ethical business practices must go hand in hand. Furthermore, the practice provides care, treatment, and services within its scope, stated mission and philosophy, and applicable law and regulation.

The practice's system of ethics supports honest and appropriate interactions with patients. The system of ethics also includes patients whenever possible in decisions about their care, treatment, and services, including ethical issues.

❑ Compliant
❑ Not Compliant

Standard RI.1.10

The practice follows ethical behavior in its business practices.

Elements of Performance for RI.1.10

1. Not applicable
2. Not applicable
3. Not applicable

B | 0 | 1 | 2 | NA |

4. Marketing materials accurately represent the practice and address the care, treatment, and services that the practice can provide, directly or by contractual arrangement.

5. Through 12. Not applicable

A | 0 | 1 | 2 | NA |

Ⓜ 13. The practice bills patients only for services and care provided.

C | 0 | 1 | 2 | NA |

Ⓜ 14. Patients are informed about who owns the practice.

❑ Compliant
❑ Not Compliant

Standard RI.1.20

The practice addresses conflicts of interest.

Elements of Performance for RI.1.20

A | 0 | 1 | 2 | NA |

1. The practice defines what constitutes a *conflict of interest.*

C | 0 | 1 | 2 | NA |

Ⓜ 2. The practice discloses existing or potential conflicts of interest for those who provide care, treatment, and services as well as governance.

B | 0 | 1 | 2 | NA |

3. The practice reviews its relationship and its staff's relationships with other care providers, educational institutions, and payers to ensure that those relationships are within law and regulation and determine if conflicts of interest exist.

Scoring Grid
0 Insufficient compliance
1 Partial compliance
2 Satisfactory compliance
NA Not applicable

Standard RI.1.30

The integrity of decisions is based on identified care, treatment, and service needs of the patients.

❑ Compliant
❑ Not Compliant

Elements of Performance for RI.1.30

1. Not applicable

Ⓜ 2. To avoid compromising the quality of care, decisions are based on the patient's identified care, treatment, and service needs and in accordance with practice policy. — C | 0 | 1 | 2 | NA

3. Information about the relationship between the use of care, treatment, and services and financial incentives are available to all patients, staff, licensed independent practitioners, and contracted providers, when requested. — B | 0 | 1 | 2 | NA

Standard RI.1.40

Not Applicable

Individual Rights

Standard RI.2.10

The practice respects the rights of patients.

❑ Compliant
❑ Not Compliant

Elements of Performance for RI.2.10

1. Not applicable

Ⓜ 2. Each patient has a right to have his or her cultural, psychosocial, spiritual, and personal values, beliefs, and preferences respected. — C | 0 | 1 | 2 | NA

Standard RI.2.20

Not applicable

Standard RI.2.30

Patients are involved in decisions about care, treatment, and services provided.

❑ Compliant
❑ Not Compliant

Elements of Performance for RI.2.30

Ⓜ 1. Patients are involved in decisions about their care, treatment, and services. — C | 0 | 1 | 2 | NA

Ⓜ 2. Patients are involved in resolving dilemmas about care, treatment, and services. — C | 0 | 1 | 2 | NA

Ⓜ 3. A surrogate decision maker, as allowed by law, is identified when a patient cannot make decisions about his or her care, treatment, and services. — C | 0 | 1 | 2 | NA

Standard RI.2.40

Informed consent is obtained.

❑ Compliant
❑ Not Compliant

Rationale for RI.2.40

Informed consent is not merely a signed document. It is an ongoing process that considers patient needs and preferences, compliance with law and regulation, and patient education.

Elements of Performance for RI.2.40

1. Not applicable

Ⓜ 2. Informed consent is obtained and documented in accordance with the practice's policy. — C | 0 | 1 | 2 | NA

RI

Scoring Grid
0 Insufficient compliance
1 Partial compliance
2 Satisfactory compliance
NA Not applicable

B 0 1 2 NA

3. A complete informed consent process includes a discussion of the following elements:*
   - The nature of the proposed care, treatment, services, medications, interventions, or procedures
   - Potential benefits, risks, or side effects, including potential problems related to recuperation
   - Reasonable alternatives to the proposed care, treatment, and services
   - The patient's condition
   - When blood or blood components may be used, the risk of and alternatives to the use of blood or blood components

❑ Compliant
❑ Not Compliant

Standard RI.2.60

Patients receive adequate information about the person(s) responsible for the delivery of their care, treatment, and services.

Elements of Performance for RI.2.60

1. Not applicable
2. Not applicable

C 0 1 2 NA

Ⓜ 3. The patient (and family, as appropriate) are given information about the following:
   - The licensed independent practitioner(s) responsible for the procedure
   - The licensed independent practitioner or staff member primarily responsible for the sedation and anesthesia
   - Others authorizing or performing procedures and treatment

C 0 1 2 NA

Ⓜ 4. At the time of initial consultation, before any surgical procedure or service is performed, the patient receives disclosure information about the licensed independent practitioner's licensure and relevant education, training, and experience in performing the planned procedure.

   Note: *This information can be provided in any written format that the practice chooses.*

C 0 1 2 NA

Ⓜ 5. The licensed independent practitioner described in the disclosure information is the licensed independent practitioner that performs the procedure.

C 0 1 2 NA

Ⓜ 6. The disclosure information also includes the qualifications of the licensed independent practitioner or clinical staff who will administer and monitor anesthesia during the procedure.

C 0 1 2 NA

Ⓜ 7. The patient signs an acknowledgement that he or she has received the disclosure information.†

C 0 1 2 NA

Ⓜ 8. Each patient has the right to be informed of any educational activities related to care and can refuse to participate in any such activity without that refusal compromising usual care.

❑ Compliant
❑ Not Compliant

Standard RI.2.70

Patients have the right to refuse care, treatment, and services in accordance with law and regulation.

Element of Performance for RI.2.70

A 0 1 2 NA

1. Patients have the right to refuse care, treatment, and services in accordance with law and regulation.

---

* Documentation of the items listed in EP 3 may be in a form, progress notes, or elsewhere in the record.

† Please *see* standards PC.6.10 and PC.6.30 and the Introduction to the education standards located in the "Provision of Care, Treatment, and Services" (PC) chapter on pages PC-13–PC-14.

Scoring Grid
0 Insufficient compliance
1 Partial compliance
2 Satisfactory compliance
NA Not applicable

Standard RI.2.80

Not applicable

Standard RI.2.90

❑ Compliant
❑ Not Compliant

Patients and, when appropriate, their families are informed about the outcomes of care, treatment, and services that have been provided, including unanticipated outcomes.

Elements of Performance for RI.2.90

At a minimum, the patient and, when appropriate, his or her family, is informed about the following (EPs 1–2):

Ⓜ 1. Outcomes of care, treatment, and services that have been provided that the patient (or family) must be knowledgeable about to participate in current and future decisions affecting the patient's care, treatment, and services — C 0 1 2 NA

Ⓜ 2. Unanticipated outcomes of care, treatment, and services that relate to sentinel events considered reviewable* by the Joint Commission. — C 0 1 2 NA

Ⓜ 3. The responsible licensed independent practitioner or his or her designee informs the patient (and when appropriate, his or her family) about those unanticipated outcomes of care, treatment, and services (*see* EP 2). — C 0 1 2 NA

RI

Standard RI.2.100

❑ Compliant
❑ Not Compliant

The practice respects the patient's right to and need for effective communication.

Elements of Performance for RI.2.100

1. Not applicable
2. Not applicable
3. Not applicable

Ⓜ 4. The practice addresses the needs of those with vision, speech, hearing, language, and cognitive impairments. — C 0 1 2 NA

Standard RI.2.110

Not applicable

Standard RI.2.120

❑ Compliant
❑ Not Compliant

The practice addresses the resolution of complaints from patients and their families.

Elements of Performance for RI.2.120

Ⓜ 1. The practice informs patients, families, and staff about the complaint resolution process. — C 0 1 2 NA

Ⓜ 2. The practice receives, reviews, and, when possible, resolves complaints from patients and their families. — C 0 1 2 NA

Standard RI.2.130

❑ Compliant
❑ Not Compliant

The practice respects the needs of patients for confidentiality, privacy, and security.

---

* *See* the "Sentinel Events" chapter of this manual for a definition of reviewable sentinel events.

Scoring Grid
0 Insufficient compliance
1 Partial compliance
2 Satisfactory compliance
NA Not applicable

Elements of Performance for RI.2.130

C | 0 | 1 | 2 | NA | Ⓜ 1. The practice protects confidentiality of information about patients.

C | 0 | 1 | 2 | NA | Ⓜ 2. The practice respects the privacy of patients.

3. Not applicable

C | 0 | 1 | 2 | NA | Ⓜ 4. The practice provides for the safety and security of patients and their property.

5. Through 20. Not applicable

A | 0 | 1 | 2 | NA | Ⓜ 21. The practice addresses the needs of those with physical and visual impairments for physical access to the facility.

Standard RI.2.140 Through RI.2.170

Not applicable

RI

❑ Compliant
❑ Not Compliant

Standard RI.2.180

The practice protects research subjects and respects their rights during research, investigation, and clinical trials involving human subjects.

Elements of Performance for RI.2.180

C | 0 | 1 | 2 | NA | Ⓜ 1. The practice reviews all research protocols in relation to its mission, values, and other guidelines and weighs the relative risks and benefits to the research subjects.

C | 0 | 1 | 2 | NA | Ⓜ 2. The practice provides patients who are potential subjects in research, investigation, and clinical trials with adequate information* to participate or refuse to participate in research.

C | 0 | 1 | 2 | NA | Ⓜ 3. Patients are informed that refusing to participate or discontinuing participation at any time will not compromise their access to care, treatment, and services not related to the research.

4. Through 8. Not applicable

C | 0 | 1 | 2 | NA | Ⓜ 9. Each patient participating in research activities is monitored to determine whether changes in his or her clinical condition or in research protocols should affect continued participation in the activities.

Individual Responsibilities

❑ Compliant
❑ Not Compliant

Standard RI.3.10

Patients are given information about their responsibilities while receiving care, treatment, and services.

Rationale for RI.3.10

The practice identifies patient and family responsibilities and educates them about these responsibilities as appropriate to the services provided. Patients are responsible for providing accurate and complete information about their symptoms or reasons for visit, past illnesses, hospitalizations, medications (including prescribed and nonprescribed medications and herbals), and other matters of care. Patients are also responsible for acknowledging when they do not understand a contemplated treatment course or care decision.

* **Adequate information** includes an explanation of the purpose of the research and expected duration of the subject's participation; a description of expected benefits, potential discomforts, and risks; alternative services that might prove advantageous to the individual; and a full explanation of the procedures to be followed.

Scoring Grid
0 Insufficient compliance
1 Partial compliance
2 Satisfactory compliance
NA Not applicable

Elements of Performance for RI.3.10

1. Not applicable
2. Not applicable

Ⓜ 3. Patients are informed about their responsibilities verbally, in writing, or both, based on practice policy. C | 0 | 1 | 2 | NA

Ⓜ 4. Patients are informed about their responsibilities initially and as needed thereafter. C | 0 | 1 | 2 | NA

5. Not applicable

Responsibilities include at least the following:

Ⓜ 6. **Providing information.** The patient is responsible for providing, to the best of his or her knowledge, accurate and complete information about present complaints, past illnesses, hospitalizations, medications, and unexpected changes in the patient's condition. C | 0 | 1 | 2 | NA

Ⓜ 7. **Asking questions.** Patients are responsible for asking questions when they do not understand what they have been told or what they are expected to do. C | 0 | 1 | 2 | NA

Ⓜ 8. **Following instructions.** The patient and family are responsible for following the preoperative and postdischarge care plan. They should express any concerns they have about their ability to follow and comply with the proposed care plan or course of treatment, including anesthesia or operative requirements. Every effort is made to adapt the plan to the patient's specific needs and limitations. C | 0 | 1 | 2 | NA

Ⓜ 9. **Accepting consequences.** The patient and family are responsible for the outcomes if they do not follow the care plan. C | 0 | 1 | 2 | NA

Ⓜ 10. **Following rules and regulations.** The patient and family are responsible for following the practice's rules and regulations concerning patient care and conduct. C | 0 | 1 | 2 | NA

Ⓜ 11. **Showing respect and consideration.** Patients and families are responsible for being considerate of the practice's staff and property. C | 0 | 1 | 2 | NA

Ⓜ 12. **Meeting financial commitments.** The patient and family are responsible for promptly meeting any financial obligation agreed to with the practice. C | 0 | 1 | 2 | NA

RI

Provision of Care, Treatment, and Services*

Overview

The goal of surgical and invasive procedures, sedation, anesthesia, and recovery activities in an office-based surgery practice is to provide for effective, appropriate, and individualized care and procedures that respond to the patient's specific needs. Before any procedure, the practice assesses the patient as an appropriate candidate for an office-based procedure. Sedation and anesthesia assessment and any necessary examinations and diagnostic testing occur, and the patient is informed about risks, benefits, alternatives, and informed consent. The surgeon gives final approval for the planned sedation or anesthesia and the invasive or surgical procedure based on these assessments. Assessment occurs throughout the pre-, peri-, and postprocedure phases, addressing not only physical and functional status, but also physiological and cognitive status as they relate to the use of sedation and anesthesia. Surgeons perform the surgical and invasive procedures. The administration and monitoring of sedation or anesthesia is performed by a qualified licensed independent practitioner or by qualified clinical staff under the supervision of a licensed independent practitioner. Discharge planning in the office-based surgery practice addresses appropriate referrals, transfers, and follow-up. The practice maintains timely and accurate documentation of all phases of care to support treatment and performance improvement.

PC

Glossary Terms
These key terms have specific Joint Commission definitions. Please access the Glossary found near the end of your manual for the Joint Commission definition and appropriate use.

abuse
- mental abuse
- physical abuse
- sexual abuse

anesthesia and sedation
- minimal sedation (anxiolysis)
- moderate sedation/analgesia (conscious sedation)
- deep sedation/analgesia

assessment
blood component
care planning (or planning of care)
CLIA '88
community
continuing care
continuity
discharge
entry
exploitation
family
invasive procedure
leader
licensed independent practitioner
loss of protective reflexes
medication
neglect
nutrition assessment
operative and other high-risk procedures
policies and procedures
practice guidelines
qualified individual
reassessment
referral
staff
transfer
waived testing

* This chapter is a compilation of the former "Surgical and Invasive Procedures, Sedation, Anesthesia, and Recovery," "Clinical Support Services," and "Education" chapters.

Standards

The following is a list of all standards for this function. They are presented here for your convenience without footnotes or other explanatory text. If you have a question about a term used here, please check the Glossary.

Note: *A revised standard numbering system is being used with the reformatted standards. The revised numbering system allows for more flexibility to add standards while maintaining the current label for each standard.*

Entry to Care, Treatment, and Services

PC.1.10 The organization accepts for care, treatment, and services only those patients whose identified needs it can meet.

Assessment

PC.2.10 Through PC.2.120 Not applicable

PC.2.130 Initial assessments are performed as defined by the practice.

PC.2.140 Not applicable

PC.2.150 Not applicable

Additional Standards for Victims of Abuse

PC.3.10 Patients who may be victims of abuse, neglect, or exploitation are assessed.

PC.3.20 Through PC.3.220 Not applicable

Diagnostic Services

PC.3.230 Diagnostic testing necessary for determining the patient's health care needs is performed.

Planning Care, Treatment, and Services

PC.4.10 Development of a plan for care, treatment, and services is individualized and appropriate to the patient's needs, strengths, limitations, and goals.

PC.4.20 Through PC.4.120 Not applicable

Providing Care, Treatment, and Services

PC.5.10 The organization provides care, treatment, and services for each patient according to the plan for care, treatment, and services.

PC.5.20 Through PC.5.50 Not applicable

PC.5.60 The practice coordinates the care, treatment, and services provided to a patient as part of the plan for care, treatment, and services and consistent with the organization's scope of care, treatment, and services.

PC.5.70 Not applicable

Education

PC.6.10 The patient receives education and training specific to the patient's needs and as appropriate to the care, treatment, and services provided.

PC.6.20 Not applicable

PC.6.30 The patient receives education and training specific to the patient's abilities as appropriate to the care, treatment, and services provided by the practice.

PC.6.40 Through PC.6.60 Not applicable

Nutritional Care

PC.7.10 The practice has a process for preparing and/or distributing food and nutrition products as appropriate.

Pain

PC.8.10 Pain is assessed in all patients.

Restorative Services

Standards PC.8.20 Through PC.8.70 Not applicable

Specific Procedures

Administering Blood and Blood Components

PC.9.10 Blood and blood components are administered safely, as appropriate to the setting.

Responding to Life-Threatening Emergencies

PC.9.20 The practice responds to medical life-threatening emergencies according to practice policy and procedure.

PC.9.30 Through PC.12.190 Not applicable

Standards for Additional Special Procedures

Operative or Other High-Risk Procedures and/or the Administration of Moderate or Deep Sedation or Anesthesia

PC.13.10 Licensed independent practitioners define the scope of assessment for operative or other procedures and/or the administration of moderate or deep sedation or anesthesia.

PC.13.20 Operative or other procedures and/or the administration of moderate or deep sedation or anesthesia are planned.

PC.13.30 Patients are monitored during the procedure and/or administration of moderate or deep sedation or anesthesia.

PC.13.40 Patients are monitored immediately after the procedure and/or administration of moderate or deep sedation or anesthesia.

PC.13.50 Through PC.14.30 Not applicable

Discharge or Transfer from the Practice

PC.15.10 A process addresses the needs for continuing care, treatment, and services after transfer.

PC.15.20 The transfer or discharge of a patient is based on the patient's assessed needs and the practice's capabilities.

PC.15.30 When patients are transferred or discharged, appropriate information related to the care, treatment, and services provided is exchanged with other service providers.

Waived Testing

PC.16.10 The practice establishes policies and procedures that define the context in which waived test results are used in patient care, treatment, and services.

PC.16.20 The practice identifies the staff responsible for performing and supervising waived testing.

PC.16.30 Staff performing tests have adequate, specific training and orientation to perform the tests and demonstrate satisfactory levels of competence.

PC.16.40 Approved policies and procedures for specific testing-related processes are current and readily available.

PC.16.50 Quality control checks, as defined by the organization, are conducted on each procedure.

PC.16.60 Appropriate quality control and test records are maintained.

Understanding the Parts of This Chapter

To help you navigate this reformatted standards chapter, it may be helpful to think of its parts this way:

- The **standard** is the "goal."
- The **rationale** explains why it's important to achieve this goal.
- The **elements of performance** identify the step(s) needed to achieve this goal.

These parts are defined as follows.

Standard A statement that defines the performance expectations and/or structures or processes that must be in place in order for a practice to provide safe, high-quality care, treatment, and services. An practice is either "compliant" or "not compliant" with a standard as reflected by the check boxes in the margin by the standard:

❑ Compliant
❑ Not Compliant

Accreditation decisions are based on simple counts of the standards that are determined to be "not compliant."

Rationale A statement that provides background, justification, or additional information about a standard. A standard's rationale is not scored. In some instances, the rationale for a standard is self-evident. Therefore, not every standard has a written rationale.

Elements of performance (EPs) The specific performance expectations and/or structures or processes that must be in place in order for a practice to provide safe, high-quality care, treatment, and services. The scoring of EP compliance determines a practice's overall compliance with a standard. EPs are evaluated on the following scale:

0 Insufficient compliance
1 Partial compliance
2 Satisfactory compliance
NA Not applicable

You will find a **measure of success** icon—Ⓜ—next to some EPs. Measures of success (MOS) need to be developed for certain EPs when a standard is judged to be out of compliance through the on-site survey. An MOS is defined as a quantifiable measure, usually related to an audit, that can be used to determine whether an action has been effective and is being sustained.*

Using the Self-Assessment Grid to Assess Your Compliance

Once you are familiar with the parts of this chapter, you can begin to assess your compliance with its requirements. A self-assessment grid (otherwise known as a scoring grid) has been provided in the margins for your convenience. If you would like to assess your practice's performance, mark your scores for the EPs on the scoring grid by following the simple steps described below. **Note:** *You are **not** required to complete this scoring grid. It is provided simply to help you assess your own performance.*

Two components are scored for each EP: (1) compliance with the requirement itself **and** (2) compliance with the track record† for that requirement. Scoring has been simplified from the past edition of the manual, and track record achievements (which have always been part of the scoring) have been appropriately modified.

---

* For more information about Measures of Success, *see* "The New Joint Commission Accreditation Process" chapter in this manual.

† **Track record** The amount of time that a practice has been in compliance with a standard, element of performance, or other requirement.

Note: *Some standards and EPs do not apply to a particular type of practice; these standards and EPs are marked "not applicable" and the related text is not included. Your practice is not expected to comply with standards and EPs marked "not applicable."*

In addition, some standards and EPs that do apply to practices may not apply to the specific care, treatment, and services that your individual practice provides. Although these standards and EPs are included in the manual, you are not expected to comply with them. If you are unsure about the standards or EPs that apply to your practice, please contact the Joint Commission's Standards Interpretation Group at 630/792-5900.

Step 1: Score Your Compliance with Each Element of Performance

Before you can determine your compliance with the standards, you must score your compliance with each EP. First look at the EP scoring criterion category listed immediately preceding the scoring scale in the margin next to the EP. There are three scoring criterion categories: A, B, and C (described below). Please note that for each EP scoring criterion category, your practice must meet the performance requirement itself and the track record achievements (*see* below).

Category A

These EPs relate to the presence or absence of the requirement(s) and are scored either yes (2) or no (0); however, score 1 for partial compliance is also possible based on track record achievements (*see* below).

If an A EP has multiple components designated by bullets, your practice must be compliant with all the bullets to receive a score of 2. If your practice does not meet one or more requirements in the bullets, you will receive a score of 0.

Category B

Category B EPs are scored in two steps:

1. As with category A EPs, category B EPs relate to the presence or absence of the requirement(s). If your practice *does not meet* the requirement(s), the EP is scored 0; there is no need to assess your compliance with the principles of good process design (*see* below).
2. If your practice *does meet* the requirement(s), but there is concern about the quality or comprehensiveness of the effort, then and only then should you assess the qualitative aspect of the EP. That is, review the applicable principles of good process design and ask how the principles were applied in the situation under discussion. Good process design has the following characteristics:
   - Is consistent with your practice's mission, values, and goals
   - Meets the needs of patients
   - Reflects the use of currently accepted practices (doing the right thing, using resources responsibly, using practice guidelines)
   - Incorporates current safety information and knowledge such as sentinel event data and National Patient Safety Goals
   - Incorporates relevant performance improvement results

This two-part evaluation applies to both simple and bulleted B EPs. First, the EPs are assessed to determine if the requirements are present. If the EP has multiple components designated by bullets, as with the category A EPs, your practice must meet the requirements in *all* the bulleted items to get a score of 2. If your practice meets *none* of the requirements in the bullets, it receives a score of 0. If your practice meets *at least one, but not all,* of the bulleted requirements, it will receive a score of 1 for the EPs.

Use the following rules to determine your EP score:

- Your EP score is 0 if your practice does not meet the requirement(s); you *do not* need to assess your compliance with the preceding applicable principles of good process design
- Your EP score is 1 if your practice does meet the requirement(s), but considered only *some* of the preceding applicable principles of good process design

- Your EP score is 2 if your practice does meet the requirement(s) *and* considered *all* the preceding principles of good process design

Category C

C EPs are scored 0, 1, or 2 based on the number of times your practice does not meet the EP. These EPs are frequency based and require totaling the number of occurrences (that is, results of performance or nonperformance) related to a particular EP. Each situation discovered by a surveyor(s) will be counted as a separate occurrence.

Note: *Multiple events of the same type related to a single patient and single practitioner/staff member are counted as* one occurrence only.

Use the following rules to determine your EP score:
- Your EP score is 2 if you find one or fewer occurrences of noncompliance with the EP
- Your EP score is 1 if you find two occurrences of noncompliance with the EP
- Your EP score is 0 if you find three or more occurrences of noncompliance with the EP

If an EP in the C category has multiple requirements designated by bullets, the following scoring guidelines apply:
- If there are fewer than 2 findings in all bullets, the EP is scored 2
- If there are three or more findings in all bullets, the EP is scored 0
- In all other combinations of findings, the EP is scored 1

PC

Track Record Achievements

In addition to meeting the requirement(s) in each EP, regardless of category, your practice must also meet the following track record achievements:

Score	Initial Survey	Full Survey
2	4 months or more	12 months or more
1	2 to 3 months	6 to 11 months
0	Fewer than 2 months	Fewer than 6 months

Sample Sizes

If during an on-site survey, your practice has been found to be not compliant with one or more standards, you must demonstrate Evidence of Standards Compliance (ESC) for each standard that is not compliant. The ESC must address compliance at the EP level; when an EP within a noncompliant standard requires an MOS, your practice must demonstrate achievement with the MOS when completing the ESC.

Note: *Not every EP requires an MOS. EPs that do require an MOS are clearly marked in this chapter. Practices are required to demonstrate achievement with an MOS* only *for EPs within a noncompliant standard that require an MOS. Practices* do not *need to demonstrate achievement with an MOS for any EP within a compliant standard.*

When demonstrating achievement with an MOS during the ESC process, your practice is **required** to use the following sample sizes, which were established because of their statistical significance, their relative simplicity in application, and their sensitivity to a practice's population size:
- For a population size of fewer than 30 cases,* sample 100% of available cases
- For a population size of 30 to 100 cases, sample 30 cases
- For a population size of 101 to 500 cases, sample 50 cases
- For a population size greater than 500 cases, sample 70 cases

When demonstrating an ESC (mandatory use), use the following percentages to determine your EP score: 90% through 100% of your sample size is in compliance = score 2; 80% through 89% of your sample size is in compliance = score 1; less than 80% of your sample size is in compliance = score 0.

---

* "Case" refers to a single instance in which a situation related to a survey finding occurs. For example, if a survey finding was related to **pain assessment,** then a "case" would be any patient record. If a survey finding was related to **pain management,** a "case" would be any patient record for patients receiving pain management.

In addition, the following information should govern your practice's selection of samples:

- The appropriate sample size should be determined by the specific population related to the survey findings.
- The sampling approach should involve either systematic random sampling (for example, your practice selects every second or third case for review) or simple random sampling (for example, your practice uses a series of random numbers generated by a computer to identify the cases to be reviewed).
- When submitting clarifying ESC, if your practice selects records as part of its sample, the records should be from a period of no more than three months before the last date of the survey.
- Assessment of MOS compliance is conducted for a four-month period following the date of ESC approval. Your practice should select records as a part of your sample following the date of ESC approval and use the required sample sizes. MOS percentage compliance rates are derived from the average of all four months.

Step 2: Use Your EP Scores to Gauge Your Compliance with the Standards

Now that you have evaluated and scored each EP for a particular standard, use these simple rules to determine your compliance with the standard itself:

- Your practice is not in compliance (that is, "not compliant") with the standard if any EP is scored 0
- Otherwise, your practice is in compliance with a standard if 65% or more of its EPs are scored 2

Scoring Grid

0 Insufficient compliance
1 Partial compliance
2 Satisfactory compliance
NA Not applicable

Standards, Rationales, Elements of Performance, and Scoring

Entry to Care, Treatment, and Services

Standard PC.1.10

The practice accepts for care, treatment, and services only those patients whose identified care, treatment, and service needs it can meet.

❑ Compliant
❑ Not Compliant

Elements of Performance for PC.1.10

1. The practice has a defined written process that includes the following: **B** | 0 | 1 | 2 | NA |
   - The information to be gathered to determine eligibility for entrance into the practice
   - The populations of patients accepted or not accepted by the practice*
   - The criteria to determine eligibility for entry into the system
   - The procedures for accepting referrals

Assessment

Standards PC.2.10 Through PC.2.120

Not applicable

Standard PC.2.130

Initial assessments are performed as defined by the practice.

❑ Compliant
❑ Not Compliant

Elements of Performance for PC.2.130

1. Through 13. Not applicable

14. Information from the patient, appropriate practitioners, and results from testing (where appropriate) is gathered and used to formulate a clinical impression or preliminary diagnosis. **B** | 0 | 1 | 2 | NA |

15. The information collected is appropriate to the patient's presenting problem or health status and the services to be rendered. **B** | 0 | 1 | 2 | NA |

16. To avoid unnecessary duplication of tests and procedures, relevant clinical information from a referring practitioner or results from previous testing may be used. **B** | 0 | 1 | 2 | NA |

17. When appropriate, information from the patient's family† is also considered. **B** | 0 | 1 | 2 | NA |

Standard PC.2.140

Not applicable

---

* For example, programs designed to treat adults that do not treat young children.

† **Family** The person(s) who plays a significant role in the individual's life. This may include a person(s) not legally related to the individual. This person(s) is often referred to as a surrogate decision maker if authorized to make care decisions for an individual if the individual loses decision-making capacity.

Standard PC.2.150

Not applicable

Additional Standard for Victims of Abuse

❑ Compliant
❑ Not Compliant

Standard PC.3.10

Patients who may be victims of abuse, neglect, or exploitation are assessed. (*See* standard RI.2.150.)

Rationale for PC.3.10

Unless possible victims of abuse are identified and assessed, they cannot receive appropriate care. Such patients have special assessment and care needs. Victims of abuse or neglect may come to the practice in a variety of ways. The patient might be unable or reluctant to speak of the abuse, and it might not be obvious to the casual observer. Staff needs to be able to identify abuse, neglect, or exploitation as well as the extent and circumstances of the abuse, neglect, or exploitation to give the patient appropriate care.

Criteria for identifying and assessing victims of abuse, neglect, or exploitation should be used throughout the practice. The assessment of the patient must be conducted within the context of the requirements of the law to preserve evidentiary materials and support future legal actions.

Elements of Performance for PC.3.10

A | 0 | 1 | 2 | NA |

1. The practice develops or adopts criteria* for identifying victims in each of the following situations:
   - Physical assault
   - Rape
   - Sexual molestation
   - Domestic abuse
   - Elder neglect or abuse
   - Child neglect or abuse

B | 0 | 1 | 2 | NA |

2. Appropriate staff[†] are educated about abuse, neglect, and exploitation and how to refer as appropriate.

A | 0 | 1 | 2 | NA |

3. A list of private and public community agencies that provide or arrange for assessment and care of abuse victims is maintained to facilitate appropriate referrals.

B | 0 | 1 | 2 | NA |

4. Victims of abuse, neglect, or exploitation are identified using the criteria developed or adopted by the practice at entry into the system and on an ongoing basis.

B | 0 | 1 | 2 | NA |

5. The practice's staff refers appropriately or conducts the assessment of victims of abuse, neglect, or exploitation.

Standard PC.3.20 Through PC.3.220

Not applicable

---

* The Family Violence Prevention Fund is one resource that can be contacted for further information at http://www.fvpf.org.

† Staff should be able to screen for abuse, neglect and exploitation as indicated by the patient's needs or conditions. The practice may define who conducts the full assessment for alleged or suspected abuse, neglect or exploitation or refer to another practice.

Scoring Grid
0 Insufficient compliance
1 Partial compliance
2 Satisfactory compliance
NA Not applicable

Diagnostic Services

Standard PC.3.230

Diagnostic testing* necessary for determining the patient's health care needs is performed.

❑ Compliant
❑ Not Compliant

Elements of Performance for PC.3.230

1. Through 5. Not applicable

6. Clinical staff determine which tests, if any, are to be performed. **A** | 0 | 1 | 2 | NA |

7. Previous diagnostic tests are used in the assessment process only if they are considered current at the time of assessment. **B** | 0 | 1 | 2 | NA |

Planning Care, Treatment, and Services

Standard PC.4.10

Development of a plan for care, treatment, and services is individualized and appropriate to the patient's needs, strengths, limitations, and goals.

❑ Compliant
❑ Not Compliant

PC

Rationale for PC.4.10

Treatment is effective, efficient, individualized, and appropriate. Each phase of care—assessment, administration of sedation or anesthesia, surgical/invasive procedure, recovery, and discharge—identifies and responds to each patient's needs, expectations, characteristics, age, and severity of disease, condition, or impairment.

Element of Performance for PC.4.10

1. Care, treatment, and services are planned to ensure that they are appropriate to the patient's needs. **B** | 0 | 1 | 2 | NA |

Standards PC.4.20 Through PC.4.120

Not applicable

Providing Care, Treatment, and Services

Standard PC.5.10

The practice provides care, treatment, and services for each patient according to the plan for care, treatment, and services.

❑ Compliant
❑ Not Compliant

Elements of Performance for PC.5.10

1. Through 3. Not applicable

4. The practice uses at least two patient identifiers (neither of which is the patient's physical location identifier) whenever taking blood samples or administering medications, or blood, or blood products. **A** | 0 | 1 | 2 | NA |

* Diagnostic testing includes laboratory, radiologic, electrodiagnostic, and other functional tests and imaging technologies.

Scoring Grid
0 Insufficient compliance
1 Partial compliance
2 Satisfactory compliance
NA Not applicable

Standards PC.5.20 Through PC.5.50

Not applicable

❑ Compliant
❑ Not Compliant

Standard PC.5.60

The practice coordinates the care, treatment, and services provided to a patient as part of the plan for care, treatment, and services and consistent with the practice's scope of care, treatment, and services.

Elements of Performance for PC.5.60

1. Through 4. Not applicable

B | 0 | 1 | 2 | NA |

5. The plan of care, treatment, and services is designed to occur in a time frame that meets the patient's health needs.

Standard PC.5.70

Not applicable

Education

PC

Introduction

The goal of patient and family education in an office-based surgery practice is to improve patient outcomes by involving the patient and, as appropriate, family in treatment decisions. This goal is met when an office-based surgery practice performs the following processes well:

- Promoting interactive communication between patients, practitioners, and staff
- Improving patients' understanding of their assessed needs, their options for procedures and anesthesia, and the anticipated risks and benefits of treatment
- Encouraging patient participation in decision making about care
- Adhering to preoperative and post-procedure instructions
- Maximizing patient self-care skills
- Enhancing patient participation in continuing care
- Informing patients about their financial responsibilities for treatment, when known

Recognizing that psychosocial, spiritual, and cultural values also affect patients' responses to and participation in education and care, the practice supports patient involvement in their own treatment and the educational process.

Note: *Although the following standards recommend a systematic approach to education, they do not require any specific structure, such as an education department, a patient education committee, or the employment of an educator. More important is a philosophy that views the educational function as in interactive one in which all parties are learners. These standards help the practice focus on how education is consistent with the patient's plan for care, the level of care, educational opportunities in this setting, and the continuity of care.*

❑ Compliant
❑ Not Compliant

Standard PC.6.10

The patient receives education and training specific to the patient's needs and as appropriate to the care, treatment, and services provided.

Elements of Performance for PC.6.10

1. Through 12. Not applicable

C | 0 | 1 | 2 | NA |

13. As appropriate to the patient's condition and assessed needs and the practice's scope of services, the patient is educated about the following:
    - Description of the procedure and options
    - Description of the sedation or anesthesia and related options

Scoring Grid
0 Insufficient compliance
1 Partial compliance
2 Satisfactory compliance
NA Not applicable

- The safe and effective use of medications
- Expected duration of the procedure
- Expected duration of recovery
- Anticipated signs and symptoms following discharge and their duration
- Preoperative preparations the patient must undertake
- The need for a responsible adult to escort the patient following discharge
- Follow-up instructions (for example, limitations on activity, surgical-site cleansing, medication use)
- Who the patient may call with any questions following discharge
- Understanding pain, the risk for pain, the importance of effective pain management, the pain assessment process, and methods for pain management, when identified as part of treatment
- Care activities appropriate to the patient's status and needs relative to habilitation or rehabilitation

Note: *These issues should be addressed as part of preoperative assessment and postoperative follow-up instructions.*

Standard PC.6.20

Not applicable

PC

Standard PC.6.30

The patient receives education and training specific to the patient's abilities as appropriate to the care, treatment, and services provided by the practice.

❑ Compliant
❑ Not Compliant

Elements of Performance for PC.6.30

1. Education provided is appropriate to the patient's abilities. — **B** | 0 | 1 | 2 | NA |

2. Through 5. Not applicable

Ⓜ 6. Staff, while imparting information to patients and families, elicits feedback to ensure that the information is understood. — **C** | 0 | 1 | 2 | NA |

7. Staff uses family or community resources as necessary to help in education, comprehension, and use of information. — **B** | 0 | 1 | 2 | NA |

Standards PC.6.40 Through PC.6.60

Not applicable

Nutritional Care

Standard PC.7.10

The practice has a process for preparing and/or distributing food and nutrition products as appropriate.

Element of Performance for PC.7.10

1. Food and nutrition products are provided for the patient as appropriate to the patient needs identified during assessment. — **B** | 0 | 1 | 2 | NA |

Scoring Grid
0 Insufficient compliance
1 Partial compliance
2 Satisfactory compliance
NA Not applicable

Pain

❑ Compliant
❑ Not Compliant

Standard PC.8.10

Pain is assessed in all patients.

Elements of Performance for PC.8.10

1. Not applicable

C 0 1 2 NA — Ⓜ 2. A referral for a comprehensive pain assessment is made or a comprehensive pain assessment is conducted when warranted by the patient's condition.

3. Not applicable

C 0 1 2 NA — Ⓜ 4. Reassessment and follow-up occur according to the criteria developed by the practice or as required by the practice assessing or treating the pain.

C 0 1 2 NA — Ⓜ 5. If conducted by the practice, the assessment and a measure of pain intensity and quality (for example, pain character, frequency, location, duration, exacerbating and relieving factors) appropriate to the patient's age are recorded.

6. Not applicable

C 0 1 2 NA — Ⓜ 7. When pain is identified, the patient is treated by the practice or referred for treatment.

Restorative Services

Standards PC.8.20 Through PC.8.70

Not applicable

Specific Procedures

Administering Blood and Blood Components

❑ Compliant
❑ Not Compliant

Standard PC.9.10

Blood and blood components are administered safely, as appropriate to the setting.

Elements of Performance for PC.9.10

1. Through 10. Not applicable

B 0 1 2 NA — 11. The practice has detailed written procedures for how to obtain blood components or blood products.

B 0 1 2 NA — 12. The procedures describe at least the following:
- The source of the materials
- The time frames for obtaining them
- Accountability for procurement
- On-site storage

Scoring Grid
0 Insufficient compliance
1 Partial compliance
2 Satisfactory compliance
NA Not applicable

Responding to Life-Threatening Emergencies

Standard PC.9.20

The practice responds to life-threatening emergencies according to practice policy and procedure.

❑ Compliant
❑ Not Compliant

Rationale for PC.9.20

The practice has the capability through sedation policies, dosage guidelines, resuscitative equipment, staff training, transfer agreements, and other measures to address the patient's potential risks or needs (for example, certain patients undergoing high volume or tumescent liposuction) and potential clinical emergencies during the procedure until the patient is discharged from the setting.

Elements of Performance for PC.9.20

1. Through 3. Not applicable

4. In the event of a patient emergency, there are at least two staff members on site at all times during which patients are undergoing procedures and until patients are discharged. **A** 0 1 2 NA

5. Staff members have been appropriately trained in their roles in the event that a patient experiences a medical emergency. **A** 0 1 2 NA

6. Staff members know when and how to use emergency medical services and other community resources to help in a patient's medical emergency. **B** 0 1 2 NA

7. Appropriate equipment for resuscitation is available. **A** 0 1 2 NA

Standards PC.9.30 Through PC.12.190

Not applicable

Standards for Additional Special Procedures

Standards for Operative or Other High-Risk Procedures and/or the Administration of Moderate or Deep Sedation or Anesthesia

The goal of surgical and invasive procedures, sedation, anesthesia, and recovery activities in an office-based surgery practice is to provide for effective, appropriate, and individualized care and procedures that respond to the patient's specific needs. Before any procedure, the practice assesses the patient as an appropriate candidate for an office-based procedure. Sedation and anesthesia assessment and any necessary examinations and diagnostic testing occur, and the patient is informed about risks, benefits, alternatives, and informed consent. The surgeon gives final approval for the planned sedation or anesthesia and the invasive or surgical procedure based on these assessments. Assessment occurs throughout the pre-, peri-, and postprocedure phases, addressing not only physical and functional status, but also physiological and cognitive status as they relate to the use of sedation and anesthesia. Surgeons perform the surgical and invasive procedures.

Because sedation is a continuum, it is not always possible to predict how an individual patient receiving sedation will respond. Therefore, each practice develops specific, appropriate protocols for the care of patients receiving sedation. These protocols are consistent with professional standards and address at least the following:

- Sufficient qualified individuals present to perform the procedure and to monitor the patient throughout administration and recovery. The individuals providing moderate or deep sedation and anesthesia have at a minimum had competency-based education, training, and experience in the following:
  1. Evaluating patients before performing moderate or deep sedation and anesthesia.

2. Performing the moderate or deep sedation and anesthesia, including rescuing patients who slip into a deeper-than-desired level of sedation or analgesia. These include the following:
   a. Moderate sedation—are qualified to rescue patients from deep sedation and are competent to manage a compromised airway and to provide adequate oxygenation and ventilation
   b. Deep sedation—are qualified to rescue patients from general anesthesia and are competent to manage an unstable cardiovascular system as well as a compromised airway and inadequate oxygenation and ventilation

- Appropriate equipment for care and resuscitation
- Appropriate monitoring of vital signs, including, but not limited to, heart rates and oxygenation using pulse oximetry equipment, respiratory frequency and adequacy of pulmonary ventilation, the monitoring of blood pressure at regular intervals, and cardiac monitoring (by EKG or use of continuous cardiac monitoring device) in patients with significant cardiovascular disease or when dysrhythmias are anticipated or detected
- Documentation of care
- Monitoring of outcomes

Discharge planning in the office-based surgery practice addresses appropriate referrals, transfers, and follow-up. The practice maintains timely and accurate documentation of all phases of care to support treatment and performance improvement.

The standards for sedation and anesthesia care apply when patients receive, in any setting, for any purpose, by any route, moderate or deep sedation as well as general, spinal, or other major regional anesthesia.

Definitions of four levels of sedation and anesthesia include the following:

- **Minimal sedation (anxiolysis)**
  A drug-induced state during which patients respond normally to verbal commands. Although cognitive function and coordination might be impaired, ventilatory and cardiovascular functions are unaffected.
- **Moderate sedation/analgesia (conscious sedation)**
  A drug-induced depression of consciousness during which patients respond purposefully to verbal commands (note, reflex withdrawal from a painful stimulus is not considered a purposeful response)—either alone or accompanied by light tactile stimulation. No interventions are required to maintain a patent airway, and spontaneous ventilation is adequate. Cardiovascular function is usually maintained.
- **Deep sedation/analgesia**
  A drug-induced depression of consciousness during which patients cannot be easily aroused but respond purposefully after repeated or painful stimulation. The ability to independently maintain ventilatory function might be impaired. Patients might require assistance in maintaining a patent airway and spontaneous ventilation might be inadequate. Cardiovascular function is usually maintained.
- **Anesthesia**
  Consists of general anesthesia and spinal or major regional anesthesia. It does *not* include local anesthesia. General anesthesia is a drug-induced loss of consciousness during which patients are not arousable, even by painful stimulation. The ability to independently maintain ventilatory function is often impaired. Patients often require assistance in maintaining a patent airway, and positive pressure ventilation might be required because of depressed spontaneous ventilation or drug-induced depression of neuromuscular function. Cardiovascular function might be impaired.

Note: *A discussion of processes to be considered for use by a practice performing moderate sedation/analgesia is found in "Practice Guidelines for Sedation and Analgesia by Non-Anesthesiologists,"* Anesthesiology *84:459–71, 1996 © 1996 American Society of Anesthesiologists, Inc. (ASA), Lippincott-Raven Publishers. It can also be located at the ASA Web site at* http://asahq.org/Practice/Sedation/Sedation.html.

Scoring Grid
- **0** Insufficient compliance
- **1** Partial compliance
- **2** Satisfactory compliance
- **NA** Not applicable

The standards for surgical and invasive procedures apply whenever a surgical or invasive procedure might have a significant (as defined by principles of standards or care and/or regulation) physiological effect, such as placing the patient at risk, whether or not anesthesia is administered. The standards focus on surgical and invasive procedures for the following:
- Diagnosis
- Cure or palliation of disease, impairment, or disability
- Restoration or improvement of function
- Relief of symptoms

These standards relate to the following processes:
- Selecting appropriate procedures
- Preparing patients for procedures
- Performing procedures and patient monitoring
- Providing postprocedure care and education

Standard PC.13.10

Licensed independent practitioners define the scope of assessment for operative or other procedures and/or the administration of moderate or deep sedation or anesthesia.

❑ Compliant
❑ Not Compliant

Rationale for PC.13.10

Established guidelines are used to assess patients undergoing surgical and invasive procedures. Guidelines may include information from state regulatory agencies, as applicable. The assessment provides all information necessary to conduct the appropriate procedure at the optimal time, perform the procedure safely, and provide a baseline for interpreting findings while monitoring the patient.

Element of Performance for PC.13.10

1. The assessment includes the following:
   - The patient's history
   - The patient's physical status
   - Diagnostic data
   - The risks and benefits of procedures

B	0	1	2	NA

Standard PC.13.20

Operative or other procedures and/or the administration of moderate or deep sedation or anesthesia are planned.

❑ Compliant
❑ Not Compliant

Rationale for PC.13.20

Because the response to procedures is not always predictable and sedation-to-anesthesia is a continuum, it is not always possible to predict how an individual patient will respond. Therefore, qualified individuals are trained in professional standards and techniques to do the following:
- Administer pharmacologic agents to predictably achieve desired levels of sedation
- Monitor patients carefully to maintain them at the desired level of sedation
- Manage patients in the case of a potentially harmful event

Assessment of all patients includes information needed to do the following:
- Plan moderate or deep sedation and anesthesia care
- Safely administer moderate or deep sedation and anesthesia
- Interpret findings during patient monitoring

Scoring Grid

0 Insufficient compliance
1 Partial compliance
2 Satisfactory compliance
NA Not applicable

Elements of Performance for PC.13.20

B 0 1 2 NA — 1. Sufficient numbers of qualified staff (in addition to the licensed independent practitioner performing the procedure) are present to evaluate the patient, help with the procedure, provide the sedation and/or anesthesia, monitor, and recover the patient.

A 0 1 2 NA — 2. Individuals administering moderate or deep sedation and anesthesia are qualified and have the appropriate credentials to manage patients at whatever level of sedation or anesthesia is achieved, either intentionally or unintentionally.

3. Not applicable

B 0 1 2 NA — 4. Appropriate equipment to monitor the patient's physiologic status is available.

B 0 1 2 NA — 5. Appropriate equipment to administer intravenous fluids and drugs, including blood and blood components, is available as needed.

B 0 1 2 NA — 6. Resuscitation capabilities are available.

The following must occur before the operative and other procedures or the administration of moderate or deep sedation or anesthesia (EPs 7–10):

C 0 1 2 NA — Ⓜ 7. The anticipated needs of the patient are assessed to plan for the appropriate level of postprocedure care.

PC

C 0 1 2 NA — Ⓜ 8. Preprocedural education, treatments, and services are provided according to the plan for care, treatment, and services.

A 0 1 2 NA — 9. The site, procedure, and patient are accurately identified and clearly communicated, using active communication techniques, during a final verification process such as a timeout before the start of any surgical or invasive procedure.

A 0 1 2 NA — 10. A presedation or preanesthesia assessment is conducted by a licensed independent practitioner, or other qualified clinical staff determines whether the patient can safely undergo the planned sedation or anesthesia.

A 0 1 2 NA — 11. Before sedating or anesthetizing a patient, a licensed independent practitioner with appropriate clinical privileges plans or concurs with the planned anesthesia.

A 0 1 2 NA — 12. The patient is reevaluated immediately before moderate or deep sedation and before anesthesia induction to identify any changes that might have occurred since the initial clinical assessment that might affect the safe and effective administration of moderate or deep sedation or anesthesia.

A 0 1 2 NA — 13. Operative and other procedures are done only after completion and documentation of appropriate history and physical examination, any indicated diagnostic tests, and the preoperative diagnosis.

C 0 1 2 NA — Ⓜ 14. A history and physical examination are completed within 30 days before an operative or other procedure.

15. Through 18. Not applicable

C 0 1 2 NA — Ⓜ 19. Durable, legible originals or reproductions of the assessment documents completed and/or authenticated by the surgeon and/or the licensed independent practitioner are included in the patient's record.

B 0 1 2 NA — 20. Any significant changes in the patient's condition subsequent to these assessments are recorded.

A 0 1 2 NA — 21. A licensed independent practitioner* performs the surgical or invasive procedure.

**See* standard RI.2.60 in the "Practice Ethics, and Patient Rights and Responsibilities" chapter for more information about the licensed independent practitioner who performs the procedure.

Scoring Grid
0 Insufficient compliance
1 Partial compliance
2 Satisfactory compliance
NA Not applicable

Standard PC.13.30

Patients are monitored during the procedure and/or administration of moderate or deep sedation or anesthesia.

❑ Compliant
❑ Not Compliant

Rationale for PC.13.30

Physiological monitoring is often the only reliable source of assessment information for patients who have lost consciousness or who undergo sedation or anesthesia. The patient's physiological status is measured and assessed throughout sedation or anesthesia to ensure appropriate physiological support. Monitoring methods depend on the patient's preprocedure status, sedation or anesthesia choice, and complexity of the procedure.

Elements of Performance for PC.13.30

1. Not applicable
2. Ⓜ The procedure and/or the administration of moderate or deep sedation or anesthesia for each patient is documented in the medical record. — C | 0 | 1 | 2 | NA
3. Heart rate and oxygenation are continuously monitored by pulse oximetry. — A | 0 | 1 | 2 | NA
4. Respiratory frequency and adequacy of pulmonary ventilation are continually monitored. — A | 0 | 1 | 2 | NA
5. Blood pressure is measured at regular intervals. — A | 0 | 1 | 2 | NA
6. EKG is monitored in patients with significant cardiovascular disease or when dysrhythmias are anticipated or detected. — A | 0 | 1 | 2 | NA

Standard PC.13.40

Patients are monitored immediately after the procedure and/or administration of moderate or deep sedation or anesthesia.

❑ Compliant
❑ Not Compliant

Rationale for PC.13.40

A patient who has recovered from moderate or deep sedation or anesthesia sufficiently to be discharged might still experience minor and temporary impairments to cognition or coordination.

Elements of Performance for PC.13.40

1. The patient's status is assessed immediately after the procedure and/or administration of moderate or deep sedation or anesthesia. — A | 0 | 1 | 2 | NA
2. Ⓜ Each patient's physiological status, mental status, and pain level are monitored. — C | 0 | 1 | 2 | NA
3. Monitoring is at a level consistent with the potential effect of the procedure and/or sedation or anesthesia. — B | 0 | 1 | 2 | NA
4. Patients are discharged from the postsedation or postanesthesia recovery phase by the qualified licensed independent practitioner responsible for the sedation or anesthesia. — B | 0 | 1 | 2 | NA
5. Ⓜ Patients who have received sedation or anesthesia are discharged in the company of a responsible, designated adult. — C | 0 | 1 | 2 | NA
6. Not applicable
7. The licensed independent practitioner who performed the procedure and the clinical staff who administered and monitored sedation or anesthesia remain on site and available until the patient is discharged from the postsedation or postanesthesia recovery phase.* — A | 0 | 1 | 2 | NA

   Note: *These might be one and the same person, although in some practices they might be two different individuals.*

* Please note the differentiation between discharge from sedation or anesthesia recovery (EP 7) and discharge from the setting (EP 8). In some cases, these processes occur simultaneously; in other cases, they are two discrete events.

PC

A | 0 | 1 | 2 | NA

8. The patient is discharged from the setting by one of the following processes:
   - The licensed independent practitioner who performed the procedure is on-site and discharges the patient from the setting.
     or
   - The licensed independent practitioner who performed the procedure has left the practice office. The licensed independent practitioner consults with the clinical staff on site, who have determined that the patient has met clinical criteria for discharge from the setting using criteria approved by the practice's licensed independent practitioner(s). The licensed independent practitioner authorizes discharge from the setting, and compliance with discharge criteria and the licensed independent practitioner's authorization are documented in the patient's medical record.
     or
   - The licensed independent practitioner who performed the procedure has left the practice office. Another licensed independent practitioner, who is on-site and has competencies equivalent to those of the licensed independent practitioner who performed the procedure, has been assigned responsibility for discharging the patient from the setting.

B | 0 | 1 | 2 | NA

9. The postdischarge assessment is appropriate to the type of procedure performed and the patient's clinical status during and following the procedure.

A | 0 | 1 | 2 | NA

10. For patients who received moderate or deep sedation or anesthesia, clinical staff members certified in advanced life support (ALS) or, when applicable, pediatric advanced life support (PALS) are on-site until all such patients have been discharged from the setting.

A | 0 | 1 | 2 | NA

11. For patients who received minimal sedation, clinical staff certified in basic life support (BLS) or, when applicable, pediatric basic life support (PBLS) are on-site until all such patients have been discharged from the setting.

Standards PC.13.50 Through PC.14.30

Not applicable

Discharge or Transfer from the Practice

❑ Compliant
❑ Not Compliant

Standard PC.15.10

A process addresses the needs for continuing care, treatment, and services after transfer.

Rationale for PC.15.10

Follow-up planning begins when the patient is first seen. The practice assesses the patient's needs for follow-up care.

Element of Performance for PC.15.10

B | 0 | 1 | 2 | NA

1. The process addresses the following:
   - The reason(s) for transfer
   - The conditions under which transfer can occur
   - Shifting responsibility for a patient's care from one clinician or organization to another
   - Mechanisms for transfer
   - The accountability and responsibility for the patient's safety during transfer of both the practice initiating the transfer and the organization receiving the patient

Scoring Grid
0 Insufficient compliance
1 Partial compliance
2 Satisfactory compliance
NA Not applicable

Standard PC.15.20

❑ Compliant
❑ Not Compliant

The transfer or discharge of a patient is based on the patient's assessed needs and the practice's capabilities.

Rationale for PC.15.20

For some patients, effective planning addresses how needs will be met as they move to the next level of care, treatment, and services. For other patients, planning consists of a clear understanding of how to access services in the future should the need arise.

Elements of Performance for PC.15.20

1\. Through 6. Not applicable

Ⓜ 7. When indicated, the patient is educated about how to obtain further care, treatment, and services to meet his or her identified needs. — C | 0 | 1 | 2 | NA |

8\. Not applicable

Ⓜ 9. Written discharge instructions in a form the patient can understand are given to the patient and/or those responsible for providing continuing care. — C | 0 | 1 | 2 | NA |

Standard PC.15.30

❑ Compliant
❑ Not Compliant

When patients are transferred or discharged, appropriate information related to the care, treatment, and services provided is exchanged with other service providers.

Elements of Performance for PC.15.30

Ⓜ 1. The practice communicates appropriate information to any practice or provider to which the patient is transferred or discharged. — C | 0 | 1 | 2 | NA |

Ⓜ 2. The information shared includes the following, as appropriate to the care, treatment, and services provided: — C | 0 | 1 | 2 | NA |
- The reason for transfer or discharge
- The patient's physical and psychosocial status
- A summary of care, treatment, and services provided

3\. Through 8. Not applicable

Ⓜ 9. When ongoing care will be provided by another practitioner (such as the patient's primary care practitioner), the practice submits relevant clinical information on services provided, procedures performed, patient status at discharge, and any postdischarge instructions and medications provided. — C | 0 | 1 | 2 | NA |

Waived Testing

The federal regulation governing laboratory testing, known as the Clinical Laboratory Improvement Amendments of 1988 (CLIA '88), classifies testing into four complexity levels: high complexity, moderate complexity, PPM (Provider Performed Microscopy, a subset of moderate complexity), and waived testing. The high, moderate, and PPM levels, otherwise called nonwaived testing, have specific and detailed requirements regarding personnel qualifications, quality assurance, quality control, and other systems. Joint Commission requirements for the tests and laboratories or sites that perform them are located in the *Comprehensive Accreditation Manual for Laboratory and Point-of-Care Testing* (*CAMLAB*).

Waived testing is the most common complexity level performed by caregivers at the patient's bedside or point of care. The same laboratory test may be available by more than one method within a practice, and those methods may be of different complexity levels. The list of methods that are approved as waived is under constant revision, so it is advisable to check the Food and Drug Administration (FDA), Centers for Disease Control and Prevention (CDC), or Center for Medicare & Medicaid Services (CMS) Web site for the most up-to-date information regarding test categorization and complete CLIA '88 requirements:

http://www.fda.gov/cdrh/clia/index.html

http://www.phppo.cdc.gov/clia

http://www.cms.hhs.gov/clia

CLIA '88 identifies laboratory testing as an activity that occurs, not defined as *occurring* at a specific location. Any activity that evaluates any substance removed from a human body and translates that evaluation to a result becomes a laboratory test. The results may be stated as a number, presence or absence of a cell or reaction, or an interpretation, such as what occurs when recording a urine color. Test results that are used to assess a patient's condition or make a clinical decision about a patient are governed by CLIA '88.

Tests that produce a result measured as a number are called *quantitative* and are usually performed with the assistance of some type of instrument. Tests that produce a negative or positive result, such as occult bloods and urine pregnancy screens, are termed *qualitative* and are usually known as manual tests. Any test with analysis steps that rely on the use of an instrument to produce a result is an instrument-based test.

When a patient performs a test on himself or herself (for example, whole blood glucose testing by a patient on his or her own meter cleared by the FDA for home use), the action is not regulated. Testing performed by one individual on another individual while carrying out professional responsibilities is an activity regulated by CLIA '88. This distinction is important when caring for patients who monitor their own glucose or prothrombin times with home devices.

❑ Compliant
❑ Not Compliant

Standard PC.16.10

The practice establishes policies and procedures that define the context in which waived test results are used in patient care, treatment, and services.

Elements of Performance for PC.16.10

B | 0 | 1 | 2 | NA |
1. Quantitative test result reports in the clinical record are accompanied by reference intervals specific to the test method used and are appropriate to the population served.

B | 0 | 1 | 2 | NA |
2. Criteria for confirmatory testing for each test, qualitative or quantitative, is specified in the written procedure as dictated by clinical usage and methodology limitations.

B | 0 | 1 | 2 | NA |
3. Actual usage is consistent with the practice 's policies and the manufacturer's recommendations for each waived test.

❑ Compliant
❑ Not Compliant

Standard PC.16.20

The practice identifies the staff responsible for performing and supervising waived testing.

Elements of Performance for PC.16.20

B | 0 | 1 | 2 | NA |
1. Staff members who perform testing are identified.

B | 0 | 1 | 2 | NA |
2. Staff members who direct or supervise testing are identified.

Note: *These individuals may be employees of the practice, contracted staff, or employees of a contracted service.*

Scoring Grid
0 Insufficient compliance
1 Partial compliance
2 Satisfactory compliance
NA Not applicable

Standard PC.16.30

Staff performing tests have adequate, specific training and orientation to perform the tests and demonstrate satisfactory levels of competence.

❑ Compliant
❑ Not Compliant

Rationale for PC.16.30

For waived tests to be performed properly, the staff performing them must be qualified to do so. Staff members who perform waived testing have specific training in each test performed. This training may be acquired through practice or other training programs, such as those provided by other health care practices or manufacturers.

Elements of Performance for PC.16.30

Ⓜ 1. Current competence of testing staff is demonstrated. C | 0 | 1 | 2 | NA

Ⓜ 2. Each staff member who performs testing has been trained specifically for each test he or she is authorized to perform. C | 0 | 1 | 2 | NA

Ⓜ 3. Each staff member who performs testing has been oriented according to the practice's specific needs.

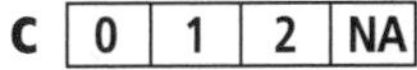

4. Testing that requires the use of an instrument is performed by staff with adequate and specific training on the use and care of that instrument.

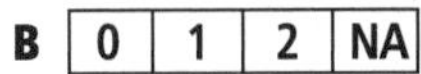

Ⓜ 5. Competence is assessed according to practice policy at defined intervals, but at least at the time of orientation and annually thereafter.

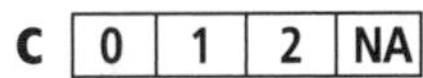

6. These assessments have considered the following:
   - The frequency by which staff members perform tests
   - The technical backgrounds of the staff
   - The complexity of the test methodology and the consequences of an inaccurate result

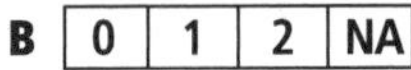

7. Methods to assess current competency include at least two of the following:
   - Performing a test on an unknown specimen
   - Having the supervisor or qualified delegate periodically observe routine work
   - Monitoring each user's quality control performance
   - Having written testing that is specific to the method assessed

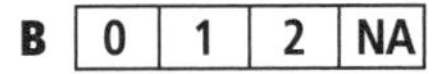

8. The practice evaluates and documents the information listed previously.

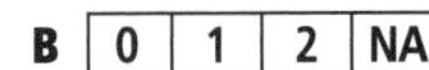

   Note: *All staff who perform instrument-based testing, including (but not limited to) physicians, licensed independent practitioners, contracted staff, and RNs, must participate in training and competence demonstrations.*

PC

Standard PC.16.40

Approved policies and procedures governing specific testing-related processes are current and readily available.

❑ Compliant
❑ Not Compliant

Rationale for PC.16.40

Current and up-to-date policies and procedures are an important reference tool in managing laboratory testing activities, particularly when individual staff members perform them infrequently. Testing policies and procedures include requirements that are in compliance with the manufacturer's recommendations regarding all the following, as applicable:

- Specimen type (for example, a method for whole blood is not used for spinal fluid)
- Storage considerations for test components (for example, compliance with directions such as *store away from direct light,* temperature requirements, open container expiration dates and so forth)
- Instrument maintenance and function checks such as calibration
- Quality control frequency and type

Scoring Grid
0 Insufficient compliance
1 Partial compliance
2 Satisfactory compliance
NA Not applicable

- Result follow-up recommendations (for example, out-of-range results' recommendation for retesting)
- Tests approved by the FDA for home use only are not used for professional purposes (for example, glucose meters cleared for home use only are not used in a hospital setting by nursing staff except as patient education)

Elements of Performance for PC.16.40

B | 0 | 1 | 2 | NA |

1. Written policies and procedures address all the following items:
   - Specimen collection, identification, and required labeling, as appropriate
   - Specimen preservation, as appropriate
   - Instrument calibration
   - Quality control and remedial action
   - Equipment performance evaluation
   - Test performance

B | 0 | 1 | 2 | NA |

2. The policies and procedures for each item are applicable to the specific practice.

   Note: *Reference to a manufacturer's manual is acceptable if appropriate modifications have been made to customize the manual's content for the practice.*

C | 0 | 1 | 2 | NA |

Ⓜ 3. Current and complete policies and procedures are readily available to the person performing the test.

A | 0 | 1 | 2 | NA |

4. The director named on the waived testing certificate or a designee approves policies and procedures at defined intervals.

❑ Compliant
❑ Not Compliant

Standard PC.16.50

Quality control checks, as defined by the practice, are conducted on each procedure.

Elements of Performance for PC.16.50

B | 0 | 1 | 2 | NA |

1. The practice has a written quality control plan that specifies how procedures will be controlled for quality, establishes timetables, and explains the rationale for choice of procedures and timetables.

B | 0 | 1 | 2 | NA |

2. Quality control procedures are performed at least as frequently as recommended by the manufacturer, according to the practice's policies.

C | 0 | 1 | 2 | NA |

Ⓜ 3. For instrument-based waived testing, quality control requirements include two levels of control, if commercially available.

C | 0 | 1 | 2 | NA |

Ⓜ 4. Quality control procedures are performed at least once each day on each instrument used for patient testing.

B | 0 | 1 | 2 | NA |

5. The documented quality control rationale is based on the following:
   - How the test is used
   - Reagent stability
   - Manufacturers' recommendations
   - The practice's experience with the test
   - Currently accepted guidelines

B | 0 | 1 | 2 | NA |

6. At a minimum, manufacturers' instructions are followed.

❑ Compliant
❑ Not Compliant

Standard PC.16.60

Appropriate quality control and test records are maintained.

Scoring Grid

0 Insufficient compliance
1 Partial compliance
2 Satisfactory compliance
NA Not applicable

Elements of Performance for PC.16.60

Ⓜ 1. All quality control test results are documented, including internal, external, liquid, and electronic. **C** | 0 | 1 | 2 | NA |

Ⓜ 2. Test results are documented. **C** | 0 | 1 | 2 | NA |

Note: *Test results may be located in the clinical record.*

3. Quality control records, instrument problems, and individual results are correlated. **B** | 0 | 1 | 2 | NA |

4. A formal log is not required, but a functional audit trail is maintained that allows retrieval of results and associated quality control values for a minimum of two years. **B** | 0 | 1 | 2 | NA |

Medication* Management

Overview

The clinical services needed to support office-based surgery may be provided on a contract basis. The following standards address both the direct provision of the clinical services as well as clinical services provided through contract.

Medication† Management

Medications are essential to patient care; however, their use and handling entail certain risks. The following standards identify significant risk points and offer a system for managing them. Medical evaluation of past and current drug treatments is conducted when medications are used. Treatment efficacy, impact on current functioning, and side effects are considered, including evaluations from the patient, family, or caregivers. These standards address the following components of medication management:

a. Availability
b. Prescribing or ordering‡
c. Preparation and dispensing
d. Administration
e. Monitoring of effect

MM

Glossary Terms

These key terms have specific Joint Commission definitions. Please access the Glossary found near the end of your manual for the Joint Commission definition and appropriate use.

adverse drug event
adverse drug reaction (ADR)
investigational medication
medication

medication management
- administration
- dispensing
- monitoring
- ordering and transcribing
- preparing
- procurement
- storage
- transcribing

* For the purpose of these standards, *medication* includes prescription medications; sample medications; herbal remedies; vitamins; nutraceuticals; over-the-counter drugs; vaccines; diagnostic and contrast agents used on or administered to persons to diagnose, treat, or prevent disease or other abnormal conditions; radioactive medications; respiratory therapy treatments; parenteral nutrition; blood derivatives; intravenous solutions (plain, with electrolytes and/or drugs); and any product designated by the Food and Drug Administration (FDA) as a drug. The definition of *medication* does not include enteral nutrition solutions (which are considered food products), oxygen, and other medical gases.

† **Medication** Any prescription medications; sample medications; herbal remedies; vitamins; nutriceuticals; over-the-counter drugs; vaccines; diagnostic and contrast agents used on or administered to persons to diagnose, treat, or prevent disease or other abnormal conditions; radioactive medications; respiratory therapy treatments; parenteral nutrition; blood derivatives; intravenous solutions (plain, with electrolytes and/or drugs); and any product designated by the FDA as a drug. This definition of medication does not include enteral nutrition solutions, oxygen, and other medical gases.

‡ **Prescribing or ordering** Directing the preparation, dispensing, or administration of a specific medication(s) to a specific patient.

Standards

The following is a list of all standards for this chapter. They are presented here for your convenience without footnotes or other explanatory text. If you have a question about a term used here, please check the Glossary.

Note: *A revised standard numbering system is being used with the reformatted standards. This revised numbering system allows for more flexibility to add standards while maintaining the current label for each standard.*

Patient-Specific Information

MM.1.10 Patient-specific information is readily accessible to those involved in the medication management system.

MM.2.10 Not applicable

Storage

MM.2.20 Medications are properly and safely stored throughout the practice.

MM.2.30 Emergency medications and/or supplies, if any, are consistently available, controlled, and secure in the practice's patient care areas.

MM.2.40 Not applicable

Ordering and Transcribing

MM.3.10 Not applicable

MM.3.20 Not applicable

Preparing and Dispensing

MM.4.10 All prescriptions or medication orders are reviewed for appropriateness.

MM.4.20 Medications are prepared safely.

MM.4.30 Medications are appropriately labeled.

MM.4.40 Medications are dispensed safely.

MM.4.50 Not applicable

MM.4.60 Not applicable

MM.4.70 Medications dispensed by the practice are retrieved when recalled or discontinued by the manufacturer or the FDA for safety reasons.

MM.4.80 Not applicable

Administering

MM.5.10 Medications are safely and accurately administered.

MM.5.20 Not applicable

MM.5.30 Prescribing and ordering medications follow established procedures.

Monitoring

MM.6.10 Not applicable

MM.6.20 Not applicable

High-Risk Medications

MM.7.10 The practice develops processes for managing high-risk or high-alert medications.

MM.7.20 Not applicable

MM.7.30 Not applicable

MM.7.40 Investigational medications are safely controlled and administered.

Evaluation

MM.8.10 The practice evaluates its medication management system.

Understanding the Parts of This Chapter

To help you navigate this reformatted standards chapter, it may be helpful to think of its parts this way:

- The **standard** is the "goal."
- The **rationale** explains why it's important to achieve this goal.
- The **elements of performance** identify the step(s) needed to achieve this goal.

These parts are defined as follows.

Standard A statement that defines the performance expectations and/or structures or processes that must be in place in order for a practice to provide safe, high-quality care, treatment, and services. An practice is either "compliant" or "not compliant" with a standard as reflected by the check boxes in the margin by the standard:

❑ Compliant
❑ Not Compliant

Accreditation decisions are based on simple counts of the standards that are determined to be "not compliant."

Rationale A statement that provides background, justification, or additional information about a standard. A standard's rationale is not scored. In some instances, the rationale for a standard is self-evident. Therefore, not every standard has a written rationale.

Elements of performance (EPs) The specific performance expectations and/or structures or processes that must be in place in order for a practice to provide safe, high-quality care, treatment, and services. The scoring of EP compliance determines a practice's overall compliance with a standard. EPs are evaluated on the following scale:

0 Insufficient compliance
1 Partial compliance
2 Satisfactory compliance
NA Not applicable

You will find a **measure of success** icon—Ⓜ—next to some EPs. Measures of success (MOS) need to be developed for certain EPs when a standard is judged to be out of compliance through the on-site survey. An MOS is defined as a quantifiable measure, usually related to an audit, that can be used to determine whether an action has been effective and is being sustained.*

Using the Self-Assessment Grid to Assess Your Compliance

Once you are familiar with the parts of this chapter, you can begin to assess your compliance with its requirements. A self-assessment grid (otherwise known as a scoring grid) has been provided in the margins for your convenience. If you would like to assess your practice's performance, mark your scores for the EPs on the scoring grid by following the simple steps described below. **Note:** *You are **not** required to complete this scoring grid. It is provided simply to help you assess your own performance.*

Two components are scored for each EP: (1) compliance with the requirement itself **and** (2) compliance with the track record† for that requirement. Scoring has been simplified from the past edition of the manual, and track record achievements (which have always been part of the scoring) have been appropriately modified.

---

* For more information about Measures of Success, *see* "The New Joint Commission Accreditation Process" chapter in this manual.

† **Track record** The amount of time that a practice has been in compliance with a standard, element of performance, or other requirement.

Note: *Some standards and EPs do not apply to a particular type of practice; these standards and EPs are marked "not applicable" and the related text is not included. Your practice is not expected to comply with standards and EPs marked "not applicable."*

In addition, some standards and EPs that do apply to practices may not apply to the specific care, treatment, and services that your individual practice provides. Although these standards and EPs are included in the manual, you are not expected to comply with them. If you are unsure about the standards or EPs that apply to your practice, please contact the Joint Commission's Standards Interpretation Group at 630/792-5900.

Step 1: Score Your Compliance with Each Element of Performance

Before you can determine your compliance with the standards, you must score your compliance with each EP. First look at the EP scoring criterion category listed immediately preceding the scoring scale in the margin next to the EP. There are three scoring criterion categories: A, B, and C (described below). Please note that for each EP scoring criterion category, your practice must meet the performance requirement itself and the track record achievements (*see* below).

Category A

These EPs relate to the presence or absence of the requirement(s) and are scored either yes (2) or no (0); however, score 1 for partial compliance is also possible based on track record achievements (*see* below).

If an A EP has multiple components designated by bullets, your practice must be compliant with all the bullets to receive a score of 2. If your practice does not meet one or more requirements in the bullets, you will receive a score of 0.

Category B

Category B EPs are scored in two steps:

1. As with category A EPs, category B EPs relate to the presence or absence of the requirement(s). If your practice *does not meet* the requirement(s), the EP is scored 0; there is no need to assess your compliance with the principles of good process design (*see* below).
2. If your practice *does meet* the requirement(s), but there is concern about the quality or comprehensiveness of the effort, then and only then should you assess the qualitative aspect of the EP. That is, review the applicable principles of good process design and ask how the principles were applied in the situation under discussion. Good process design has the following characteristics:
   - Is consistent with your practice's mission, values, and goals
   - Meets the needs of patients
   - Reflects the use of currently accepted practices (doing the right thing, using resources responsibly, using practice guidelines)
   - Incorporates current safety information and knowledge such as sentinel event data and National Patient Safety Goals
   - Incorporates relevant performance improvement results

This two-part evaluation applies to both simple and bulleted B EPs. First, the EPs are assessed to determine if the requirements are present. If the EP has multiple components designated by bullets, as with the category A EPs, your practice must meet the requirements in *all* the bulleted items to get a score of 2. If your practice meets *none* of the requirements in the bullets, it receives a score of 0. If your practice meets *at least one, but not all,* of the bulleted requirements, it will receive a score of 1 for the EPs.

Use the following rules to determine your EP score:

- Your EP score is 0 if your practice does not meet the requirement(s); you *do not* need to assess your compliance with the preceding applicable principles of good process design
- Your EP score is 1 if your practice does meet the requirement(s), but considered only *some* of the preceding applicable principles of good process design

MM

- Your EP score is 2 if your practice does meet the requirement(s) *and* considered *all* the preceding principles of good process design

Category C

C EPs are scored 0, 1, or 2 based on the number of times your practice does not meet the EP. These EPs are frequency based and require totaling the number of occurrences (that is, results of performance or nonperformance) related to a particular EP. Each situation discovered by a surveyor(s) will be counted as a separate occurrence.

Note: *Multiple events of the same type related to a single patient and single practitioner/staff member are counted as* one occurrence only.

Use the following rules to determine your EP score:

- Your EP score is 2 if you find one or fewer occurrences of noncompliance with the EP
- Your EP score is 1 if you find two occurrences of noncompliance with the EP
- Your EP score is 0 if you find three or more occurrences of noncompliance with the EP

If an EP in the C category has multiple requirements designated by bullets, the following scoring guidelines apply:

- If there are fewer than 2 findings in all bullets, the EP is scored 2
- If there are three or more findings in all bullets, the EP is scored 0
- In all other combinations of findings, the EP is scored 1

Track Record Achievements

In addition to meeting the requirement(s) in each EP, regardless of category, your practice must also meet the following track record achievements:

Score	Initial Survey	Full Survey
2	4 months or more	12 months or more
1	2 to 3 months	6 to 11 months
0	Fewer than 2 months	Fewer than 6 months

Sample Sizes

If during an on-site survey, your practice has been found to be not compliant with one or more standards, you must demonstrate Evidence of Standards Compliance (ESC) for each standard that is not compliant. The ESC must address compliance at the EP level; when an EP within a noncompliant standard requires an MOS, your practice must demonstrate achievement with the MOS when completing the ESC.

Note: *Not every EP requires an MOS. EPs that do require an MOS are clearly marked in this chapter Practices are required to demonstrate achievement with an MOS* only *for EPs within a noncompliant standard that require an MOS. Practices* do not *need to demonstrate achievement with an MOS for any EP within a compliant standard.*

When demonstrating achievement with an MOS during the ESC process, your practice is **required** to use the following sample sizes, which were established because of their statistical significance, their relative simplicity in application, and their sensitivity to a practice's population size:

- For a population size of fewer than 30 cases,* sample 100% of available cases
- For a population size of 30 to 100 cases, sample 30 cases
- For a population size of 101 to 500 cases, sample 50 cases
- For a population size greater than 500 cases, sample 70 cases

When demonstrating an ESC (mandatory use), use the following percentages to determine your EP score: 90% through 100% of your sample size is in compliance = score 2; 80% through 89% of your sample size is in compliance = score 1; less than 80% of your sample size is in compliance = score 0.

* "Case" refers to a single instance in which a situation related to a survey finding occurs. For example, if a survey finding was related to **pain assessment,** then a "case" would be any patient record. If a survey finding was related to **pain management,** a "case" would be any patient record for patients receiving pain management.

In addition, the following information should govern your practice's selection of samples:

- The appropriate sample size should be determined by the specific population related to the survey findings.
- The sampling approach should involve either systematic random sampling (for example, your practice selects every second or third case for review) or simple random sampling (for example, your practice uses a series of random numbers generated by a computer to identify the cases to be reviewed).
- When submitting clarifying ESC, if your practice selects records as part of its sample, the records should be from a period of no more than three months before the last date of the survey.
- Assessment of MOS compliance is conducted for a four-month period following the date of ESC approval. Your practice should select records as a part of your sample following the date of ESC approval and use the required sample sizes. MOS percentage compliance rates are derived from the average of all four months.

Step 2: Use Your EP Scores to Gauge Your Compliance with the Standards

Now that you have evaluated and scored each EP for a particular standard, use these simple rules to determine your compliance with the standard itself:

- Your practice is not in compliance (that is, "not compliant") with the standard if any EP is scored 0
- Otherwise, your practice is in compliance with a standard if 65% or more of its EPs are scored 2

Standards, Rationales, Elements of Performance, and Scoring

Patient-Specific Information

❑ Compliant
❑ Not Compliant

Standard MM.1.10

Patient-specific information is readily accessible to those involved in the medication management system.

Rationale for MM.1.10

A major cause of medication-related sentinel events and medication errors is a lack of information. Licensed independent practitioners, appropriate health care professionals, and staff who participate in the medication management system need access to important information about each patient to:

- Facilitate continuity of care, treatment, and services
- Create an accurate medication history and a current list of medications (also known as a drug profile)
- Safely order, prepare, dispense, administer, and monitor medications, as appropriate
- Supplement monitoring of adverse medication events*

Element of Performance for MM.1.10

1. Not applicable

A | 0 | 1 | 2 | NA

2. At a minimum, the information includes the following:
   - The patient's current medications
   - The patient's relevant laboratory values
   - The patient's allergies and past sensitivities

   As appropriate to the patient, the practice also includes information regarding the following:
   - Weight and height
   - Pregnancy and lactation status
   - Any other information required by the practice for safe medication management

Standard MM.2.10

Not applicable

Storage

❑ Compliant
❑ Not Compliant

Standard MM.2.20

Medications are properly and safely stored throughout the practice.

Note: *This standard is applicable only to practices that store medications in their facility.*

Note: *The following EPs also apply to emergency medications. Additional requirements for emergency medications are addressed at standard MM.2.30.*

Elements of Performance for MM.2.20

1. Not applicable

---

* *See* the "Improving Practice Performance" (PI) chapter in this manual.

Scoring Grid
0 Insufficient compliance
1 Partial compliance
2 Satisfactory compliance
NA Not applicable

Ⓜ 2. Medications are stored under necessary conditions to ensure stability. — A 0 1 2 NA

3. Not applicable

4. Controlled substances are stored to prevent diversion and according to state and federal laws and regulations. — A 0 1 2 NA

5. All expired, damaged, and/or contaminated medications are segregated until they are removed from the organization. — A 0 1 2 NA

6. Medications that are easy to confuse (for example, sound-alike and look-alike drugs or reagents and chemicals that may be mistaken for medications) are segregated. — B 0 1 2 NA

7. Not applicable

8. Drug concentrations available in the practice are standardized and limited in number. — A 0 1 2 NA

Ⓜ 9. Concentrated electrolytes are removed from care units or areas, unless patient safety is at risk if the concentrated electrolyte is not immediately available on a specific care unit or area and specific precautions are taken to prevent inadvertent administration. — A 0 1 2 NA

Standard MM.2.30

❑ Compliant
❑ Not Compliant

Emergency medications and/or supplies, if any, are consistently available, controlled, and secure in the practice's patient care areas.

Note: *The following requirements for emergency medications are in addition to the requirements at standard MM.2.20, which are also applicable to emergency medications.*

Elements of Performance for MM.2.30

1. Through 3. Not Applicable

Ⓜ 4. Emergency medications are sealed or stored in containers (for example, crash carts, tackle boxes, emergency drug kits, closed bags that are clearly labeled, and so forth) in such a way that staff can readily determine that the contents are complete and have not expired. — A 0 1 2 NA

5. Through 8. Not applicable

Ⓜ 9. Emergency medications are available, controlled, and secured in the procedure areas. — A 0 1 2 NA

Standard MM.2.40 Through MM.3.30

Not applicable

Preparing and Dispensing

Standard MM.4.10

❑ Compliant
❑ Not Compliant

All prescriptions or medication orders are reviewed for appropriateness.

Note: *This standard is applicable only to practices that dispense medications.*

Elements of Performance for MM.4.10

1. Through 4. Not applicable

Scoring Grid
0 Insufficient compliance
1 Partial compliance
2 Satisfactory compliance
NA Not applicable

B | 0 | 1 | 2 | NA |

5. The practice has a process to review all prescriptions for the following:
   - The appropriateness of the drug, dose, frequency, and route of administration
   - Therapeutic duplication
   - Real or potential allergies or sensitivities
   - Real or potential interactions between the prescription and other medications, food, and laboratory values
   - Other contraindications
   - Other relevant medication-related issues or concerns

❑ Compliant
❑ Not Compliant

Standard MM.4.20

Medications are prepared safely.

Elements of Performance for MM.4.20

1. Not applicable

C | 0 | 1 | 2 | NA |

Ⓜ 2. Wherever medications are prepared, staff use safety materials and equipment while preparing hazardous medications.

C | 0 | 1 | 2 | NA |

Ⓜ 3. Wherever medications are prepared, staff use techniques to assure accuracy in medication preparation.

C | 0 | 1 | 2 | NA |

Ⓜ 4. Wherever medications are prepared, staff use appropriate techniques to avoid contamination during medication preparation, which include, but are not limited to, the following:
   - Using clean or sterile techniques as appropriate
   - Maintaining clean, uncluttered, and functionally separate areas for product preparation to minimize the possibility of contamination
   - Using a laminar airflow hood or other class 100 environment while preparing any intravenous (IV) admixture in the pharmacy, any sterile product made from non sterile ingredients, or any sterile product that will not be used within 24 hours
   - Visually inspecting the integrity of the medications

MM

❑ Compliant
❑ Not Compliant

Standard MM.4.30

Medications are appropriately labeled.

Elements of Performance for MM.4.30

B | 0 | 1 | 2 | NA |

1. Medications are labeled in a standardized manner according to practice policy, applicable law and regulation, and standards of practice.

B | 0 | 1 | 2 | NA |

2. Any time one or more medications are prepared but are not administered immediately, the medication container* must be appropriately labeled.

   Note: *A practice that exclusively uses a single medication in an area can draw up or prepare multiple doses for later use as long as the medication is segregated and secured from all other medications in the practice (for example, a vaccine or flu shot) and the container enclosing the individual doses is labeled.*

A | 0 | 1 | 2 | NA |

3. At a minimum, all medications are labeled with the following:
   - Drug name, strength, amount (if not apparent from the container)
   - Expiration date† when not used within 24 hours
   - Expiration time when expiration occurs in less than 24 hours
   - The date prepared and the diluent for all compounded IV admixtures

* A container can be any storage device such as a plastic bag, syringe, bottle, or box, which can be labeled and secured in such a way that it can be readily determined that the contents are intact and have not expired.

† Expiration date, also called the *beyond use date,* refers to the last date that the product should be used by the patient.

Scoring Grid
- **0** Insufficient compliance
- **1** Partial compliance
- **2** Satisfactory compliance
- **NA** Not applicable

4. When preparing individualized medications for multiple specific patients, or when the person preparing the individualized medications is not the person administering the medication, the label also includes the following:
   - Patient name
   - Directions for use and any applicable cautionary statements either on the label or attached as an accessory label (for example, "requires refrigeration," "for IM use only")

   A | 0 | 1 | 2 | NA |

Standard MM.4.40

❑ Compliant
❑ Not Compliant

Medications are dispensed safely.

Note: *This standard is applicable to all practices that dispense medications.*

Element of Performance for MM.4.40

1. Quantities of medications are dispensed that minimize diversion yet are still consistent with the patient's needs.

   B | 0 | 1 | 2 | NA |

Standards MM.4.50 Through MM.4.60

Not applicable

Standard MM.4.70

❑ Compliant
❑ Not Compliant

Medications dispensed by the practice are retrieved when recalled or discontinued by the manufacturer or the FDA for safety reasons.

Note: *This standard is applicable to all practices that dispense medications, including sample medications.*

Elements of Performance for MM.4.70

1. Through 3. Not applicable

4. The practice has procedures for retrieving and safely disposing of recalled medications including the following:
   - Identifying each patient who is receiving or has received recalled medications
   - Identifying the source of the medication
   - Providing for the retrieval and safe disposal of medications subject to recall
   - Providing for external reporting of medication product defects

   B | 0 | 1 | 2 | NA |

Standard MM.4.80

Not applicable

Scoring Grid
0 Insufficient compliance
1 Partial compliance
2 Satisfactory compliance
NA Not applicable

Administering

❑ Compliant
❑ Not Compliant

Standard MM.5.10
Medications are safely and accurately administered.

Elements of Performance for MM.5.10
Policies and procedures address the following (EPs 1–2):

B | 0 | 1 | 2 | NA | 1. Health care staff who may administer medications, with or without supervision, consistent with law and regulation and practice policy. (The practice's policy may address an individual's qualification to administer by medication, medication class, or route of administration.)

2. Not applicable

Before administering a medication, the licensed independent practitioner or appropriate health care professional administering the medication does the following (EPs 3–5):

C | 0 | 1 | 2 | NA | Ⓜ 3. Verifies that the medication selected for administration is the correct one based on the medication order and product label

C | 0 | 1 | 2 | NA | Ⓜ 4. Verifies that the medication is stable based on visual examination for particulates or discoloration and that the medication has not expired

C | 0 | 1 | 2 | NA | Ⓜ 5. Verifies that there is no contraindication for administering the medication

6. Through 14. Not applicable

C | 0 | 1 | 2 | NA | 15. Medications are administered by or under the supervision of appropriately licensed staff consistent with law, regulation, and practice procedures.

MM

Standard MM.5.20
Not applicable

❑ Compliant
❑ Not Compliant

Standard MM.5.30
Prescribing and ordering medications follow established procedures.

Elements of Performance for MM.5.30
Procedures supporting safe medication prescribing or ordering address the following:

B | 0 | 1 | 2 | NA | 1. Ordering, procuring, storing, controlling, labeling, preparing, and dispensing medications according to law and regulation

B | 0 | 1 | 2 | NA | 2. Distributing and administering controlled medications, including adequate documentation and record keeping required by law

B | 0 | 1 | 2 | NA | 3. Properly storing, distributing, and controlling investigational and clinical trial medications

B | 0 | 1 | 2 | NA | 4. Identifying situations in which all or some of a patient's medications must be permanently or temporarily canceled, and mechanisms for reinstating them

B | 0 | 1 | 2 | NA | 5. Utilizing as needed (PRN) prescriptions or orders and times of dose administration

B | 0 | 1 | 2 | NA | 6. Appropriately using intravenous administration of medications and other pain management techniques used to care for patients in pain

B | 0 | 1 | 2 | NA | 7. Appropriately controlling sample drugs

B | 0 | 1 | 2 | NA | 8. Procuring, storing, controlling, and distributing prepackaged medications obtained from outside sources

Scoring Grid
0 Insufficient compliance
1 Partial compliance
2 Satisfactory compliance
NA Not applicable

9. Procuring, storing, controlling, distributing, and administering radioactive medications — **B** 0 | 1 | 2 | NA
10. Procuring, storing, controlling, distributing, administering, and monitoring all blood derivatives* — **B** 0 | 1 | 2 | NA
11. Procuring, storing, controlling, distributing, administering, and monitoring all radiographic contrast media — **B** 0 | 1 | 2 | NA
12. Counseling and educating the patient about effectively and safely using the medication — **B** 0 | 1 | 2 | NA

Monitoring

Standards MM.6.10 Through MM.6.20

Not applicable

High-Risk Medications

High-risk or high-alert drugs are those drugs involved in a high percentage of medication errors and/or sentinel events and medications that carry a higher risk for abuse, errors, or other adverse outcomes. Lists of high-risk or high-alert drugs are available from such organizations as the ISMP, the USP, and so forth, based on national data about medication use. However, the organization needs to develop its own list of high-risk or high-alert drugs based on its unique utilization patterns or drugs and its own internal data about medication errors and sentinel events. Examples of high-risk drugs include investigational drugs, controlled medications, medications not on the approved FDA list, medications with a narrow therapeutic range, psychotherapeutic medications, and look-alike/sound-alike medications. Medications that are new to the market or new to the practice should also be considered.

Standard MM.7.10

The practice develops processes for managing high-risk or high-alert medications.

❏ Compliant
❏ Not Compliant

Elements of Performance for MM.7.10

1. The practice identifies the high-risk or high-alert medications used within the organization, if any. — **A** 0 | 1 | 2 | NA
2. As appropriate to the services provided, the practice develops processes for procuring, storing, ordering, transcribing, preparing, dispensing, administering, and/or monitoring high-risk or high-alert medications. — **B** 0 | 1 | 2 | NA

Standard MM.7.20 Through MM.7.30

Not applicable

* **blood derivative** A pooled blood product such, as albumin, gamma globulin, or Rh immune globulin, whose use is considered significantly lower in risk than that of blood or blood components.

Scoring Grid
0 Insufficient compliance
1 Partial compliance
2 Satisfactory compliance
NA Not applicable

❑ Compliant
❑ Not Compliant

Standard MM.7.40

Investigational medications are safely controlled and administered.

Elements of Performance for MM.7.40

B | 0 | 1 | 2 | NA |

1. Procedures for the use of investigational medications, when used, are implemented and maintained including the following:
   - Having a written process for reviewing, approving, supervising, and monitoring investigational medication use
   - Specifying that when an investigational medication protocol is being conducted independent of the organization, the practice reviews and accommodates, as appropriate, the patient's continued participation in the protocol (*see* standard RI.2.180)
   - Specifying that when pharmacy services are provided, the pharmacy controls the storage, dispensing, labeling, and distribution of the investigational medication

B | 0 | 1 | 2 | NA |

2. Procedures address proper storage, distribution, and control of investigational and clinical trial medications.

Evaluation

❑ Compliant
❑ Not Compliant

Standard MM.8.10

The practice evaluates its medication management system.

Elements of Performance for MM.8.10

B | 0 | 1 | 2 | NA |

1. The practice evaluates its medication management system for risk points and identifies areas to improve safety.

2. Through 6. Not applicable

B | 0 | 1 | 2 | NA |

7. Procedures address appropriate use of intravenous administration of medications and other pain management techniques used to care for patients in pain.

Surveillance, Prevention, and Control of Infection

Overview

Infections can be acquired within any care, treatment, or service setting, and be transferred between settings or brought in from the community. Therefore, prevention of health care–associated infections (HAIs) represents one of the major safety initiatives that a practice can undertake.

The goal of an effective infection control (IC) program (hereafter referred to as the "IC program") is to reduce the risk of acquisition and transmission of HAIs. To achieve this goal, office-based surgery practices must do the following:

1. The practice incorporates its IC program as a major component of its safety and performance improvement programs.
2. The practice performs an ongoing assessment to identify its risks for the acquisition and transmission of infectious agents.
3. The practice effectively conducts surveillance, collects data, and interprets the data.
4. The practice effectively implements infection prevention and control processes.
5. The practice educates and collaborates with leaders across the practice to effectively participate in the design and implementation of the IC program.
6. The practice integrates its efforts with health care and community leaders to the extent practicable, recognizing that infection prevention and control is a communitywide effort.
7. The practice plans for responding to infections that might overwhelm its resources.

A program with aims of such broad scope and depth requires the direct involvement of practice leaders. Only with the ongoing attention and direction of the practice's leadership can the appropriate scope of the IC program be determined and adequately resourced.

The standards in this chapter, which focus on development and implementation of plans to prevent and control infections, are supported by standards in other chapters, such as "Management of the Environment of Care," "Management of Human Resources," "Improving Practice Performance," and "Practice Leadership," to produce a comprehensive approach to IC.

Glossary Terms

These key terms have specific Joint Commission definitions. Please access the Glossary found near the end of your manual for the Joint Commission definition and appropriate use.

infection
– endemic infection
– health care–associated infection
infection control program
plan
policies and procedures
practice guidelines
program
staff

Standards

The following is a list of all standards for this function. They are presented here for your convenience without footnotes or other explanatory text. If you have a question about a term used here, please check the Glossary.

Note: *A revised standard numbering system is being used with the reformatted standards. The revised numbering system allows for more flexibility to add standards while maintaining the current label for each standard.*

The IC Program and Its Components

IC.1.10 The risk of development of an HAI is minimized through a practicewide infection control program.

IC.2.10 The IC program identifies risks for the acquisition and transmission of infectious agents on an ongoing basis.

IC.3.10 Based on risks, the practice establishes priorities and sets goals for preventing the development of HAIs within the practice.

IC.4.10 After the practice has prioritized its goals, strategies must be implemented to achieve those goals.

IC.5.10 The IC program evaluates the effectiveness of the IC interventions and, as necessary, redesigns the IC interventions.

IC.6.10 Not applicable

Structure and Resources for the IC Program

IC.7.10 The IC program is managed effectively.

IC.8.10 Representatives from relevant components/functions within the practice collaborate to implement the IC program.

IC.9.10 Practice leaders allocate adequate resources for the IC program.

Understanding the Parts of This Chapter

To help you navigate this reformatted standards chapter, it may be helpful to think of its parts this way:

- The **standard** is the "goal."
- The **rationale** explains why it's important to achieve this goal.
- The **elements of performance** identify the step(s) needed to achieve this goal.

These parts are defined as follows.

Standard A statement that defines the performance expectations and/or structures or processes that must be in place in order for a practice to provide safe, high-quality care, treatment, and services. An practice is either "compliant" or "not compliant" with a standard as reflected by the check boxes in the margin by the standard:

❑ Compliant
❑ Not Compliant

Accreditation decisions are based on simple counts of the standards that are determined to be "not compliant."

Rationale A statement that provides background, justification, or additional information about a standard. A standard's rationale is not scored. In some instances, the rationale for a standard is self-evident. Therefore, not every standard has a written rationale.

Elements of performance (EPs) The specific performance expectations and/or structures or processes that must be in place in order for a practice to provide safe, high-quality care, treatment, and services. The scoring of EP compliance determines a practice's overall compliance with a standard. EPs are evaluated on the following scale:

0 Insufficient compliance
1 Partial compliance
2 Satisfactory compliance
NA Not applicable

You will find a **measure of success** icon—Ⓜ—next to some EPs. Measures of success (MOS) need to be developed for certain EPs when a standard is judged to be out of compliance through the on-site survey. An MOS is defined as a quantifiable measure, usually related to an audit, that can be used to determine whether an action has been effective and is being sustained.*

Using the Self-Assessment Grid to Assess Your Compliance

Once you are familiar with the parts of this chapter, you can begin to assess your compliance with its requirements. A self-assessment grid (otherwise known as a scoring grid) has been provided in the margins for your convenience. If you would like to assess your practice's performance, mark your scores for the EPs on the scoring grid by following the simple steps described below. **Note:** *You are **not** required to complete this scoring grid. It is provided simply to help you assess your own performance.*

Two components are scored for each EP: (1) compliance with the requirement itself **and** (2) compliance with the track record† for that requirement. Scoring has been simplified from the past edition of the manual, and track record achievements (which have always been part of the scoring) have been appropriately modified.

* For more information about Measures of Success, *see* "The New Joint Commission Accreditation Process" chapter in this manual.

† **Track record** The amount of time that a practice has been in compliance with a standard, element of performance, or other requirement.

Note: *Some standards and EPs do not apply to a particular type of practice; these standards and EPs are marked "not applicable" and the related text is not included. Your practice is not expected to comply with standards and EPs marked "not applicable."*

In addition, some standards and EPs that do apply to practices may not apply to the specific care, treatment, and services that your individual practice provides. Although these standards and EPs are included in the manual, you are not expected to comply with them. If you are unsure about the standards or EPs that apply to your practice, please contact the Joint Commission's Standards Interpretation Group at 630/792-5900.

Step 1: Score Your Compliance with Each Element of Performance

Before you can determine your compliance with the standards, you must score your compliance with each EP. First look at the EP scoring criterion category listed immediately preceding the scoring scale in the margin next to the EP. There are three scoring criterion categories: A, B, and C (described below). Please note that for each EP scoring criterion category, your practice must meet the performance requirement itself and the track record achievements (*see* below).

Category A

These EPs relate to the presence or absence of the requirement(s) and are scored either yes (2) or no (0); however, score 1 for partial compliance is also possible based on track record achievements (*see* below).

If an A EP has multiple components designated by bullets, your practice must be compliant with all the bullets to receive a score of 2. If your practice does not meet one or more requirements in the bullets, you will receive a score of 0.

IC

Category B

Category B EPs are scored in two steps:

1. As with category A EPs, category B EPs relate to the presence or absence of the requirement(s). If your practice *does not meet* the requirement(s), the EP is scored 0; there is no need to assess your compliance with the principles of good process design (*see* below).
2. If your practice *does meet* the requirement(s), but there is concern about the quality or comprehensiveness of the effort, then and only then should you assess the qualitative aspect of the EP. That is, review the applicable principles of good process design and ask how the principles were applied in the situation under discussion. Good process design has the following characteristics:
   - Is consistent with your practice's mission, values, and goals
   - Meets the needs of patients
   - Reflects the use of currently accepted practices (doing the right thing, using resources responsibly, using practice guidelines)
   - Incorporates current safety information and knowledge such as sentinel event data and National Patient Safety Goals
   - Incorporates relevant performance improvement results

This two-part evaluation applies to both simple and bulleted B EPs. First, the EPs are assessed to determine if the requirements are present. If the EP has multiple components designated by bullets, as with the category A EPs, your practice must meet the requirements in *all* the bulleted items to get a score of 2. If your practice meets *none* of the requirements in the bullets, it receives a score of 0. If your practice meets *at least one, but not all,* of the bulleted requirements, it will receive a score of 1 for the EPs.

Use the following rules to determine your EP score:

- Your EP score is 0 if your practice does not meet the requirement(s); you *do not* need to assess your compliance with the preceding applicable principles of good process design
- Your EP score is 1 if your practice does meet the requirement(s), but considered only *some* of the preceding applicable principles of good process design

- Your EP score is 2 if your practice does meet the requirement(s) *and* considered *all* the preceding principles of good process design

Category C

C EPs are scored 0, 1, or 2 based on the number of times your practice does not meet the EP. These EPs are frequency based and require totaling the number of occurrences (that is, results of performance or nonperformance) related to a particular EP. Each situation discovered by a surveyor(s) will be counted as a separate occurrence.

Note: *Multiple events of the same type related to a single patient and single practitioner/staff member are counted as* one occurrence only.

Use the following rules to determine your EP score:
- Your EP score is 2 if you find one or fewer occurrences of noncompliance with the EP
- Your EP score is 1 if you find two occurrences of noncompliance with the EP
- Your EP score is 0 if you find three or more occurrences of noncompliance with the EP

If an EP in the C category has multiple requirements designated by bullets, the following scoring guidelines apply:
- If there are fewer than 2 findings in all bullets, the EP is scored 2
- If there are three or more findings in all bullets, the EP is scored 0
- In all other combinations of findings, the EP is scored 1

Track Record Achievements

In addition to meeting the requirement(s) in each EP, regardless of category, your practice must also meet the following track record achievements:

Score	Initial Survey	Full Survey
2	4 months or more	12 months or more
1	2 to 3 months	6 to 11 months
0	Fewer than 2 months	Fewer than 6 months

Sample Sizes

If during an on-site survey, your practice has been found to be not compliant with one or more standards, you must demonstrate Evidence of Standards Compliance (ESC) for each standard that is not compliant. The ESC must address compliance at the EP level; when an EP within a noncompliant standard requires an MOS, your practice must demonstrate achievement with the MOS when completing the ESC.

Note: *Not every EP requires an MOS. EPs that do require an MOS are clearly marked in this chapter Practices are required to demonstrate achievement with an MOS* only *for EPs within a noncompliant standard that require an MOS. Practices* do not *need to demonstrate achievement with an MOS for any EP within a compliant standard.*

When demonstrating achievement with an MOS during the ESC process, your practice is **required** to use the following sample sizes, which were established because of their statistical significance, their relative simplicity in application, and their sensitivity to a practice's population size:
- For a population size of fewer than 30 cases,* sample 100% of available cases
- For a population size of 30 to 100 cases, sample 30 cases
- For a population size of 101 to 500 cases, sample 50 cases
- For a population size greater than 500 cases, sample 70 cases

When demonstrating an ESC (mandatory use), use the following percentages to determine your EP score: 90% through 100% of your sample size is in compliance = score 2; 80% through 89% of your sample size is in compliance = score 1; less than 80% of your sample size is in compliance = score 0.

---

* "Case" refers to a single instance in which a situation related to a survey finding occurs. For example, if a survey finding was related to **pain assessment,** then a "case" would be any patient record. If a survey finding was related to **pain management,** a "case" would be any patient record for patients receiving pain management.

In addition, the following information should govern your practice's selection of samples:

- The appropriate sample size should be determined by the specific population related to the survey findings.
- The sampling approach should involve either systematic random sampling (for example, your practice selects every second or third case for review) or simple random sampling (for example, your practice uses a series of random numbers generated by a computer to identify the cases to be reviewed).
- When submitting a clarifying ESC, if your practice selects records as part of its sample, the records should be from a period of no more than three months before the last date of the survey.
- Assessment of MOS compliance is conducted for a four-month period following the date of ESC approval. Your practice should select records as a part of your sample following the date of ESC approval and use the required sample sizes. MOS percentage compliance rates are derived from the average of all four months.

Step 2: Use Your EP Scores to Gauge Your Compliance with the Standards

Now that you have evaluated and scored each EP for a particular standard, use these simple rules to determine your compliance with the standard itself:

- Your practice is not in compliance (that is, "not compliant") with the standard if any EP is scored 0
- Otherwise, your practice is in compliance with a standard if 65% or more of its EPs are scored 2

Scoring Grid
0 Insufficient compliance
1 Partial compliance
2 Satisfactory compliance
NA Not applicable

Standards, Rationales, Elements of Performance, and Scoring

The IC Program and Its Components

Standard IC.1.10

The risk of development of an HAI is minimized through a practicewide IC program.

❑ Compliant
❑ Not Compliant

Rationale for IC.1.10

The risk of HAIs exists throughout the practice. An effective IC program that can systematically identify risks and respond appropriately must involve all relevant programs and settings within the practice.

Elements of Performance for IC.1.10

1. A practicewide IC program is implemented.

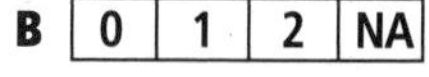

2. Through 3. Not applicable

4. Systems are in place to communicate with licensed independent practitioners, staff, students/trainees, and (as appropriate), visitors, and patients about infection prevention and control issues, including their responsibilities in preventing the spread of infection within the practice.

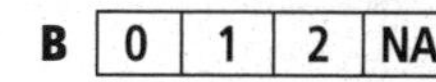

5. The practice has systems for reporting identified infections to the following:
   - The appropriate staff within the practice
   - Federal, state, and local public health authorities in accordance with law and regulation
   - Accrediting bodies (*see* SE-6–SE-8, and NPSG-3)

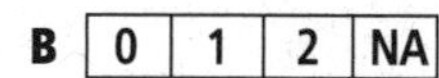

6. Not applicable

7. Applicable policies and procedures are in place throughout the practice.

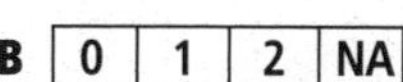

8. Not applicable

9. The practice has a written IC plan* that includes the following:
   - A description of prioritized risks
   - A statement of the goals of the IC program
   - A description of the practice's strategies to minimize, reduce, or eliminate the prioritized risks
   - A description of how the strategies will be evaluated

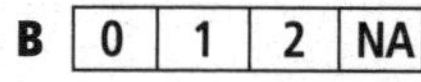

10. At a minimum, defined protocols and schedules for IC in the procedure and recovery areas include the following:
    - Only authorized and properly attired staff is allowed in procedure areas.
    - Suitable equipment and cleaning agents are provided for regular cleaning of all interior surfaces.
    - Suitable equipment is available for rapid and routine sterilization of procedure room materials.

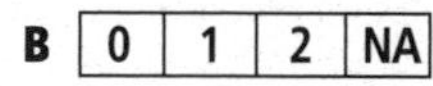

* **Written plan** A succinct, useful document, formulated beforehand, that identifies needs, lists strategies to meet those needs, and sets goals and objectives. The format of the plan may include narratives, policies and procedures, protocols, practice guidelines, clinical paths, care maps, or a combination of these.

Scoring Grid
0 Insufficient compliance
1 Partial compliance
2 Satisfactory compliance
NA Not applicable

- Sterilized materials are packaged and labeled consistently to maintain sterility.
- All individuals in procedure areas use acceptable aseptic techniques.
- Appropriate ventilation and humidity control are provided to minimize the risk of infection and provide for the patient's safety.
- Procedure areas are appropriately cleaned after each procedure.
- When patients are known or suspected to have an infectious disease, the use of isolation precautions or, when indicated, immediate transfer, is made available or provided for.

❑ Compliant
❑ Not Compliant

Standard IC.2.10

The IC program identifies risks for the acquisition and transmission of infectious agents on an ongoing basis.

Rationale for IC.2.10

A practice's risks of infection vary based on the practice's geographic location, the community environment, the types of programs/services provided, and the characteristics and behaviors of the population served. As these risks change over time—sometimes rapidly—risk assessment must be an ongoing process.

Elements of Performance for IC.2.10

B | 0 | 1 | 2 | NA |

1. The practice identifies risks for the transmission and acquisition of infectious agents throughout the practice based on the following factors:
   - The program/services provided and the characteristics of the population served
   - The results of the analysis of the practice's infection prevention and control data
   - The care, treatment, and services provided

IC

A | 0 | 1 | 2 | NA |

2. The risk analysis is formally reviewed at least annually and whenever significant changes occur in any of the preceding factors.

B | 0 | 1 | 2 | NA |

3. Surveillance activities, including data collection and analysis, are used to identify infection prevention and control risks pertaining to the following:
   - Patients
   - Licensed independent practitioners staff, and student/trainees
   - Visitors as warranted

❑ Compliant
❑ Not Compliant

Standard IC.3.10

Based on risks, the practice establishes priorities and sets goals for preventing the development of HAIs within the practice.

Rationale for IC.3.10

The risks of HAIs within a practice are many while resources are limited. An effective IC program requires a thoughtful prioritization of the most important risks to be addressed. Priorities and goals related to the identified risks guide the choice and design of strategies for infection prevention and control in a practice. These priorities and goals provide a framework for evaluating the strategies.

Elements of Performance for IC.3.10

B | 0 | 1 | 2 | NA |

1. Priorities are established and goals related to preventing the acquisition and transmission of potentially infectious agents are developed based on the risks identified.

These goals include, but are not limited to, the following:

A | 0 | 1 | 2 | NA |

2. Limiting unprotected exposure to pathogens throughout the practice

A | 0 | 1 | 2 | NA |

3. Enhancing hand hygiene
4. Not applicable

Scoring Grid
0 Insufficient compliance
1 Partial compliance
2 Satisfactory compliance
NA Not applicable

5. Minimizing the risk of transmitting infections associated with the use of procedures, medical equipment, and medical devices.

A | 0 | 1 | 2 | NA |

Standard IC.4.10

After the practice has set its goals, strategies must be implemented to achieve those goals.

❑ Compliant
❑ Not Compliant

Rationale for IC.4.10

The practice plans and implements interventions to address the IC issues that it finds important based on prioritized risks and associated surveillance data.

Elements of Performance for IC.4.10

1. Interventions are designed to incorporate relevant guidelines* for infection prevention and control activities.

B | 0 | 1 | 2 | NA |

Interventions are implemented that include the following (EPs 2 and 3):

2. An organizationwide hand hygiene program that complies with current Centers for Disease Control and Prevention (CDC) hand hygiene guidelines (National Patient Safety Goal 7, requirement 7a†)

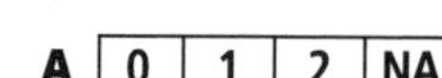

3. Methods to reduce the risks associated with procedures, medical equipment,‡ and medical devices, including the following:
    - Appropriate storage, cleaning, disinfection, sterilization, and/or disposal of supplies and equipment
    - Reuse of equipment designated by the manufacturer as disposable in a manner that is consistent with regulatory and professional standards
    - The appropriate use of personal protective equipment

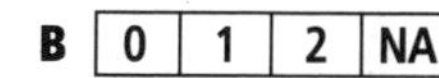

IC

4. Implementation of applicable precautions, as appropriate, is based on the following:
    - The potential for transmission
    - The mechanism of transmission
    - The care, treatment, and service setting

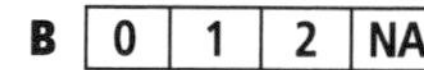

Interventions are implemented that include the following (EPs 5–7):

Ⓜ 5. Screening for exposure (for example, tuberculosis testing) and/or immunity to infectious diseases that licensed independent practitioners, staff, and student/trainees might come in contact with in their work is available as warranted.

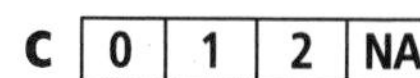

Ⓜ 6. Referral for assessment, potential testing, immunization and/or prophylaxis/treatment, and counseling (as appropriate) of licensed independent practitioners, staff, and students/trainees who are identified as potentially having an infectious disease or risk of infectious disease that might put the population they serve at risk.

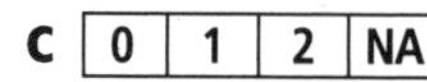

Ⓜ 7. Referral for assessment, potential testing, immunization and/or prophylaxis/treatment, and counseling (as appropriate) of patients and students/trainees, licensed independent practitioners or staff who are occupationally exposed.

C | 0 | 1 | 2 | NA |

8. Not applicable

* Examples of guidelines include those offered by the CDC, Healthcare Infection Control Practices Advisory Committee (HICPAC), and National Quality Forum (NQF).

† Organizations are required to comply with all 1A, 1B, and 1C CDC recommendations.

‡ **Medical equipment** Fixed and portable equipment used for the diagnosis, treatment, monitoring, and direct care of individuals.

Scoring Grid
0 Insufficient compliance
1 Partial compliance
2 Satisfactory compliance
NA Not applicable

IC

❑ Compliant
❑ Not Compliant

Standard IC.5.10

The IC program evaluates the effectiveness of the IC interventions and, as necessary, redesigns the IC interventions.

Rationale for IC.5.10

The evaluation of the effectiveness of interventions helps to identify which activities of the IC program are effective and which activities need to be changed to improve outcomes.

Elements of Performance for IC.5.10

A | 0 | 1 | 2 | NA

1. The practice formally evaluates and revises the goals and program (or portions of the program) at least annually and whenever risks significantly change.

B | 0 | 1 | 2 | NA

2. The evaluation addresses changes in the scope of the IC program (for example, resulting from the introduction of new services or new sites of care).

3. Through 4. Not applicable

B | 0 | 1 | 2 | NA

5. The evaluation addresses the assessment of the success or failure of interventions for preventing and controlling infection.

6. Not applicable

B | 0 | 1 | 2 | NA

7. The evaluation addresses the evolution of relevant infection prevention and control guidelines that are based on evidence or, in the absence of evidence, expert consensus.

Standard IC.6.10

Not applicable

Structure and Resources for the IC Program

❑ Compliant
❑ Not Compliant

Standard IC.7.10

The IC program is managed effectively.

Rationale for IC.7.10

The IC program requires management by an individual (or individuals) with knowledge that is appropriate to the risks identified by the practice, as well as knowledge of the analysis of infection risks, principles of infection prevention and control, and data analysis. This individual may be employed by the practice or the practice may contract with this individual. The number of individuals and their qualifications are based on the practice's size, complexity, and needs.

Elements of Performance for IC.7.10

A | 0 | 1 | 2 | NA

1. The practice assigns responsibility for managing IC program activities to one or more individuals whose number, competency, and skill mix are determined by the goals and objectives of the IC activities.

B | 0 | 1 | 2 | NA

2. Qualifications of the individual(s) responsible for managing the IC program are determined by the risks entailed in the care, treatment, and services provided; the practice's patient population(s); and the complexity of the activities that are carried out.

Scoring Grid
0 Insufficient compliance
1 Partial compliance
2 Satisfactory compliance
NA Not applicable

Note: *Qualifications may be met through ongoing education, training, experience, and/or certification (such as that offered by the Certification Board for Infection Control [CBIC]) in the prevention and control of infections).*

3. This individual(s) coordinates all infection prevention and control activities within the practice. **B** | 0 | 1 | 2 | NA |
4. This individual(s) facilitates ongoing monitoring of the effectiveness of prevention and/or control activities and interventions. **B** | 0 | 1 | 2 | NA |

Standard IC.8.10

Representatives from relevant functions within the practice collaborate to implement the IC program.

❑ Compliant
❑ Not Compliant

Rationale for IC.8.10

The successful creation of a practicewide IC program requires collaboration with all relevant functions. This collaboration is vital to successful data gathering and interpretation, design of interventions, and effective implementation of interventions.

Element of Performance for IC.8.10

1. Practice leaders, with licensed independent practitioners and other direct and indirect patient care staff collaborate on an ongoing basis with the qualified individual(s) managing the IC program. **B** | 0 | 1 | 2 | NA |

Standard IC.9.10

Practice leaders allocate adequate resources for the IC program.

❑ Compliant
❑ Not Compliant

Rationale for IC.9.10

Adequate resources are needed to effectively plan and successfully implement a program of this scope.

Elements of Performance for IC.9.10

1. The effectiveness of the practice's infection prevention and control activities is reviewed on an ongoing basis, and findings are reported to the integrated patient safety program at least annually. **A** | 0 | 1 | 2 | NA |
2. Adequate systems to access information are provided to support infection prevention and control activities. **B** | 0 | 1 | 2 | NA |
3. Not applicable
4. Adequate equipment and supplies are provided to support infection prevention and control activities. **B** | 0 | 1 | 2 | NA |

Improving Practice Performance

Overview

The goal of improving practice performance in an office-based surgery practice is to enhance the delivery of service and to maximize good patient outcomes by systematically monitoring, analyzing, and improving performance. The practice's approach to improving its performance includes designing and implementing processes that support the following essential activities:

- Monitoring performance through data collection
- Analyzing current performance
- Improving and sustaining improved performance

Value in health care is the appropriate balance between good outcomes, excellent services and care, and cost. To add value to services and care provided, practices need to understand the relation among procedures, outcomes, and costs and how these three elements are affected by processes carried out by the practice. The dimensions of performance described below define these relationships in the context of performance improvement:

Dimensions of Performance

Performance is *what* is done and *how well* it is done to provide health care. The level of performance in health care is

- the degree to which *what* is done is *efficacious* and *appropriate* to the individual patient and
- the degree to which it is *available* in a *timely* manner to patients who need it, *effective, continuous* with other care and care providers (as appropriate), *safe, efficient,* and *caring* and *respectful* to the patient.

PI

Data Collection

Monitoring Performance Through Data Collection

Monitoring performance through data collection is the foundation of all performance improvement activities. Collecting data about current performance provides for such information and allows the practice to do the following:

- Make informed judgments about the consistency of existing processes (for example, undesirable process variation)
- Identify opportunities for incrementally improving processes;
- Identify the need to redesign processes
- Decide if improvements or redesign of processes meet objectives

Because most practices have limited resources, they cannot collect data to monitor everything they want to monitor. The practice leaders must therefore decide which processes to monitor and the data to be collected. They determine the importance of the practice's processes in relation to its goals and values, available resources, and scope of service as well as concerns of patients, their families, staff, payers, and other customers.

Glossary Terms

These key terms have specific Joint Commission definitions. Please access the Glossary found near the end of your manual for the Joint Commission definition and appropriate use.

effectiveness	performance improvement (PI)
hazardous condition	quality control
leader	quality of care
medication error	root cause analysis
near miss	safety
operative and other high-risk procedures	sentinel event

Data collection focuses on the following:

- Processes, particularly those that are high-risk, high-volume, or problem-prone
- Outcomes
- Targeted areas of study
- Comprehensive performance measures (indicators)
- Other gauges of performance, such as
  - patients' and others' needs, expectations, and feedback
  - results of ongoing infection control activities
  - safety of the environment
  - quality control and risk management findings
- The dimensions of performance important to a process or an outcome, including
  - efficiency of process, procedure or service
  - appropriateness
  - availability
  - timeliness
  - effectiveness
  - continuity
  - safety
  - efficiency
  - respect and caring toward patient

The practice's leaders decide the scope and focus of performance monitoring and data collection activities. In determining the scope, the leaders identify and consider the important care and services performed. The important functions common to all health care practices and organizations are identified by the chapter titles in this manual and represent logical starting points. The leaders determine the focus of data collection monitoring when they set priorities for monitoring. In setting priorities, they consider and are guided by various concerns, such as identified high-risk or problem-prone processes or regulatory requirements. A practice wide approach to monitoring performance will, over time, include measures that relate to each of the important functions described in this manual.

Once the leaders determine the scope and focus of monitoring and data collection, they decide the following

- How to organize those activities into a systematic approach
- The frequency and intensity of data collection
- The relevant dimensions of performance to be monitored
- The incorporation of data collection activities into daily work processes

The standards in this chapter allow each practice to develop its own approach and therefore equally apply to approaches that organize monitoring and data collection around procedure codes, clinical paths, or important functions. Finally, some processes are measured on a periodic, ongoing basis while other processes are measured more intensively.

Standards

The following is a list of all standards for this function. They are presented here for your convenience without footnotes or other explanatory text. If you have a question about a term used here, please check the Glossary.

Note: *A new standard numbering system is being used with the standards. The revised numbering system allows for more flexibility to add standards while maintaining the current label for each standard.*

PI.1.10 The practice collects data to monitor its performance.

PI.1.20 Not applicable

Aggregation and Analysis

PI.2.10 Data are systematically aggregated and analyzed.

PI.2.20 Undesirable patterns or trends in performance are analyzed.

PI.2.30 Processes for identifying and managing sentinel events are defined and implemented.

Performance Improvement

PI.3.10 Information from data analysis is used to make changes that improve performance and patient safety and reduce the risk of sentinel events.

PI.3.20 An ongoing, proactive program for identifying and reducing unanticipated adverse events and safety risks to patients is defined and implemented.

Understanding the Parts of This Chapter

To help you navigate this reformatted standards chapter, it may be helpful to think of its parts this way:

- The **standard** is the "goal."
- The **rationale** explains why it's important to achieve this goal.
- The **elements of performance** identify the step(s) needed to achieve this goal.

These parts are defined as follows.

Standard A statement that defines the performance expectations and/or structures or processes that must be in place in order for a practice to provide safe, high-quality care, treatment, and services. An practice is either "compliant" or "not compliant" with a standard as reflected by the check boxes in the margin by the standard:

❑ Compliant
❑ Not Compliant

Accreditation decisions are based on simple counts of the standards that are determined to be "not compliant."

Rationale A statement that provides background, justification, or additional information about a standard. A standard's rationale is not scored. In some instances, the rationale for a standard is self-evident. Therefore, not every standard has a written rationale.

Elements of performance (EPs) The specific performance expectations and/or structures or processes that must be in place in order for a practice to provide safe, high-quality care, treatment, and services. The scoring of EP compliance determines a practice's overall compliance with a standard. EPs are evaluated on the following scale:

0 Insufficient compliance
1 Partial compliance
2 Satisfactory compliance
NA Not applicable

You will find a **measure of success** icon—Ⓜ—next to some EPs. Measures of success (MOS) need to be developed for certain EPs when a standard is judged to be out of compliance through the on-site survey. An MOS is defined as a quantifiable measure, usually related to an audit, that can be used to determine whether an action has been effective and is being sustained.*

Using the Self-Assessment Grid to Assess Your Compliance

Once you are familiar with the parts of this chapter, you can begin to assess your compliance with its requirements. A self-assessment grid (otherwise known as a scoring grid) has been provided in the margins for your convenience. If you would like to assess your practice's performance, mark your scores for the EPs on the scoring grid by following the simple steps described below. **Note:** *You are **not** required to complete this scoring grid. It is provided simply to help you assess your own performance.*

Two components are scored for each EP: (1) compliance with the requirement itself **and** (2) compliance with the track record† for that requirement. Scoring has been simplified from the past edition of the manual, and track record achievements (which have always been part of the scoring) have been appropriately modified.

---

* For more information about Measures of Success, *see* "The New Joint Commission Accreditation Process" chapter in this manual.

† **Track record** The amount of time that a practice has been in compliance with a standard, element of performance, or other requirement.

Note: *Some standards and EPs do not apply to a particular type of practice; these standards and EPs are marked "not applicable" and the related text is not included. Your practice is not expected to comply with standards and EPs marked "not applicable."*

In addition, some standards and EPs that do apply to practices may not apply to the specific care, treatment, and services that your individual practice provides. Although these standards and EPs are included in the manual, you are not expected to comply with them. If you are unsure about the standards or EPs that apply to your practice, please contact the Joint Commission's Standards Interpretation Group at 630/792-5900.

Step 1: Score Your Compliance with Each Element of Performance

Before you can determine your compliance with the standards, you must score your compliance with each EP. First look at the EP scoring criterion category listed immediately preceding the scoring scale in the margin next to the EP. There are three scoring criterion categories: A, B, and C (described below). Please note that for each EP scoring criterion category, your practice must meet the performance requirement itself and the track record achievements (*see* below).

Category A

These EPs relate to the presence or absence of the requirement(s) and are scored either yes (2) or no (0); however, score 1 for partial compliance is also possible based on track record achievements (*see* below).

If an A EP has multiple components designated by bullets, your practice must be compliant with all the bullets to receive a score of 2. If your practice does not meet one or more requirements in the bullets, you will receive a score of 0.

Category B

Category B EPs are scored in two steps:

1. As with category A EPs, category B EPs relate to the presence or absence of the requirement(s). If your practice *does not meet* the requirement(s), the EP is scored 0; there is no need to assess your compliance with the principles of good process design (*see* below).
2. If your practice *does meet* the requirement(s), but there is concern about the quality or comprehensiveness of the effort, then and only then should you assess the qualitative aspect of the EP. That is, review the applicable principles of good process design and ask how the principles were applied in the situation under discussion. Good process design has the following characteristics:
   - Is consistent with your practice's mission, values, and goals
   - Meets the needs of patients
   - Reflects the use of currently accepted practices (doing the right thing, using resources responsibly, using practice guidelines)
   - Incorporates current safety information and knowledge such as sentinel event data and National Patient Safety Goals
   - Incorporates relevant performance improvement results

This two-part evaluation applies to both simple and bulleted B EPs. First, the EPs are assessed to determine if the requirements are present. If the EP has multiple components designated by bullets, as with the category A EPs, your practice must meet the requirements in *all* the bulleted items to get a score of 2. If your practice meets *none* of the requirements in the bullets, it receives a score of 0. If your practice meets *at least one, but not all,* of the bulleted requirements, it will receive a score of 1 for the EPs.

Use the following rules to determine your EP score:

- Your EP score is 0 if your practice does not meet the requirement(s); you *do not* need to assess your compliance with the preceding applicable principles of good process design
- Your EP score is 1 if your practice does meet the requirement(s), but considered only *some* of the preceding applicable principles of good process design

- Your EP score is 2 if your practice does meet the requirement(s) *and* considered *all* the preceding principles of good process design

Category C

C EPs are scored 0, 1, or 2 based on the number of times your practice does not meet the EP. These EPs are frequency based and require totaling the number of occurrences (that is, results of performance or nonperformance) related to a particular EP. Each situation discovered by a surveyor(s) will be counted as a separate occurrence.

Note: *Multiple events of the same type related to a single patient and single practitioner/staff member are counted as* one occurrence only.

Use the following rules to determine your EP score:

- Your EP score is 2 if you find one or fewer occurrences of noncompliance with the EP
- Your EP score is 1 if you find two occurrences of noncompliance with the EP
- Your EP score is 0 if you find three or more occurrences of noncompliance with the EP

If an EP in the C category has multiple requirements designated by bullets, the following scoring guidelines apply:

- If there are fewer than 2 findings in all bullets, the EP is scored 2
- If there are three or more findings in all bullets, the EP is scored 0
- In all other combinations of findings, the EP is scored 1

Track Record Achievements

In addition to meeting the requirement(s) in each EP, regardless of category, your practice must also meet the following track record achievements:

Score	Initial Survey	Full Survey
2	4 months or more	12 months or more
1	2 to 3 months	6 to 11 months
0	Fewer than 2 months	Fewer than 6 months

Sample Sizes

If during an on-site survey, your practice has been found to be not compliant with one or more standards, you must demonstrate Evidence of Standards Compliance (ESC) for each standard that is not compliant. The ESC must address compliance at the EP level; when an EP within a noncompliant standard requires an MOS, your practice must demonstrate achievement with the MOS when completing the ESC.

Note: *Not every EP requires an MOS. EPs that do require an MOS are clearly marked in this chapter. Practices are required to demonstrate achievement with an MOS* only *for EPs within a noncompliant standard that require an MOS. Practices* do not *need to demonstrate achievement with an MOS for any EP within a compliant standard.*

When demonstrating achievement with an MOS during the ESC process, your practice is **required** to use the following sample sizes, which were established because of their statistical significance, their relative simplicity in application, and their sensitivity to a practice's population size:

- For a population size of fewer than 30 cases,* sample 100% of available cases
- For a population size of 30 to 100 cases, sample 30 cases
- For a population size of 101 to 500 cases, sample 50 cases
- For a population size greater than 500 cases, sample 70 cases

When demonstrating an ESC (mandatory use), use the following percentages to determine your EP score: 90% through 100% of your sample size is in compliance = score 2; 80% through 89% of your sample size is in compliance = score 1; less than 80% of your sample size is in compliance = score 0.

---

* "Case" refers to a single instance in which a situation related to a survey finding occurs. For example, if a survey finding was related to **pain assessment,** then a "case" would be any patient record. If a survey finding was related to **pain management,** a "case" would be any patient record for patients receiving pain management.

Scoring Grid
0 Insufficient compliance
1 Partial compliance
2 Satisfactory compliance
NA Not applicable

In addition, the following information should govern your practice's selection of samples:

- The appropriate sample size should be determined by the specific population related to the survey findings.
- The sampling approach should involve either systematic random sampling (for example, your practice selects every second or third case for review) or simple random sampling (for example, your practice uses a series of random numbers generated by a computer to identify the cases to be reviewed).
- If your practice chooses not to use these sample sizes while conducting Periodic Performance Review (PPR) options 1 or 2, you should make sure that your sample size is sufficiently large enough to ensure statistical significance.
- When submitting a clarifying ESC, if your practice selects records as part of its sample, the records should be from a period of no more than three months before the last date of the survey.
- Assessment of MOS compliance is conducted for a four-month period following the date of ESC approval. Your practice should select records as a part of your sample following the date of ESC approval and use the required sample sizes. MOS percentage compliance rates are derived from the average of all four months.

Step 2: Use Your EP Scores to Gauge Your Compliance with the Standards

Now that you have evaluated and scored each EP for a particular standard, use these simple rules to determine your compliance with the standard itself:

- Your practice is not in compliance (that is, "not compliant") with the standard if any EP is scored 0
- Otherwise, your practice is in compliance with a standard if 65% or more of its EPs are scored 2

Scoring Grid
0 Insufficient compliance
1 Partial compliance
2 Satisfactory compliance
NA Not applicable

Standards, Rationales, Elements of Performance, and Scoring

❑ Compliant
❑ Not Compliant

Standard PI.1.10

The practice collects data to monitor its performance.

Rationale for PI.1.10

Data help determine performance improvement priorities. The data collected for high-priority and required areas are used to monitor the stability of existing processes, identify opportunities for improvement, identify changes that lead to improvement, or sustain improvement. Data collection helps identify specific areas that require further study. These areas are determined by considering the information provided by the data about process stability, risks, and sentinel events, and priorities set by the leaders. In addition, the practice identifies those areas needing improvement and identifies desired changes. Performance measures are used to determine whether the changes result in desired outcomes. The practice identifies the frequency and detail of data collection.

Elements of Performance for PI.1.10

B | 0 | 1 | 2 | NA |
1. The practice collects data for priorities identified by leaders (*see* standard LD.4.50).
2. Not applicable

B | 0 | 1 | 2 | NA |
3. The practice collects data on the perceptions of care, treatment, and services* of patients, including the following:
   - Their specific needs and expectations
   - How well the practice meets these needs and expectations

PI

The practice collects data that measure the performance of each of the following potentially high-risk processes, when provided:

A | 0 | 1 | 2 | NA |
4. Medication management

A | 0 | 1 | 2 | NA |
5. Blood and blood product use

6. Through 10. Not applicable

A | 0 | 1 | 2 | NA |
11. Operative and other procedures that place patients at risk
12. Not applicable

Relevant information developed from the following activities is integrated into performance improvement initiatives. This occurs in a way consistent with any practice policies or procedures intended to preserve any confidentiality or privilege of information established by applicable law.

13. Not applicable
14. Not applicable
15. Not applicable

B | 0 | 1 | 2 | NA |
16. Infection control, surveillance, and reporting

17. Through 26. Not applicable

* The Joint Commission is moving from the phrase *satisfaction with care, treatment, and services* toward the more inclusive phrase *perception of care, treatment, and services* to better measure the performance of practices meeting the needs, expectations, and concerns of clients. By using this term, the practice will be prompted to assess not only patients' and/or families' satisfaction with care, treatment, and services, but also whether the practice meets their needs and expectations.

Scoring Grid
0 Insufficient compliance
1 Partial compliance
2 Satisfactory compliance
NA Not applicable

27. The practice collects data that measures clinical outcomes, including the following: **B** | 0 | 1 | 2 | NA |
    - Adverse clinical events during procedures
    - Complications following procedures
    - Complications requiring transfer to an acute care facility
    - Unplanned, prolonged, or frequent extended stays in recovery
    - Procedures that once begun are stopped prematurely

28. Data that the practice considers for collection to monitor performance include the following: **B** | 0 | 1 | 2 | NA |
    - Care or services provided to high-risk populations
    - Appropriateness of surgery and anesthesia

Standard PI.1.20

Not applicable

Aggregation and Analysis

Aggregating and analyzing data means transforming that data into information. The practice can use this information to draw conclusions about its performance of a process or the nature of the outcome. Data analysis can answer questions such as the following:

- What is our current level of performance?
- How consistent are our current processes?
- Are there areas that could be improved?
- Was a strategy to stabilize or improve performance effective?
- Did we meet performance expectations for processes?

The goal is to develop an analysis process that incorporates four basic comparisons: with itself, with other comparable practices, with standards, and with best practices. How often the practice aggregates and analyzes data depends on the process being measured and the practice's priorities. For example, a practice might analyze data about adverse anesthesia reactions every month and data about staff education needs every six months.

Conclusions about current performance based on data analysis might indicate a need for targeted study or more intense analysis of processes or outcomes. Such conclusions are based on comparison with the following:

- Expected clinical outcomes
- Benchmarks from external sources (such as professional societies)
- Sentinel events
- Control limits*
- Pre-established criteria
- Review of all occurrences
- Other interpretation methods

Data analysis includes all staff when appropriate for the process or outcome under review. When the analysis focuses on an individual's clinical performance, the practice leaders take appropriate action.

Standard PI.2.10

Data are systematically aggregated and analyzed.

❑ Compliant
❑ Not Compliant

---

* **Control limits** The expected limits (upper or lower) of common-cause variation (or a source of variation that is always present and is part of the random variation inherent in all processes) statistically calculated based on deviations from a process's average. Control limits are not specification or tolerance limits.

PI

Scoring Grid
0 Insufficient compliance
1 Partial compliance
2 Satisfactory compliance
NA Not applicable

Rationale for PI.2.10

Aggregating and analyzing data means transforming data into information. Aggregating data at points in time enables the practice to judge a particular process's stability or a particular outcome's predictability in relation to performance expectations. Accumulated data are analyzed in such a way that current performance levels, patterns, or trends can be identified.

Elements of Performance for PI.2.10

1. Not applicable
2. B | 0 | 1 | 2 | NA | Data are aggregated at the frequency appropriate to the activity or process being studied.
3. Not applicable
4. B | 0 | 1 | 2 | NA | Data are analyzed and compared internally over time and externally* with other sources of information when available.

❑ Compliant
❑ Not Compliant

Standard PI.2.20

Undesirable patterns or trends in performance are analyzed.

Elements of Performance for PI.2.20

1. B | 0 | 1 | 2 | NA | Analysis is performed when data comparisons indicate that levels of performance, patterns, or trends vary substantially from those expected.
2. B | 0 | 1 | 2 | NA | Analysis occurs for those topics chosen by leaders as performance improvement priorities.
3. Not applicable

An analysis is performed for the following:

4. Not applicable
5. A | 0 | 1 | 2 | NA | All serious adverse drug events, if applicable and as defined by the practice
6. A | 0 | 1 | 2 | NA | All significant medication errors, if applicable and as defined by the practice
7. A | 0 | 1 | 2 | NA | All major discrepancies between preoperative and postoperative (including pathologic) diagnoses
8. A | 0 | 1 | 2 | NA | Adverse events or patterns of adverse events during moderate or deep sedation and anesthesia use

9. Through 10. Not applicable

11. Not applicable

An analysis is performed for the following:

12. A | 0 | 1 | 2 | NA | Errors and omissions in patient assessment for surgery and anesthesia resulting in significant adverse clinical events

❑ Compliant
❑ Not Compliant

Standard PI.2.30

Processes for identifying and managing sentinel events are defined and implemented.

* External sources of information include recent scientific, clinical, and management literature, including sentinel event alerts; well-formulated practice guidelines or parameters; performance measures; reference databases; other practices with similar processes; and standards that are periodically reviewed and revised.

PI

Scoring Grid
0 Insufficient compliance
1 Partial compliance
2 Satisfactory compliance
NA Not applicable

Elements of Performance for PI.2.30

Processes for identifying and managing sentinel events include the following:

1. Defining sentinel event and communicating this definition throughout the practice. (At a minimum, the practice's definition includes those events subject to review under the Joint Commission's Sentinel Event Policy as published in this manual and may include any process variation that does not affect the outcome or result in an adverse event, but for which a recurrence carries a significant chance of a serious adverse outcome or result in an adverse event, often referred to as a near miss.) **A** 0 | 1 | 2 | NA
2. Reporting sentinel events through established channels in the practice and, as appropriate, to external agencies in accordance with law and regulation. **A** 0 | 1 | 2 | NA
3. Conducting thorough and credible root cause analyses that focus on process and system factors. **B** 0 | 1 | 2 | NA
4. Creating, documenting, and implementing a risk-reduction strategy and action plan that includes measuring the effectiveness of process and system improvements to reduce risk. **B** 0 | 1 | 2 | NA
5. The processes are implemented. **B** 0 | 1 | 2 | NA

Performance Improvement

The purpose of the PI function is to improve processes and outcomes and then sustain the improved performance. This can be accomplished by incrementally improving existing processes, redesigning an existing process, or designing or introducing an essentially new process.

Standard PI.3.10

❑ Compliant
❑ Not Compliant

Information from data analysis is used to make changes that improve performance and patient safety and reduce the risk of sentinel events.

Elements of Performance for PI.3.10

1. Not applicable
2. The practice identifies and implements changes that reduce the risk of sentinel events. **B** 0 | 1 | 2 | NA
3. Not applicable
4. Changes made to improve processes or outcomes are evaluated to ensure that they achieve the expected results. **B** 0 | 1 | 2 | NA
5. Appropriate actions are undertaken when planned improvements are not achieved or sustained. **B** 0 | 1 | 2 | NA
6. Not applicable
7. Corrective action is taken when necessary to improve medical record documentation. **B** 0 | 1 | 2 | NA

Standard PI.3.20

❑ Compliant
❑ Not Compliant

An ongoing, proactive program for identifying and reducing unanticipated adverse events and safety risks to patients is defined and implemented.

Rationale for PI.3.20

Practices should proactively seek to identify and reduce risks to the safety of patients. Such initiatives have the obvious advantage of *preventing* adverse events rather than simply *reacting* when they occur. This approach also avoids the barriers to understanding created by hindsight bias and the fear of disclosure, embarrassment, blame, and punishment that can happen after an event.

Elements of Performance for PI.3.20

The following proactive activities to reduce risks to patients are conducted:

A	0	1	2	NA	1. Selecting a high-risk process* to be analyzed (At least one high-risk process is chosen annually—the choice should be based in part on information published periodically by the Joint Commission about the most frequent sentinel events and risks.)
B	0	1	2	NA	2. Describing the chosen process (for example, through the use of a flowchart)
B	0	1	2	NA	3. Identifying the ways in which the process could break down† or fail to perform its desired function
B	0	1	2	NA	4. Identifying the possible effects that a breakdown or failure of the process could have on patients and the seriousness of the possible effects
B	0	1	2	NA	5. Prioritizing the potential process breakdowns or failures
B	0	1	2	NA	6. Determining why the prioritized breakdowns or failures could occur, which may include performing a hypothetical root cause analysis
B	0	1	2	NA	7. Redesigning the process and/or underlying systems to minimize the risk of the effects on patients
B	0	1	2	NA	8. Testing and implementing the redesigned process
B	0	1	2	NA	9. Monitoring the effectiveness of the redesigned process

PI

* **High-risk process** A process that if not planned and/or implemented correctly, has a significant potential for impacting the safety of the patient.

† The ways in which processes could break down or fail to perform their desired function are many times referred to as *the failure modes.*

Practice Leadership

Overview

The goal of planning and directing practice services in an office-based surgery practice is to provide a framework of decision making, accountability, and responsibility for delivering effective, efficient, and safe patient care services. Planning and directing practice services encompass a broad range of activities that affect all areas of the practice and should involve a collaborative process among all staff. As such, these activities are represented throughout this manual, with reference to appropriate staff. However, those whom the practice defines as its leaders are accountable for decision making in the following areas:

- Planning and designing services. Practice leaders provide a collaborative process to develop operational, strategic, and long-range plans; service design; resource allocation; and practice protocols and procedures.
- Directing services. Practice leaders provide practice direction and staffing for patient care and support services according to the scope of services offered, either directly or through delegated activities or contracted staff. Practice leaders communicate objectives and facilitate coordination of services.
- Improving performance. Practice leaders establish expectations, plans, and priorities and manage the performance improvement process, ensuring implementation of processes to measure, assess, and improve the performance of the practice's clinical and support services.

Office-based surgery practices to which this accreditation manual applies are owned or operated by surgeons. As such, the practice leadership is composed of surgeons and, as appropriate, other administrative and clinical staff.

LD

Glossary Terms

These key terms have specific Joint Commission definitions. Please access the Glossary found near the end of your manual for the Joint Commission definition and appropriate use.

administration
community
contract
contracted services
governance
leader
licensed independent practitioner
mission statement
performance improvement (PI)
plan
policies and procedures
practice guidelines
qualified individual
quality of care
safety management
scope of care, treatment, and services
sentinel event

Standards

The following is a list of all standards for this function. They are presented here for your convenience without footnotes or other explanatory text. If you have a question about a term used here, please check the Glossary.

Note: *A revised standard numbering system is being used with the reformatted standards. This revised numbering system allows for more flexibility to add standards while maintaining the current label for each standard.*

LD.1.10 Not applicable

LD.1.20 Governance responsibilities are defined in writing, as applicable.

LD.1.30 The practice complies with applicable law and regulation.

LD.2.10 Not applicable

LD.2.20 The practice has effective leadership.

LD.2.30 Through LD.2.40 Not applicable

LD.2.50 The leaders develop and monitor an annual operating budget and, as appropriate, a long-term capital expenditure plan.

LD.2.60 Through LD.2.200 Not applicable

LD.3.10 The leaders engage in both short-term and long-term planning.

LD.3.15 Not applicable

LD.3.20 Patients with comparable needs receive the same standard of care, treatment, and services throughout the practice.

LD.3.30 Through LD.3.40 Not applicable

LD.3.50 Services provided by consultation, contractual arrangements, or other agreements are provided safely and effectively.

LD.3.60 Communication is effective throughout the practice.

LD.3.70 The leaders define the required qualifications and competence of those staff who provide care, treatment, and services and recommend a sufficient number of qualified and competent staff to provide care, treatment, and services.

LD.3.80 The leaders provide for adequate space, equipment, and other resources.

LD.3.90 The leaders develop and implement policies and procedures for care, treatment, and services.

LD.3.100 Through LD.3.150 Not applicable

LD.4.10 The leaders set expectations, plan, and manage processes to measure, assess, and improve the practice's governance, management, clinical, and support activities.

LD.4.20 New or modified services or processes are designed well.

LD.4.30 Not applicable

LD.4.40 The leaders ensure that an integrated patient safety program is implemented throughout the practice.

LD.4.50 The leaders set performance improvement priorities and identify how the practice adjusts priorities in response to unusual or urgent events.

LD.4.60 The leaders allocate adequate resources for measuring, assessing, and improving the practice's performance and improving patient safety.

LD.4.70 Through LD.5.40 Not applicable

LD.5.50 Clinical practice guidelines are used in designing or improving processes that evaluate and treat specific diagnoses, conditions, and/or symptoms.

LD.5.60 The leaders identify criteria for selecting and implementing clinical practice guidelines.

LD.5.70 Appropriate leaders, practitioners, and health care professionals in the practice review and approve clinical practice guidelines selected for implementation.

LD.5.80 The leaders evaluate the outcomes related to clinical practice guidelines and refine the guidelines to improve processes.

Understanding the Parts of This Chapter

To help you navigate this reformatted standards chapter, it may be helpful to think of its parts this way:

- The **standard** is the "goal."
- The **rationale** explains why it's important to achieve this goal.
- The **elements of performance** identify the step(s) needed to achieve this goal.

These parts are defined as follows.

Standard A statement that defines the performance expectations and/or structures or processes that must be in place in order for a practice to provide safe, high-quality care, treatment, and services. An practice is either "compliant" or "not compliant" with a standard as reflected by the check boxes in the margin by the standard:

❏ Compliant
❏ Not Compliant

Accreditation decisions are based on simple counts of the standards that are determined to be "not compliant."

Rationale A statement that provides background, justification, or additional information about a standard. A standard's rationale is not scored. In some instances, the rationale for a standard is self-evident. Therefore, not every standard has a written rationale.

Elements of performance (EPs) The specific performance expectations and/or structures or processes that must be in place in order for a practice to provide safe, high-quality care, treatment, and services. The scoring of EP compliance determines a practice's overall compliance with a standard. EPs are evaluated on the following scale:

0 Insufficient compliance
1 Partial compliance
2 Satisfactory compliance
NA Not applicable

LD

You will find a **measure of success** icon—Ⓜ—next to some EPs. Measures of success (MOS) need to be developed for certain EPs when a standard is judged to be out of compliance through the on-site survey. An MOS is defined as a quantifiable measure, usually related to an audit, that can be used to determine whether an action has been effective and is being sustained.*

Using the Self-Assessment Grid to Assess Your Compliance

Once you are familiar with the parts of this chapter, you can begin to assess your compliance with its requirements. A self-assessment grid (otherwise known as a scoring grid) has been provided in the margins for your convenience. If you would like to assess your practice's performance, mark your scores for the EPs on the scoring grid by following the simple steps described below. **Note:** *You are **not** required to complete this scoring grid. It is provided simply to help you assess your own performance.*

Two components are scored for each EP: (1) compliance with the requirement itself **and** (2) compliance with the track record† for that requirement. Scoring has been simplified from the past edition of the manual, and track record achievements (which have always been part of the scoring) have been appropriately modified.

---

* For more information about Measures of Success, *see* "The New Joint Commission Accreditation Process" chapter in this manual.

† **Track record** The amount of time that a practice has been in compliance with a standard, element of performance, or other requirement.

Note: *Some standards and EPs do not apply to a particular type of practice; these standards and EPs are marked "not applicable" and the related text is not included. Your practice is not expected to comply with standards and EPs marked "not applicable."*

In addition, some standards and EPs that do apply to practices may not apply to the specific care, treatment, and services that your individual practice provides. Although these standards and EPs are included in the manual, you are not expected to comply with them. If you are unsure about the standards or EPs that apply to your practice, please contact the Joint Commission's Standards Interpretation Group at 630/792-5900.

Step 1: Score Your Compliance with Each Element of Performance

Before you can determine your compliance with the standards, you must score your compliance with each EP. First look at the EP scoring criterion category listed immediately preceding the scoring scale in the margin next to the EP. There are three scoring criterion categories: A, B, and C (described below). Please note that for each EP scoring criterion category, your practice must meet the performance requirement itself and the track record achievements (*see* below).

Category A

These EPs relate to the presence or absence of the requirement(s) and are scored either yes (2) or no (0); however, score 1 for partial compliance is also possible based on track record achievements (*see* below).

If an A EP has multiple components designated by bullets, your practice must be compliant with all the bullets to receive a score of 2. If your practice does not meet one or more requirements in the bullets, you will receive a score of 0.

Category B

Category B EPs are scored in two steps:

1. As with category A EPs, category B EPs relate to the presence or absence of the requirement(s). If your practice *does not meet* the requirement(s), the EP is scored 0; there is no need to assess your compliance with the principles of good process design (*see* below).
2. If your practice *does meet* the requirement(s), but there is concern about the quality or comprehensiveness of the effort, then and only then should you assess the qualitative aspect of the EP. That is, review the applicable principles of good process design and ask how the principles were applied in the situation under discussion. Good process design has the following characteristics:
   - Is consistent with your practice's mission, values, and goals
   - Meets the needs of patients
   - Reflects the use of currently accepted practices (doing the right thing, using resources responsibly, using practice guidelines)
   - Incorporates current safety information and knowledge such as sentinel event data and National Patient Safety Goals
   - Incorporates relevant performance improvement results

This two-part evaluation applies to both simple and bulleted B EPs. First, the EPs are assessed to determine if the requirements are present. If the EP has multiple components designated by bullets, as with the category A EPs, your practice must meet the requirements in *all* the bulleted items to get a score of 2. If your practice meets *none* of the requirements in the bullets, it receives a score of 0. If your practice meets *at least one, but not all,* of the bulleted requirements, it will receive a score of 1 for the EPs.

Use the following rules to determine your EP score:

- Your EP score is 0 if your practice does not meet the requirement(s); you *do not* need to assess your compliance with the preceding applicable principles of good process design
- Your EP score is 1 if your practice does meet the requirement(s), but considered only *some* of the preceding applicable principles of good process design

- Your EP score is 2 if your practice does meet the requirement(s) *and* considered *all* the preceding principles of good process design

Category C

C EPs are scored 0, 1, or 2 based on the number of times your practice does not meet the EP. These EPs are frequency based and require totaling the number of occurrences (that is, results of performance or nonperformance) related to a particular EP. Each situation discovered by a surveyor(s) will be counted as a separate occurrence.

Note: *Multiple events of the same type related to a single patient and single practitioner/staff member are counted as* one occurrence only.

Use the following rules to determine your EP score:

- Your EP score is 2 if you find one or fewer occurrences of noncompliance with the EP
- Your EP score is 1 if you find two occurrences of noncompliance with the EP
- Your EP score is 0 if you find three or more occurrences of noncompliance with the EP

If an EP in the C category has multiple requirements designated by bullets, the following scoring guidelines apply:

- If there are fewer than 2 findings in all bullets, the EP is scored 2
- If there are three or more findings in all bullets, the EP is scored 0
- In all other combinations of findings, the EP is scored 1

Track Record Achievements

In addition to meeting the requirement(s) in each EP, regardless of category, your practice must also meet the following track record achievements:

Score	Initial Survey	Full Survey
2	4 months or more	12 months or more
1	2 to 3 months	6 to 11 months
0	Fewer than 2 months	Fewer than 6 months

Sample Sizes

If during an on-site survey, your practice has been found to be not compliant with one or more standards, you must demonstrate Evidence of Standards Compliance (ESC) for each standard that is not compliant. The ESC must address compliance at the EP level; when an EP within a noncompliant standard requires an MOS, your practice must demonstrate achievement with the MOS when completing the ESC.

Note: *Not every EP requires an MOS. EPs that do require an MOS are clearly marked in this chapter Practices are required to demonstrate achievement with an MOS* only *for EPs within a noncompliant standard that require an MOS. Practices* do not *need to demonstrate achievement with an MOS for any EP within a compliant standard.*

When demonstrating achievement with an MOS during the ESC process, your practice is **required** to use the following sample sizes, which were established because of their statistical significance, their relative simplicity in application, and their sensitivity to a practice's population size:

- For a population size of fewer than 30 cases,* sample 100% of available cases
- For a population size of 30 to 100 cases, sample 30 cases
- For a population size of 101 to 500 cases, sample 50 cases
- For a population size greater than 500 cases, sample 70 cases

When demonstrating an ESC (mandatory use), use the following percentages to determine your EP score: 90% through 100% of your sample size is in compliance = score 2; 80% through 89% of your sample size is in compliance = score 1; less than 80% of your sample size is in compliance = score 0.

---

* "Case" refers to a single instance in which a situation related to a survey finding occurs. For example, if a survey finding was related to **pain assessment,** then a "case" would be any patient record. If a survey finding was related to **pain management,** a "case" would be any patient record for patients receiving pain management.

In addition, the following information should govern your practice's selection of samples:

- The appropriate sample size should be determined by the specific population related to the survey findings.
- The sampling approach should involve either systematic random sampling (for example, your practice selects every second or third case for review) or simple random sampling (for example, your practice uses a series of random numbers generated by a computer to identify the cases to be reviewed).
- When submitting a clarifying ESC, if your practice selects records as part of its sample, the records should be from a period of no more than three months before the last date of the survey.
- Assessment of MOS compliance is conducted for a four-month period following the date of ESC approval. Your practice should select records as a part of your sample following the date of ESC approval and use the required sample sizes. MOS percentage compliance rates are derived from the average of all four months.

Step 2: Use Your EP Scores to Gauge Your Compliance with the Standards

Now that you have evaluated and scored each EP for a particular standard, use these simple rules to determine your compliance with the standard itself:

- Your practice is not in compliance (that is, "not compliant") with the standard if any EP is scored 0
- Otherwise, your practice is in compliance with a standard if 65% or more of its EPs are scored 2

Scoring Grid

0 Insufficient compliance
1 Partial compliance
2 Satisfactory compliance
NA Not applicable

Standards, Rationales, Elements of Performance, and Scoring

Standard LD.1.10

Not applicable

❑ Compliant
❑ Not Compliant

Standard LD.1.20

Governance responsibilities are defined in writing, as applicable.

Elements of Performance for LD.1.20

A | 0 | 1 | 2 | NA |

1. Governance defines its responsibilities in writing, as applicable.

2. Through 3. Not applicable

A | 0 | 1 | 2 | NA |

4. The practice's scope of services is defined in writing and approved by the practice leaders.

❑ Compliant
❑ Not Compliant

Standard LD.1.30

The practice complies with applicable law and regulation.

Element of Performance for LD.1.30

A | 0 | 1 | 2 | NA |

1. The practice provides all care, treatment, and services in accordance with applicable licensure requirements, law, rules, and regulation.

Standard LD.2.10

Not applicable

❑ Compliant
❑ Not Compliant

Standard LD.2.20

The practice has effective leadership.

Element of Performance for LD.2.20

B | 0 | 1 | 2 | NA |

1. Leaders ensure that operations are effective and efficient.

Standard LD.2.30 Through LD.2.40

Not applicable

❑ Compliant
❑ Not Compliant

Standard LD.2.50

The leaders develop and monitor an annual operating budget and, as appropriate, a long-term capital expenditure plan.

Element of Performance for LD.2.50

A | 0 | 1 | 2 | NA |

1. An operating budget is developed annually and approved by the practice leaders.

Scoring Grid
0 Insufficient compliance
1 Partial compliance
2 Satisfactory compliance
NA Not applicable

Standards LD.2.60 Through LD.2.200

Not applicable

Standard LD.3.10

❑ Compliant
❑ Not Compliant

The leaders engage in both short-term and long-term planning.

Rationale for LD.3.10

These standards do not require the practice leaders to use a computer-assisted process or any other specific structure for planning and designing.

Elements of Performance for LD.3.10

1. Leaders create vision, mission, and goal statements. **A** | 0 | 1 | 2 | NA |

2\. Through 26. Not applicable

27. Leaders determine which surgical and invasive procedures are performed. **A** | 0 | 1 | 2 | NA |

Standard LD.3.15

Not applicable

Standard LD.3.20

❑ Compliant
❑ Not Compliant

Patients with comparable needs receive the same standard of care, treatment, and services throughout the practice.

Rationale for LD.3.20

Factors such as different individuals providing care, treatment, and services; different insurers; or different settings of care do not intentionally negatively influence the outcome.

LD

Elements of Performance for LD.3.20

1. Patients with comparable needs receive the same standard of care, treatment, and services throughout the practice. **B** | 0 | 1 | 2 | NA |
2. The practice plans, designs, and monitors care, treatment, and services so that they are consistent with the mission, vision, and goals. **B** | 0 | 1 | 2 | NA |

Standards LD.3.30 Through LD.3.40

Not applicable

Scoring Grid
0 Insufficient compliance
1 Partial compliance
2 Satisfactory compliance
NA Not applicable

❑ Compliant
❑ Not Compliant

Standard LD.3.50

Services provided by consultation, contractual arrangements, or other agreements are provided safely and effectively.

Rationale for LD.3.50

The practice leaders may choose to provide some services through consultation, contractual arrangements, or other agreements, while retaining overall responsibility and authority for the level of safety and quality of the patient care provided. These services might include the following:

- Diagnostic radiology services
- Pathology and clinical laboratory services*
- Pharmaceutical services
- Anesthesia services

Elements of Performance for LD.3.50

A | 0 | 1 | 2 | NA
1. The leaders approve sources for the practice's services that are provided by consultation, contractual arrangements, or other agreements.

A | 0 | 1 | 2 | NA
2. The clinical leaders advise the practice's leaders on the sources of clinical services to be provided by consultation, contractual arrangements, or other agreements.

3. Not applicable

A | 0 | 1 | 2 | NA
4. The nature and scope of services provided by consultation, contractual arrangements, or other agreements are defined in writing.†

5. Through 6. Not applicable

A | 0 | 1 | 2 | NA
7. The practice retains overall responsibility and authority for services furnished under a contract.

A | 0 | 1 | 2 | NA
8. All reference and contract lab services‡ meet the applicable federal regulations for clinical laboratories and maintain evidence of the same.

LD

❑ Compliant
❑ Not Compliant

Standard LD.3.60

Communication is effective throughout the practice.

Element of Performance for LD.3.60

B | 0 | 1 | 2 | NA
1. The leaders ensure processes are in place for communicating relevant information throughout the practice in a timely manner.

---

* A practice's services include those provided by a central laboratory and any ancillary, near-patient-testing, hospital-based, and point-of-care laboratories.

† When a practice contracts for patient care, treatment, or services rendered outside the practice but under the control of a Joint Commission–accredited practice, the primary practice can do the following:

- Specify in the contract that the contracting entity ensures that all services provided by contracted individuals who are licensed independent practitioners is within the scope of his or her privleges
  or
- Verify that all contracted individuals who are licensed independent practitioners and who will be providing patient care, treat ment, and services have appropriate privileges, for example by obtaining a copy of the list of privileges

When a practice contracts for patient care, treatment, or services rendered outside the practice and under the control of a non–Joint Commission–accredited practice, all licensed independent practitioners who will be providing services are privileged by the Joint Commission–accredited practice through the process described in the "Management of Human Resources"(HR) chapter in this manual.

‡ A written agreement (such as a formal contract) is not required for reference laboratories; however, it is required for a contract service where a major portion of laboratory testing is provided by an outside laboratory.

Scoring Grid
- **0** Insufficient compliance
- **1** Partial compliance
- **2** Satisfactory compliance
- **NA** Not applicable

Standard LD.3.70

The leaders define the required qualifications and competence of those staff who provide care, treatment, and services and recommend a sufficient number of qualified and competent staff to provide care, treatment, and services.

❑ Compliant
❑ Not Compliant

Element of Performance for LD.3.70

1. The leaders provide for the allocation of competent, qualified staff. **B** 0 | 1 | 2 | NA

Standard LD.3.80

The leaders provide for adequate space, equipment, and other resources.

❑ Compliant
❑ Not Compliant

Elements of Performance for LD.3.80

1. The leaders provide for the arrangement and allocation of space to facilitate efficient, effective delivery of care, treatment, and services. **B** 0 | 1 | 2 | NA
2. The leaders provide for the appropriateness of interior and exterior space for the care, treatment, and services offered and for the ages and other characteristics of the patients. **B** 0 | 1 | 2 | NA

Standard LD.3.90

The leaders develop and implement policies and procedures for care, treatment, and services.

❑ Compliant
❑ Not Compliant

Rationale for LD.3.90

To determine topics that need to be addressed in policies and procedures, look at processes that individuals would be trained on and where consistency would be of value.

Elements of Performance for LD.3.90

1. The leaders develop policies and procedures that guide and support patient care, treatment, and services. **B** 0 | 1 | 2 | NA

Ⓜ 2. Policies and procedures are consistently implemented.

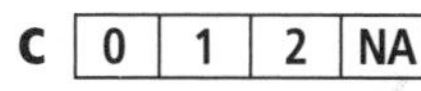

3. Through 6. Not applicable

7. These policies and procedures describe how specific patient groups' care needs are assessed and met with specific services.

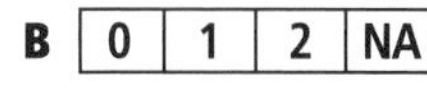

8. The following elements are addressed: **B** 0 | 1 | 2 | NA
   - The type(s) and age(s) of patients served
   - The scope and complexity of patients' care needs
   - How well the level of care provided will meet patient's needs
   - The appropriateness, clinical necessity, and timeliness of support services provided directly or through referral
   - The availability of necessary staff
   - The recognized practice standards or guidelines, when available
   - The methods used to assess and meet patient care needs

Standards LD.3.100 Through LD.3.150

Not applicable

Standard LD.4.10

The leaders set expectations, plan, and manage processes to measure, assess, and improve the practice's management, clinical, and support activities.

❑ Compliant
❑ Not Compliant

LD

Scoring Grid
0 Insufficient compliance
1 Partial compliance
2 Satisfactory compliance
NA Not applicable

Elements of Performance for LD.4.10

B 0 1 2 NA 1. The leaders set expectations for performance improvement.

B 0 1 2 NA 2. The leaders develop plans for performance improvement.

B 0 1 2 NA 3. The leaders manage processes to improve practice performance.

❑ Compliant
❑ Not Compliant

Standard LD.4.20

New or modified services or processes are designed well.

Elements of Performance for LD.4.20

The design of new or modified services or processes incorporates the following:

1. Through 5. Not applicable

B 0 1 2 NA 6. Testing and analysis to determine whether the proposed design or redesign is an improvement

Standard LD.4.30

Not applicable

❑ Compliant
❑ Not Compliant

Standard LD.4.40

The leaders ensure that an integrated patient safety program is implemented throughout the practice.

Rationale for LD.4.40

The leaders should work to foster a safe environment throughout the practice by integrating safety priorities into all relevant practice processes, functions, and services. In pursuit of this effort, a patient safety program can work to improve safety by reducing the risk of system or process failures. As part of its responsibility to communicate objectives and coordinate efforts to integrate patient care and support services throughout the practice and with contracted services, leadership takes the lead in developing, implementing, and overseeing a patient safety program.

The standard does not require the creation of new structures or offices in the practice; rather, the standard emphasizes the need to integrate all patient safety activities, both existing and newly created, with the practice's leadership identified as accountable for this integration.

Elements of Performance for LD.4.40

The patient safety program includes the following:

A 0 1 2 NA 1. One or more qualified individuals or an interdisciplinary group assigned to manage the practice wide safety program

B 0 1 2 NA 2. Definition of the scope of the program's oversight, typically ranging from no-harm, frequently occurring slips to sentinel events with serious adverse outcomes

B 0 1 2 NA 3. Integration into and participation of all components of the practice into the practice wide program

B 0 1 2 NA 4. Procedures for immediately responding to system or process failures, including care, treatment, or services for the affected individual(s), containing risk to others, and preserving factual information for subsequent analysis

B 0 1 2 NA 5. Clear systems for internal and external reporting of information about system or process failures

B 0 1 2 NA 6. Defined responses to various types of unanticipated adverse events and processes for conducting proactive risk assessment/risk reduction activities

Scoring Grid
0 Insufficient compliance
1 Partial compliance
2 Satisfactory compliance
NA Not applicable

7. Defined support systems* for staff members who have been involved in a sentinel event — B | 0 | 1 | 2 | NA
8. Reports, at least annually, to the practice's governance or authority on system or process failures and actions taken to improve safety, both proactively and in response to actual occurrences — A | 0 | 1 | 2 | NA

Standard LD.4.50

The leaders set performance improvement priorities and identify how the practice adjusts priorities in response to unusual or urgent events.

❑ Compliant
❑ Not Compliant

Rationale for LD.4.50

The practice leaders consider changing priorities when the practice expands, adds new services, and soon.

Elements of Performance for LD.4.50

1. The leaders set priorities for performance improvement for practice wide activities and patient health outcomes. — B | 0 | 1 | 2 | NA
2. The leaders give high priority to high-volume, high-risk, or problem-prone processes. — B | 0 | 1 | 2 | NA
3. Performance improvement activities are reprioritized in response to significant changes in the internal or external environment. — B | 0 | 1 | 2 | NA

Standard LD.4.60

The leaders allocate adequate resources for measuring, assessing, and improving the practice's performance and improving patient safety.

❑ Compliant
❑ Not Compliant

Elements of Performance for LD.4.60

1. Sufficient staff is assigned to conduct activities for performance improvement and safety improvement. — B | 0 | 1 | 2 | NA
2. Adequate time is provided for staff to participate in activities for performance improvement and safety improvement. — B | 0 | 1 | 2 | NA
3. Adequate information systems are provided to support activities for performance improvement and safety improvement. — B | 0 | 1 | 2 | NA
4. Staff is trained in performance improvement and safety improvement approaches and methods. — B | 0 | 1 | 2 | NA

LD

Standards LD.4.70 Through LD.5.40

Not applicable

Standard LD.5.50

Clinical practice guidelines are used in designing or improving processes that evaluate and treat specific diagnoses, conditions, and/or symptoms.

❑ Compliant
❑ Not Compliant

Rationale for LD.5.50

Clinical practice guidelines can improve quality, appropriate utilization of health care services, and the value of health care services. Clinical practice guidelines help practitioners in making decisions

* Support systems provide individuals with additional help and support as well as additional resources through the human resources function or an employee assistance program. Support systems recognize that conscientious health care workers who are involved in sentinel events are themselves victims of the event and require support. Support systems also focus on the process rather than blaming the involved individuals.

Scoring Grid

0 Insufficient compliance
1 Partial compliance
2 Satisfactory compliance
NA Not applicable

about preventing, diagnosing, treating, and managing selected conditions. Clinical practice guidelines can also be used in designing processes or checking the design of existing processes. The leaders identify and consider for implementation clinical practice guidelines from such sources as the Agency for Healthcare Research and Quality, National Guideline Clearinghouse, and professional practices.

Element of Performance for LD.5.50

B 0 | 1 | 2 | NA

1. The leaders have used clinical practice guidelines in designing or improving processes.

❏ Compliant
❏ Not Compliant

Standard LD.5.60

The leaders identify criteria for selecting and implementing clinical practice guidelines.

Rationale for LD.5.60

Selecting and implementing clinical practice guidelines that are appropriate to the practice are critical. Therefore, the leaders set criteria to guide the selection and implementation of guidelines that are consistent with the practice's mission and priorities. The leaders also consider the steps and changes or variations needed to encourage use, dissemination, and implementation of chosen guidelines throughout the practice. This includes staff communication, training, implementation, feedback, and evaluation.

Elements of Performance for LD.5.60

B 0 | 1 | 2 | NA

1. The leaders identify criteria to guide the selection and implementation of guidelines.

B 0 | 1 | 2 | NA

2. The practice manages, evaluates, and learns from variation.

❏ Compliant
❏ Not Compliant

LD

Standard LD.5.70

Appropriate leaders, practitioners, and health care professionals in the practice review and approve clinical practice guidelines selected for implementation.

Rationale for LD.5.70

To be successfully implemented, clinical practice guidelines should be reviewed, revised, or adapted by the providers using them and approved by the practice's leaders.

Element of Performance for LD.5.70

A 0 | 1 | 2 | NA

1. Appropriate practice leaders review and approve the clinical practice guidelines selected for use.

❏ Compliant
❏ Not Compliant

Standard LD.5.80

The leaders evaluate the outcomes related to clinical practice guidelines and refine the guidelines to improve processes.

Rationale for LD.5.80

To fully benefit from the use of clinical practice guidelines, the outcomes of patients treated using clinical practice guidelines are evaluated, and refinements are made in how the guidelines are used, if necessary.

Element of Performance for LD.5.80

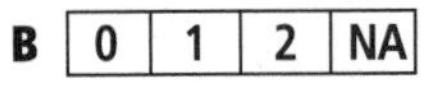

1. Clinical practice guidelines are monitored and reviewed for effectiveness and modified as appropriate.

Management of the Environment of Care

Overview

Environment of Care Process Overview

Practices, whether in owned or leased spaces, are responsible for compliance with the standards in this chapter. Methods of compliance can include the following in any combination:

- Direct management and implementation of the environment of care by the practice
- Contracted relationships with external entities that provide or maintain such service
- Leasing and service arrangements with the building owner or manager
- Documentation of licensing or inspections by appropriate authorities (for example, fire marshal, municipal building department, and so forth)

Please note that some standards contain requirements that are applicable to some, but not all, office-based surgical practices. Specific standards language addresses the following:

- Practices where electrical life support equipment or assisted mechanical ventilation are used
- Practices with fire detection equipment
- Practices that have emergency power systems
- Practices that have emergency generators
- Practices that simultaneously render four or more patients incapable of self-preservation in emergencies
- Practices that have a patient stay beyond regular business hours*

Office-based surgery practices that simultaneously render *four or more patients* incapable of self-preservation in emergencies must demonstrate compliance with provisions of the *Life Safety Code*® (*LSC*)†, *NFPA 101*® in the following manner:

Conduct a Self-Assessment

This assessment should address key elements of the Statement of Conditions™ (SOC). Documentation of compliance may include appropriate legal attestations from local authorities (for example, fire marshal, municipal building department, insurance company inspections, and so forth), which confirm compliance with the identified elements of the SOC.

The review of this self-assessment will result in one of the following outcomes:

1. Compliance with the *LSC*
2. Identification of deficiencies, which can be addressed through one of the following:
   a. The practice repairing the deficiency
   b. The practice requesting an equivalency from the Joint Commission, which will allow them to demonstrate that they have implemented alternative, effective means and processes for compliance
   c. The practice documenting the repair process in a plan for improvement

The thoroughness of the self-assessment is verified during the on-site survey process.

---

* Practices surveyed under these standards can retain no more than one patient in extended recovery beyond regular business hours. Practices that retain more than one patient in recovery beyond regular business hours must be surveyed under the *Comprehensive Accreditation Manual for Ambulatory Care.* "Beyond regular business hours" is considered as the time at which the earlier of these two situations occurs:

a. The business hours of the practice have concluded. Most staff is free to leave for the day. Most records, systems, supplies, and pharmaceuticals are secured for the evening. No routine external calls are being taken.

b. For practices not in freestanding buildings, the building in which the practice operates has closed for routine business. Lighting, ventilation, and other utilities are reduced. Most staff has left for the day. Many corridors and exits are locked.

† Life Safety Code® is a registered trademark of the National Fire Protection Association, Quincy, MA.

EC

Management of the Environment of Care Overview

The goal of management of the environment of care in an office-based surgery practice is to provide a safe, functional, and effective environment for patients, staff, and others, which is crucial to providing patient care and achieving good outcomes. Achieving this goal depends on performing the following processes:

- Planning by the practice leadership for the space, equipment, and resources needed to safely and effectively support the services provided. Planning should be consistent with the practice's goals and priorities.
- Educating staff about the role of the environment in safely and effectively supporting patient care. The practice educates staff about the environment, including equipment use and the processes for promoting safety while reducing risk in the practice.
- Implementing actions to create and safely manage the practice's environment of care, including actions to identify opportunities to improve the status of the environment of care.

The environment of care is made up of three basic components: building(s), equipment, and people. Effectively managing the environment of care includes using processes and activities to do the following:

- Reduce and control environmental hazards and risks
- Prevent accidents and injuries
- Maintain safe conditions for patients, staff, and others

The standards in this chapter focus on how everyone in the practice participates in the activities that make the care environment safe and effective. Practices carry out most of these functions directly, but in some cases carry them out through contractual or leasing relationships.

Glossary Terms

These key terms have specific Joint Commission definitions. Please access the Glossary found near the end of your manual for the Joint Commission definition and appropriate use.

emergency
emergency management plan
environmental tours
hazard vulnerability analysis
mitigation activities
occupancy
preparedness activities

Standards

The following is a list of all standards for this function. They are presented here for your convenience without footnotes or other explanatory text. If you have a question about a term used here, please check the Glossary.

Note: *A revised standard numbering system is being used with the reformatted standards. The revised numbering system allows for more flexibility to add standards while maintaining the current label for each standard.*

Planning and Implementation Activities

EC.1.10 The practice manages safety risks.

EC.1.20 The practice maintains a safe environment.

EC.1.25 Not applicable

EC.1.27 The practice provides for staff safety.

EC.1.30 The practice develops and implements a policy to prohibit smoking except in specified circumstances.

EC.2.10 The practice identifies and manages its security risks.

EC.3.10 The practice manages its hazardous materials and waste risks.

EC.4.10 The practice addresses emergency management.

EC.4.20 The practice conducts drills regularly to test emergency management.

EC.5.10 The practice manages fire safety risks.

EC.5.20 Newly constructed and existing environments of care are designed and maintained to comply with the *LSC*®.

EC.5.30 The practice conducts fire drills regularly.

EC.5.40 The practice maintains fire-safety equipment and building features.

EC.5.50 Not applicable

EC.6.10 The practice manages medical equipment risks.

EC.6.20 Medical equipment is maintained, tested, and inspected.

EC.6.30 Through EC.6.130 Not applicable

EC.7.10 The practice manages its utility risks.

EC.7.20 The practice provides a reliable emergency electrical power source.

EC.7.30 The practice maintains, tests, and inspects its utility systems.

EC

EC.7.40 The practice maintains, tests, and inspects its emergency power systems.

EC.7.50 Not applicable

EC.8.10 The practice establishes and maintains an appropriate environment.

Understanding the Parts of This Chapter

To help you navigate this reformatted standards chapter, it may be helpful to think of its parts this way:

- The **standard** is the "goal."
- The **rationale** explains why it's important to achieve this goal.
- The **elements of performance** identify the step(s) needed to achieve this goal.

These parts are defined as follows.

Standard A statement that defines the performance expectations and/or structures or processes that must be in place in order for a practice to provide safe, high-quality care, treatment, and services. An practice is either "compliant" or "not compliant" with a standard as reflected by the check boxes in the margin by the standard:

❑ Compliant
❑ Not Compliant

Accreditation decisions are based on simple counts of the standards that are determined to be "not compliant."

Rationale A statement that provides background, justification, or additional information about a standard. A standard's rationale is not scored. In some instances, the rationale for a standard is self-evident. Therefore, not every standard has a written rationale.

Elements of performance (EPs) The specific performance expectations and/or structures or processes that must be in place in order for a practice to provide safe, high-quality care, treatment, and services. The scoring of EP compliance determines a practice's overall compliance with a standard. EPs are evaluated on the following scale:

0 Insufficient compliance
1 Partial compliance
2 Satisfactory compliance
NA Not applicable

You will find a **measure of success** icon—Ⓜ—next to some EPs. Measures of success (MOS) need to be developed for certain EPs when a standard is judged to be out of compliance through the on-site survey. An MOS is defined as a quantifiable measure, usually related to an audit, that can be used to determine whether an action has been effective and is being sustained.*

Using the Self-Assessment Grid to Assess Your Compliance

Once you are familiar with the parts of this chapter, you can begin to assess your compliance with its requirements. A self-assessment grid (otherwise known as a scoring grid) has been provided in the margins for your convenience. If you would like to assess your practice's performance, mark your scores for the EPs on the scoring grid by following the simple steps described below. **Note:** *You are **not** required to complete this scoring grid. It is provided simply to help you assess your own performance.*

Two components are scored for each EP: (1) compliance with the requirement itself **and** (2) compliance with the track record† for that requirement. Scoring has been simplified from the past edition of the manual, and track record achievements (which have always been part of the scoring) have been appropriately modified.

---

* For more information about Measures of Success, *see* "The New Joint Commission Accreditation Process" chapter in this manual.

† **Track record** The amount of time that a practice has been in compliance with a standard, element of performance, or other requirement.

EC

Note: *Some standards and EPs do not apply to a particular type of practice; these standards and EPs are marked "not applicable" and the related text is not included. Your practice is not expected to comply with standards and EPs marked "not applicable."*

In addition, some standards and EPs that do apply to practices may not apply to the specific care, treatment, and services that your individual practice provides. Although these standards and EPs are included in the manual, you are not expected to comply with them. If you are unsure about the standards or EPs that apply to your practice, please contact the Joint Commission's Standards Interpretation Group at 630/792-5900.

Step 1: Score Your Compliance with Each Element of Performance

Before you can determine your compliance with the standards, you must score your compliance with each EP. First look at the EP scoring criterion category listed immediately preceding the scoring scale in the margin next to the EP. There are three scoring criterion categories: A, B, and C (described below). Please note that for each EP scoring criterion category, your practice must meet the performance requirement itself and the track record achievements (*see* below).

Category A

These EPs relate to the presence or absence of the requirement(s) and are scored either yes (2) or no (0); however, score 1 for partial compliance is also possible based on track record achievements (*see* below).

If an A EP has multiple components designated by bullets, your practice must be compliant with all the bullets to receive a score of 2. If your practice does not meet one or more requirements in the bullets, you will receive a score of 0.

Category B

Category B EPs are scored in two steps:

1. As with category A EPs, category B EPs relate to the presence or absence of the requirement(s). If your practice *does not meet* the requirement(s), the EP is scored 0; there is no need to assess your compliance with the principles of good process design (*see* below).
2. If your practice *does meet* the requirement(s), but there is concern about the quality or comprehensiveness of the effort, then and only then should you assess the qualitative aspect of the EP. That is, review the applicable principles of good process design and ask how the principles were applied in the situation under discussion. Good process design has the following characteristics:
   - Is consistent with your practice's mission, values, and goals
   - Meets the needs of patients
   - Reflects the use of currently accepted practices (doing the right thing, using resources responsibly, using practice guidelines)
   - Incorporates current safety information and knowledge such as sentinel event data and National Patient Safety Goals
   - Incorporates relevant performance improvement results

This two-part evaluation applies to both simple and bulleted B EPs. First, the EPs are assessed to determine if the requirements are present. If the EP has multiple components designated by bullets, as with the category A EPs, your practice must meet the requirements in *all* the bulleted items to get a score of 2. If your practice meets *none* of the requirements in the bullets, it receives a score of 0. If your practice meets *at least one, but not all,* of the bulleted requirements, it will receive a score of 1 for the EPs.

Use the following rules to determine your EP score:

- Your EP score is 0 if your practice does not meet the requirement(s); you *do not* need to assess your compliance with the preceding applicable principles of good process design
- Your EP score is 1 if your practice does meet the requirement(s), but considered only *some* of the preceding applicable principles of good process design

- Your EP score is 2 if your practice does meet the requirement(s) *and* considered *all* the preceding principles of good process design

Category C

C EPs are scored 0, 1, or 2 based on the number of times your practice does not meet the EP. These EPs are frequency based and require totaling the number of occurrences (that is, results of performance or nonperformance) related to a particular EP. Each situation discovered by a surveyor(s) will be counted as a separate occurrence.

Note: *Multiple events of the same type related to a single patient and single practitioner/staff member are counted as* one occurrence only.

Use the following rules to determine your EP score:
- Your EP score is 2 if you find one or fewer occurrences of noncompliance with the EP
- Your EP score is 1 if you find two occurrences of noncompliance with the EP
- Your EP score is 0 if you find three or more occurrences of noncompliance with the EP

If an EP in the C category has multiple requirements designated by bullets, the following scoring guidelines apply:
- If there are fewer than 2 findings in all bullets, the EP is scored 2
- If there are three or more findings in all bullets, the EP is scored 0
- In all other combinations of findings, the EP is scored 1

Track Record Achievements

In addition to meeting the requirement(s) in each EP, regardless of category, your practice must also meet the following track record achievements:

Score	Initial Survey	Full Survey
2	4 months or more	12 months or more
1	2 to 3 months	6 to 11 months
0	Fewer than 2 months	Fewer than 6 months

Sample Sizes

If during an on-site survey, your practice has been found to be not compliant with one or more standards, you must demonstrate Evidence of Standards Compliance (ESC) for each standard that is not compliant. The ESC must address compliance at the EP level; when an EP within a noncompliant standard requires an MOS, your practice must demonstrate achievement with the MOS when completing the ESC.

Note: *Not every EP requires an MOS. EPs that do require an MOS are clearly marked in this chapter. Practices are required to demonstrate achievement with an MOS* only *for EPs within a noncompliant standard that require an MOS. Practices* do not *need to demonstrate achievement with an MOS for any EP within a compliant standard.*

When demonstrating achievement with an MOS during the ESC process, your practice is **required** to use the following sample sizes, which were established because of their statistical significance, their relative simplicity in application, and their sensitivity to a practice's population size:
- For a population size of fewer than 30 cases,* sample 100% of available cases
- For a population size of 30 to 100 cases, sample 30 cases
- For a population size of 101 to 500 cases, sample 50 cases
- For a population size greater than 500 cases, sample 70 cases

When demonstrating an ESC (mandatory use), use the following percentages to determine your EP score: 90% through 100% of your sample size is in compliance = score 2; 80% through 89% of your sample size is in compliance = score 1; less than 80% of your sample size is in compliance = score 0.

* "Case" refers to a single instance in which a situation related to a survey finding occurs. For example, if a survey finding was related to **pain assessment,** then a "case" would be any patient record. If a survey finding was related to **pain management,** a "case" would be any patient record for patients receiving pain management.

In addition, the following information should govern your practice's selection of samples:

- The appropriate sample size should be determined by the specific population related to the survey findings.
- The sampling approach should involve either systematic random sampling (for example, your practice selects every second or third case for review) or simple random sampling (for example, your practice uses a series of random numbers generated by a computer to identify the cases to be reviewed).
- When submitting clarifying ESC, if your practice selects records as part of its sample, the records should be from a period of no more than three months before the last date of the survey.
- Assessment of MOS compliance is conducted for a four-month period following the date of ESC approval. Your practice should select records as a part of your sample following the date of ESC approval and use the required sample sizes. MOS percentage compliance rates are derived from the average of all four months.

Step 2: Use Your EP Scores to Gauge Your Compliance with the Standards

Now that you have evaluated and scored each EP for a particular standard, use these simple rules to determine your compliance with the standard itself:

- Your practice is not in compliance (that is, "not compliant") with the standard if any EP is scored 0
- Otherwise, your practice is in compliance with a standard if 65% or more of its EPs are scored 2

Scoring Grid
0 Insufficient compliance
1 Partial compliance
2 Satisfactory compliance
NA Not applicable

Standards, Rationales, Elements of Performance, and Scoring

Standard EC.1.10

The practice manages safety risks.

❏ Compliant
❏ Not Compliant

Elements of Performance for EC.1.10

1. The practice plans for processes it implements to effectively manage the environmental safety of patients, staff, and other people coming to the practice's facilities. — **B** 0 1 2 NA
2. Not applicable
3. Not applicable
4. The practice conducts comprehensive, proactive risk assessments that evaluate the potential adverse impact of buildings, grounds, equipment, and internal physical systems on the safety and health of patients, staff, and other people coming to the practice's facilities. — **B** 0 1 2 NA

5. Through 8. Not applicable

9. The practice ensures that all grounds and equipment are maintained appropriately. — **B** 0 1 2 NA

Standard EC.1.20

The practice maintains a safe environment.

❏ Compliant
❏ Not Compliant

Elements of Performance for EC.1.20

1. The practice conducts environmental tours to identify environmental deficiencies, hazards, and unsafe practices. — **B** 0 1 2 NA
2. Ⓜ The practice conducts environmental tours at least every six months in all areas where patients are served. — **C** 0 1 2 NA
3. Ⓜ The practice conducts environmental tours at least annually in areas where patients are not served. — **C** 0 1 2 NA

EC

Standard EC.1.25

Not applicable

Standard EC.1.27

The practice provides for staff safety.

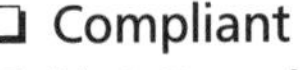

❏ Compliant
❏ Not Compliant

Elements of Performance for EC.1.27

1. Safety planning and implementation include identifying processes for staff to report all incidents of occupational illness and staff injury in a timely manner to practice leadership. — **B** 0 1 2 NA
2. The practice investigates all incidents of occupational illness and staff injury. — **B** 0 1 2 NA

Standard EC.1.30

The practice develops and implements a policy to prohibit smoking except in specified circumstances.

❏ Compliant
❏ Not Compliant

Scoring Grid
0 Insufficient compliance
1 Partial compliance
2 Satisfactory compliance
NA Not applicable

Rationale for EC.1.30
This standard is intended to reduce the following risks:
- To people who smoke, including possible adverse effects on care, treatment, and services
- Of passive smoking for others
- Of fire

Element of Performance for EC.1.30
B | 0 | 1 | 2 | NA
1. The practice develops a policy regarding smoking in all areas of all building(s) under the practice's control.

❑ Compliant
❑ Not Compliant

Standard EC.2.10
The practice identifies and manages its security risks.

Rationale for EC.2.10
The practice identifies processes for the following:
- Addressing security issues concerning patients, visitors, staff, and property
- Reporting and investigating all security incidents involving patients, visitors, staff, and property
- Identifying patients, staff, and visitors
- Controlling access to sensitive areas as determined by the practice

Elements of Performance for EC.2.10
B | 0 | 1 | 2 | NA
1. The practice plans for describing the processes it implements to effectively manage the security of patients, staff, and other people coming to the practice's facilities.
2. Not applicable
3. Not applicable

C | 0 | 1 | 2 | NA
Ⓜ 4. The practice implements procedures to reduce security risks.

B | 0 | 1 | 2 | NA
5. The practice identifies, as appropriate, patients, staff, and other people entering the practice's facilities.

C | 0 | 1 | 2 | NA
Ⓜ 6. The practice controls access to and egress from security-sensitive areas, as determined by the practice.

B | 0 | 1 | 2 | NA
7. The practice implements security procedures that address actions taken in the event of a security incident.

❑ Compliant
❑ Not Compliant

Standard EC.3.10
The practice manages its hazardous materials and waste* risks.

Elements of Performance for EC.3.10
1. Not applicable
2. Not applicable

The practice establishes and implements processes for selecting, handling, storing, transporting, using, and disposing of hazardous materials and waste from receipt or generation through use and/or final disposal, including managing the following (EPs 3–6):

* **Hazardous materials (HAZMAT) and waste** Materials whose handling, use, and storage are guided or regulated by local, state, or federal regulation. Examples include OSHA's Regulations for Bloodborne Pathogens (regarding the blood, other infectious materials, contaminated items that release blood or other infectious materials, or contaminated sharps), the Nuclear Regulatory Commission's regulations for handling and disposal of radioactive waste, management of hazardous vapors (such as glutaraldehyde, ethylene oxide, and nitrous oxide), chemicals regulated by the EPA, Department of Transportation requirements, and hazardous energy sources (for example, ionizing or nonionizing radiation, lasers, microwaves, and ultrasound).

Scoring Grid
0 Insufficient compliance
1 Partial compliance
2 Satisfactory compliance
NA Not applicable

Ⓜ 3. Chemicals — C 0 1 2 NA

4. Chemotherapeutic materials — A 0 1 2 NA

5. Radioactive materials — A 0 1 2 NA

Ⓜ 6. Infectious and regulated medical wastes, including sharps — C 0 1 2 NA

7. The practice provides adequate and appropriate space and equipment for safely handling and storing hazardous materials and waste. — B 0 1 2 NA

8. The practice monitors and disposes of hazardous gases and vapors. — B 0 1 2 NA

9. Through 14. Not applicable

15. The practice reports (internally, as appropriate, and externally) and investigates all spills, exposures, and other incidents related to hazardous materials and waste. — B 0 1 2 NA

Standard EC.4.10

The practice addresses emergency management.

❑ Compliant
❑ Not Compliant

Elements of Performance for EC.4.10

1. Not applicable

2. Not applicable

3. The practice develops and maintains an emergency management plan describing the process for disaster readiness and emergency management, and implements it when appropriate.

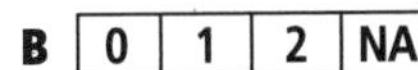

4. Through 25. Not applicable

26. The plan provides processes for the following: — B 0 1 2 NA
    - Identifying specific procedures in response to a variety of disasters*
    - Notifying external authorities of emergencies
    - Managing space, supplies, and security
    - Evacuating the building (both horizontally and, when applicable, vertically) when the environment cannot support adequate patient care, treatment, and services
    - Managing patients during emergencies, including scheduling, modifying, or discontinuing services, control of patient information, and patient transportation
    - Having a back-up communication system in the event of failure during disasters and emergencies (for example, two-way radios, cell phones)

EC

Standard EC.4.20

The practice conducts drills regularly to test emergency management.

❑ Compliant
❑ Not Compliant

Elements of Performance for EC.4.20

1. The practice tests the response phase of its emergency management plan once a year, either in response to an actual emergency or in planned drills.†

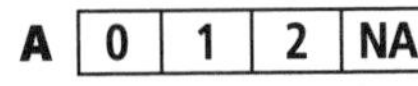

---

* **Disasters** Natural or man-made events that significantly disrupt the environment of care, such as damage to the practice's building(s) and grounds due to severe winds, storms, tornadoes, hurricanes, or earthquakes. Also, events that disrupt patient care, treatment, and services, such as loss of utilities (power, water, or telephones) due to floods, civil disturbances, accidents, or emergencies within the practice or in the surrounding community; or events that result in sudden, significantly changed, or increased demands for the practice's services (for example, bioterrorist attack, building collapse, or plane crash in the practice's community).

† **Note:** *Drills that involve packages of information that simulate patients, their families, and the public are acceptable.*

Scoring Grid
0 Insufficient compliance
1 Partial compliance
2 Satisfactory compliance
NA Not applicable

Note 1: *Staff in each freestanding building classified as a business occupancy (as defined by the LSC) that does not offer emergency services nor is community-designated as a disaster-receiving station need to participate in only one emergency management drill annually. Staff in areas of the building that the practice occupies must participate in this drill.*

Note 2: *Tabletop exercises, though useful in planning or training, are not acceptable substitutes for drills.*

2. Through 7. Not applicable

A | 0 | 1 | 2 | NA — 8. A practice that offers emergency services performs an additional test each year of the response phase of its emergency management plan, either in response to an actual emergency or in planned drills.

A | 0 | 1 | 2 | NA — 9. A practice that offers emergency services performs at least one exercise yearly that includes an influx of volunteer or simulated patients.

❑ Compliant
❑ Not Compliant

Standard EC.5.10

The practice manages fire safety risks.

Elements of Performance for EC.5.10

1. Not applicable

B | 0 | 1 | 2 | NA — 2. The practice identifies proactive processes for protecting patients, staff, and others coming to the practice's facilities, as well as protecting property from fire, smoke, and other products of combustion.

B | 0 | 1 | 2 | NA — 3. The practice identifies processes for regularly inspecting, testing, and maintaining fire protection and fire safety systems, equipment, and components.

B | 0 | 1 | 2 | NA — 4. The practice develops and implements a fire response plan that addresses the following:
- Facilitywide fire response
- Area-specific needs including fire evacuation routes
- Specific roles and responsibilities of staff, licensed independent practitioners, and volunteers at a fire's point of origin
- Specific roles and responsibilities of staff, licensed independent practitioners, and volunteers away from a fire's point of origin
- Specific roles and responsibilities of staff, licensed independent practitioners, and volunteers in preparing for building evacuation

EC

❑ Compliant
❑ Not Compliant

Standard EC.5.20

Newly constructed and existing environments are designed and maintained to comply with the *Life Safety Code*®*.

Note 1: *This standard applies only to office-based surgery practices that provide services or treatment that simultaneously renders four or more patients incapable of taking action for self-preservation under emergency situations without the help of others.*

Rationale for EC.5.20

The *LSC* requires that a building is designed, constructed, and maintained with the capability of being fire safe. When undertaking the design of a newly remodeled building, the practice should also satisfy any requirements of others (local, state, or federal) that might be more stringent than the *LSC*.

Note 2: *This standard does not apply to the following facilities:*
- *Classified as a business occupancy by the LSC that are freestanding buildings*

Scoring Grid
0 Insufficient compliance
1 Partial compliance
2 Satisfactory compliance
NA Not applicable

- *Classified as a business occupancy by the* LSC *that are connected to a health care occupancy, but are separated by a two-hour rated fire barrier and do not serve as a required means of egress from the health care occupancy*
- *Housing three or fewer patients*

Elements of Performance for EC.5.20

1. Each building in which patients are housed or receive care, treatment, and services complies with the *LSC,* NFPA 101® 2000; — **B** 0 1 2 NA

   or

   Each building in which patients are housed or receive care, treatment, and services does not comply with the *LSC,* but the resolution of all deficiencies is evidenced through the following:
   - An equivalency approved by the Joint Commission
     Or
   - Continued progress in completing an acceptable Plan For Improvement (SOC, Part 4)
2. A current, practicewide SOC compliance document* has been prepared. — **A** 0 1 2 NA

   Note: *You can obtain a copy of the SOC from our Web site at http://www.jcaho.org or by calling Customer Service at 630/792-5800. You may make as many copies of the SOC as you wish. However, remember to keep the original blank for future copying.*
3. Not applicable
4. Not applicable
5. The practice is making sufficient progress† toward the corrective actions described in a previously approved SOC. — **A** 0 1 2 NA

Standard EC.5.30

The practice conducts fire drills regularly.

❑ Compliant
❑ Not Compliant

Elements of Performance for EC.5.30

Ⓜ 1. Fire drills are conducted quarterly in each building defined by the *LSC* as the following: — **C** 0 1 2 NA
   - Ambulatory health care occupancy

2. Fire drills are conducted annually in all freestanding buildings classified as a business occupancy as defined by the *LSC* where patients are seen or treated. — **A** 0 1 2 NA

   Note: *In leased or rented facilities, only staff in areas of the building that the practice occupies must participate in such drills.*
3. Not applicable
4. Not applicable
5. Not applicable
6. All fire drills are critiqued to identify deficiencies and opportunities for improvement. — **B** 0 1 2 NA
7. The effectiveness of fire response training is evaluated at least annually. — **A** 0 1 2 NA

---

* **SOC compliance document** A proactive document that helps a practice perform a critical self-assessment of its current level of compliance and describe how to resolve any *LSC* deficiencies. The SOC was created to be a living, ongoing management tool that should be used in a management process that continually identifies, assesses, and resolves *LSC* deficiencies.

† **Sufficient progress** Failure to make sufficient progress toward the corrective actions described in an approved SOC, Part 4, Plan For Improvement, would result in a recommendation of Conditional Accreditation (*see* Conditional Accreditation rule CON04).

Scoring Grid
0 Insufficient compliance
1 Partial compliance
2 Satisfactory compliance
NA Not applicable

B 0 1 2 NA

8. During fire drills, staff knowledge is evaluated including the following:
   - When and how to sound fire alarms (where such alarms are available)
   - When and how to transmit for off-site fire responders
   - Containment of smoke and fire
   - Transfer of patients to areas of refuge
   - Fire extinguishment
   - Specific fire response duties
   - Preparation for building evacuation

A 0 1 2 NA

9. Fire drills are unannounced.

❑ Compliant
❑ Not Compliant

Standard EC.5.40

The practice maintains fire-safety equipment and building features.

Note 1: *This standard does not require practices to have the types of fire-safety equipment and building features discussed in the following. However, if these types of equipment or features exist within the practice, then the following maintenance, testing, and inspection requirements apply.*

Note 2: *Practices that offer care, treatment, and services in leased facilities need to communicate maintenance expectations for building equipment not under their control to their landlord through contractual language, lease agreements, memos, and so forth. These practices are not required to possess maintenance documentation, but must only have access to such documentation as needed and during survey. It is also important that the landlord communicate to the practice any building equipment problems identified that could negatively affect the safety or health of patients, staff, and other people coming to the practice, as well as the landlord's plan to resolve such issues.*

Elements of Performance for EC.5.40

C 0 1 2 NA

Ⓜ 1. Initiating devices and fire detection and alarm equipment are tested as follows:*
   - All supervisory signal devices (except valve tamper switches) are tested at least quarterly.
   - All valve tamper switches and water flow devices are tested at least semiannually.
   - All duct detectors, electromechanical releasing devices, heat detectors, manual fire alarm boxes, and smoke detectors are tested at least annually.

EC

C 0 1 2 NA

Ⓜ 2. Occupant alarm notification devices, including all audible devices, speakers, and visible devices, are tested at least annually.

A 0 1 2 NA

3. Off-premises emergency services notification transmission equipment is tested at least quarterly.

C 0 1 2 NA

Ⓜ 4. For water-based automatic fire-extinguishing systems, all fire pumps are tested at least weekly under no-flow condition.†

C 0 1 2 NA

Ⓜ 5. For water-based automatic fire-extinguishing systems, all water-storage tank high- and low-water level alarms are tested at least semiannually.

C 0 1 2 NA

Ⓜ 6. For water-based automatic fire-extinguishing systems, all water-storage tank low-water temperature alarms (during cold weather only) are tested at least monthly.

C 0 1 2 NA

Ⓜ 7. For water-based automatic fire-extinguishing systems, main drain tests are conducted at least annually at all system risers.

C 0 1 2 NA

Ⓜ 8. For water-based automatic fire-extinguishing systems, all fire department connections are inspected quarterly.

---

* For additional guidance, *see* NFPA 72-1999 edition (Table 7-3.2).

† For additional guidance, *see* NFPA 25-1998 edition.

Scoring Grid
0 Insufficient compliance
1 Partial compliance
2 Satisfactory compliance
NA Not applicable

Note for EPs 4–8: *EPs 4–8 apply only to office-based surgery practices that provide care, treatment, or services that simultaneously render four or more patients incapable of taking action for self-preservation under emergency situations without the help of others.*

9. Not applicable
10. Not applicable
11. Not applicable
12. Ⓜ All portable fire extinguishers* are clearly identified, inspected at least monthly, and maintained at least annually. — C 0 1 2 NA
13. Not applicable
14. Ⓜ All fire and smoke dampers are operated at least every four years (with fusible links removed where applicable) to verify that they fully close.† — C 0 1 2 NA
15. All automatic smoke-detection shutdown devices for air-handling equipment are tested at least annually.‡ — A 0 1 2 NA
16. Ⓜ All horizontal and vertical sliding and rolling fire doors are tested for proper operation and full closure at least annually.§ — C 0 1 2 NA

Note for EPs 14–16: *EPs 14–16 apply only to office-based surgery practices that provide care, treatment, or services that simultaneously render four or more patients incapable of taking action for self-preservation under emergency situations without the help of others.*

Standard EC.5.50

Not applicable

Standard EC.6.10

The practice manages medical equipment risks.

❑ Compliant
❑ Not Compliant

Elements of Performance for EC.6.10

1. Not applicable
2. The practice identifies and implements a process(es) for selecting and acquiring medical equipment. ‖ — B 0 1 2 NA
3. Not applicable
4. Not applicable
5. The practice defines intervals for inspecting, testing, and maintaining appropriate equipment (that is, those pieces of equipment benefiting from scheduled activities to minimize the clinical and physical risks) that are based upon criteria such as manufacturers' recommendations, risk levels, Clinical Laboratory Improvement Amendments of 1988 (CLIA '88), and current practice experience. — B 0 1 2 NA

* For additional guidance, *see* NFPA 10-1998 edition (sections 1-6, 4-3, and 4-4).

† For additional guidance, *see* NFPA 90A-1999 edition (section 3-4.7).

‡ For additional guidance, *see* NFPA 90A-1999 edition (section 4-4.1).

§ For additional guidance, *see* NFPA 80-1999 edition (section 15-2.4).

‖ **Note:** *The acquisition process includes initially evaluating the condition and function of the equipment when received and evaluating the training of users before use on patients.*

EC

Scoring Grid
0 Insufficient compliance
1 Partial compliance
2 Satisfactory compliance
NA Not applicable

B 0 1 2 NA
6. The practice identifies and implements processes for monitoring and acting on equipment hazard notices and recalls.

B 0 1 2 NA
7. The practice identifies and implements processes for monitoring and reporting incidents in which a medical device is suspected or attributed to the death, serious injury, or serious illness of any individual, as required by the Safe Medical Devices Act of 1990.

A 0 1 2 NA
8. The practice identifies and implements processes for emergency procedures that address the following:
   - What to do in the event of equipment disruption or failure
   - When and how to perform emergency clinical interventions when medical equipment fails
   - Availability of backup equipment
   - How to obtain repair services

A 0 1 2 NA
9. At a minimum, defined protocols and schedules for infection control in the procedure and recovery areas include the following:
   - Anesthetic apparatus is inspected and tested before each use by the practitioner who will administer the anesthetic. If found defective, the equipment is not used until the fault is repaired; repair of the equipment is documented.
   - Temperature control for sterilizers, refrigerators, and other machines is monitored.
   - A preventive maintenance schedule is established and maintained that includes periodic calibration, cleaning, and adjustment of all equipment, as appropriate.

❑ Compliant
❑ Not Compliant

Standard EC.6.20

Medical equipment is maintained, tested, and inspected.

Rationale for EC.6.20

The practice ensures performance and safety testing of all medical equipment that may pose a risk to patient safety or adversely impact the delivery of patient care.

Elements of Performance for EC.6.20

1. Not applicable

A 0 1 2 NA
2. The practice documents performance and safety testing of all equipment before initial use.
3. Not applicable
4. Not applicable

A 0 1 2 NA
Ⓜ 5. The practice documents performance testing of all sterilizers used.

6. Through 14. Not applicable

C 0 1 2 NA
Ⓜ 15. The practice ensures preventive maintenance and inspection of medical equipment according to a schedule based on manufacturer's recommendations, with time frames modified by current practice experience.

Standards EC.6.30 Through EC.6.130

Not applicable

❑ Compliant
❑ Not Compliant

Standard EC.7.10

The practice manages its utility risks.

Scoring Grid
0 Insufficient compliance
1 Partial compliance
2 Satisfactory compliance
NA Not applicable

Rationale for EC.7.10

Utility systems* are essential to the proper operation of the environment of care and significantly contribute to effective, safe, and reliable provision of care to patients in health care organizations. It is important that health care organizations establish and maintain a utility systems management program to promote a safe, controlled, and comfortable environment that does the following:

- Ensures operational reliability of utility systems
- Reduces the potential for organization–acquired illness to be transmitted through the utility systems
- Assesses the reliability and minimizes potential risks of utility system failures

Elements of Performance for EC.7.10

1. Through 8. Not applicable

9. The practice establishes risk criteria† for identifying, evaluating, and creating an inventory of operating components of systems before the equipment is used.

   B | 0 | 1 | 2 | NA |

   These criteria address the following:
   - Life support
   - Infection control
   - Support of the environment
   - Equipment support
   - Communication

   Note: *This EP applies only to office-based surgery practices using electrical life support equipment, or whose patients are provided assisted mechanical ventilation, or if the practice has blood, bone, and tissue storage units.*

10. Not applicable

11. The practice defines intervals for inspecting, testing, and maintaining appropriate utility systems equipment (that is, those pieces of equipment benefiting from scheduled activities to minimize the clinical and physical risks) that are based upon criteria such as manufacturers' recommendations, risk levels, and current practice experience.

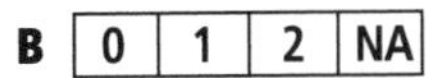

12. The practice identifies and implements emergency procedures for responding to utility system disruptions or failures that address the following:
    - What to do if utility systems malfunction
    - Identification of an alternative source of practice-defined essential utilities
    - Shutting off the malfunctioning systems and notifying staff in affected areas
    - How and when to perform emergency clinical interventions when utility systems fail
    - Obtaining repair services

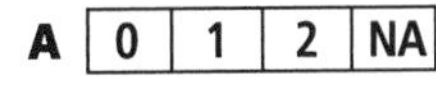

EC

13. The practice maps the distribution of utility systems.

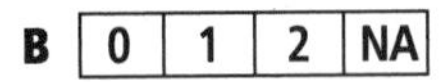

   Note: *This EP applies only to office-based surgery practices using electrical life support equipment, or whose patients are provided assisted mechanical ventilation, or if the practice has blood, bone, and tissue storage units.*

Ⓜ 14. The practice labels controls for a partial or complete emergency shutdown.

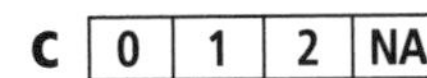

   Note: *This EP applies only to office-based surgery practices using electrical life support equipment, or whose patients are provided assisted mechanical ventilation or if the practice has blood, bone, and tissue storage units.*

15. Not applicable

---

* **Utility systems** May include electrical distribution; emergency power; vertical and horizontal transport; heating, ventilating, and air conditioning; plumbing, boiler, and steam; piped gases; vacuum systems; or communication systems including data-exchange systems.

† **Note:** *The practice may choose not to use risk criteria to limit the types of utility systems to be included in the utility management plan, but rather include all utility systems.*

Scoring Grid
0 Insufficient compliance
1 Partial compliance
2 Satisfactory compliance
NA Not applicable

A 0 1 2 NA

16. The practice designs, installs, and maintains ventilation equipment to provide appropriate pressure relationships, air-exchange rates, and filtration efficiencies for ventilation systems serving areas specially designed to control airborne contaminants (such as biological agents, gases, fumes, and dust).

❑ Compliant
❑ Not Compliant

Standard EC.7.20

The practice provides an emergency electrical power source.

Note: *EC.7.20 applies only to office-based surgery practices using electrical life support equipment, or whose patients are provided assisted mechanical ventilation, or if the practice has blood, bone, and tissue storage units.*

Elements of Performance for EC.7.20

The practice provides a reliable emergency power system*, as required by the *LSC* occupancy requirements, that supplies electricity to the following areas when normal electricity is interrupted:

1. Through 4. Not applicable

The practice provides a reliable emergency power system, as required by the services provided and patients served, that supplies electricity to the following areas when normal electricity is interrupted (EPs 5–18):

A 0 1 2 NA
5. Blood, bone, and tissue storage units
6. Not applicable
7. Not applicable
8. Not applicable

A 0 1 2 NA
9. Medical air compressors

A 0 1 2 NA
10. Medical and surgical vacuum systems
11. Not applicable
12. Not applicable
13. Not applicable

A 0 1 2 NA
14. Operating rooms

A 0 1 2 NA
15. Postoperative recovery rooms
16. Not applicable
17. Not applicable

A 0 1 2 NA
18. An emergency back-up power unit is available to provide at least 90 minutes of power to all life safety devices and resuscitative equipment when normal electricity is interrupted.

❑ Compliant
❑ Not Compliant

Standard EC.7.30

The practice maintains, tests, and inspects its utility systems.

* **Reliable emergency power system** For guidance in establishing a reliable emergency power system (that is, an Essential Electrical Distribution System), *see* NFPA 99-2002 edition (Chapters 13 and 14).

Scoring Grid
- **0** Insufficient compliance
- **1** Partial compliance
- **2** Satisfactory compliance
- **NA** Not applicable

Note: *Practices that offer care, treatment, and services in leased facilities need to communicate maintenance expectations for building equipment not under their control to their landlord through contractual language, lease agreements, memos, and so forth. These practices are not required to possess maintenance documentation, but must have access to such documentation as needed and during survey. It is also important that the landlord communicate to the practice any building equipment problems identified that could negatively affect the safety or health of patients, staff, and other people coming to the practice, as well as the landlord's plan to resolve such issues.*

Elements of Performance for EC.7.30

1. Not applicable

Ⓜ 2. The practice maintains documentation of performance and safety testing of each critical component before initial use. **A** | 0 | 1 | 2 | NA |

3. Not applicable

4. Not applicable

5. Not applicable

Ⓜ 6. The practice ensures preventive maintenance and inspection, and performance and safety testing of each critical utility component that might pose a risk to patient safety or adversely impact the delivery of patient care. **A** | 0 | 1 | 2 | NA |

Standard EC.7.40

❑ Compliant
❑ Not Compliant

The practice maintains, tests, and inspects its emergency power systems.

Note: *This standard does not require practices to have the types of emergency power systems discussed in the following EPs. However, if a practice has these types of systems, then the following maintenance, testing, and inspection requirements apply.*

Elements of Performance for EC.7.40

Ⓜ 1. The practice tests each generator 12 times a year, with testing intervals not less than 20 days and not more than 40 days apart. These tests shall be conducted for at least 30 continuous minutes under a dynamic load that is at least 30% of the name plate rating of the generator. **C** | 0 | 1 | 2 | NA |

Note: *Organizations may choose to test to less than 30% of the emergency generator's nameplate. However, these practices shall (in addition to performing a test for 30 continuous minutes under operating temperature at the intervals described in EP 1) revise their existing documented management plan to conform to current NFPA 99 and NFPA 110 testing and maintenance activities. These activities shall include inspection procedures for assessing the prime movers' exhaust gas temperature against the minimum temperature recommended by the manufacturer.*

If diesel-powered generators do not meet the minimum exhaust gas temperatures as determined during these tests, they shall be exercised for 30 continuous minutes at the intervals described in EP 1 with available Emergency Power Supply Systems (EPSS) load, and exercised annually with supplemental loads of
- *25% of name plate rating for 30 minutes, followed by*
- *50% of name plate rating for 30 minutes, followed by*
- *75% of name plate rating for 60 minutes for a total of two continuous hours.*

2. Not applicable

Ⓜ 3. The practice tests all battery-powered lights required for egress. Testing includes (a) a functional test at 30-day intervals for a minimum of 30 seconds and (b) an annual test for a duration of 1.5 hours.

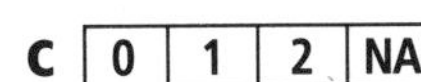

EC

Scoring Grid
0 Insufficient compliance
1 Partial compliance
2 Satisfactory compliance
NA Not applicable

C | 0 | 1 | 2 | NA

Ⓜ 4. The practice tests Stored Emergency Power Supply Systems (SEPSS) whose malfunction might severely jeopardize the occupants' life and safety.* Testing includes (a) a quarterly functional test for 5 minutes or as specified for its class,† whichever is less, and (b) an annual test at full load for 60% of the full duration of its class.

Standard EC.7.50

Not applicable

❑ Compliant
❑ Not Compliant

Standard EC.8.10

The practice establishes and maintains an appropriate environment.

Elements of Performance for EC.8.10

B | 0 | 1 | 2 | NA

1. Interior spaces should be the following:
   - Appropriate to the care, treatment, and services provided and the needs of the patients related to age and other characteristics
2. Not applicable
3. Not applicable

C | 0 | 1 | 2 | NA

Ⓜ 4. Areas used by the patient are safe, clean, functional, and comfortable.

B | 0 | 1 | 2 | NA

5. Lighting is suitable for care, treatment, and services and the specific activities being conducted.

6. Through 31. Not applicable

A | 0 | 1 | 2 | NA

32. The building in which the practice is located must be accessible after normal operating hours through an elevator, when appropriate, and properly functioning doors.

A | 0 | 1 | 2 | NA

33. Each patient bed must be equipped with a call button or alert signal device or be under direct supervision.

B | 0 | 1 | 2 | NA

34. Appropriate patient and staff restrooms are available.

EC

* **Stored Emergency Power Supply Systems (SEPSS)** Are intended to automatically supply illumination or power to critical areas and equipment essential for safety to human life. Included are systems that supply emergency power for such functions as illumination for safe exiting, ventilation where it is essential to maintain life, fire detection and alarm systems, public safety communications systems, and processes where the current interruption would produce serious life safety or health hazards to patients, the public, or staff. **Note:** *Other non-SEPSS battery back-up emergency power systems that a practice has determined to be critical for operations during a power failure (for example, laboratory equipment, electronic medical records) should be properly tested and maintained in accordance with manufacturer's recommendations.*

† **Class** Defines the minimum time for which the SEPSS is designed to operate at its rated load without being recharged (for additional guidance, *see* NFPA 111 [1996 edition] *Standard on Stored Electrical Energy Emergency and Standby Power Systems*).

Management of Human Resources

Overview

The goal of staff development, training, and competence activities in an office-based surgery practice is to identify and provide the right number of competent staff to meet the needs of patients served by the practice. The practice leader(s)* facilitates the following activities:

- **Planning.** The planning process defines the qualifications, competencies, and staffing necessary to provide for the practice's existing and new procedures, techniques, and services.
- **Providing competent staff.** Such staffing is achieved either through traditional employer/employee arrangements or contractual arrangements with other entities.
- **Assessing, maintaining, and improving staff competence.** Ongoing, periodic competence assessment evaluates staff members' continuing abilities to perform throughout their association with the practice.
- **Promoting self-development and learning.** Staff is encouraged to pursue ongoing professional development goals and provide feedback about the work environment.

Glossary Terms

These key terms have specific Joint Commission definitions. Please access the Glossary found near the end of your manual for the Joint Commission definition and appropriate use.

clinical privileges
credentialing
licensed independent practitioner
licensure
primary source
privileging
run chart
staff

* Office-based surgery practices to which this accreditation manual applies are owned or operated by surgeons. As such, the practice leadership is composed of surgeons and, as appropriate, other clinical and administrative personnel.

Standards

The following is a list of all standards for this function. They are presented here for your convenience without footnotes or other explanatory text. If you have a question about a term used here, please check the Glossary.

Note: *A revised standard numbering system is being used with the reformatted standards. The revised numbering system allows for more flexibility to add standards while maintaining the current label for each standard.*

Planning

HR.1.10 The practice provides an adequate number and mix of staff consistent with the practice's staffing plan.

HR.1.20 The practice has a process to ensure that a person's qualifications are consistent with his or her job responsibilities.

HR.1.30 Not applicable

Orientation, Training, and Education

HR.2.10 Orientation provides initial job training and information.

HR.2.20 Staff members, licensed independent practitioners, students, and volunteers, as appropriate, can describe or demonstrate their roles and responsibilities, based on specific job duties or responsibilities, relative to safety.

HR.2.30 Ongoing education, including in-services, training, and other activities, maintains and improves competence.

Assessing Competence

HR.3.10 Competence to perform job responsibilities is assessed, demonstrated, and maintained.

HR.3.20 Through HR.3.60 Not applicable

Credentialing and Assignment of Clinical Responsibilities of Licensed Independent Practitioners

Credentialing and Privileging

HR.4.10 There is a process for ensuring the competence of all practitioners permitted by law and the practice to practice independently.

HR.4.20 Individuals permitted by law and the practice to practice independently are granted clinical privileges.

HR.4.30 Through HR.4.50 Not applicable

HR.4.60 Individual surgeons' and licensed independent practitioners' credentials information that is subject to change is reverified at least every two years and reevaluated in the event of a change in services, an unexpected adverse outcome, or a sentinel event.

Understanding the Parts of This Chapter

To help you navigate this reformatted standards chapter, it may be helpful to think of its parts this way:

- The **standard** is the "goal."
- The **rationale** explains why it's important to achieve this goal.
- The **elements of performance** identify the step(s) needed to achieve this goal.

These parts are defined as follows.

Standard A statement that defines the performance expectations and/or structures or processes that must be in place in order for a practice to provide safe, high-quality care, treatment, and services. An practice is either "compliant" or "not compliant" with a standard as reflected by the check boxes in the margin by the standard:

❑ Compliant
❑ Not Compliant

Accreditation decisions are based on simple counts of the standards that are determined to be "not compliant."

Rationale A statement that provides background, justification, or additional information about a standard. A standard's rationale is not scored. In some instances, the rationale for a standard is self-evident. Therefore, not every standard has a written rationale.

Elements of performance (EPs) The specific performance expectations and/or structures or processes that must be in place in order for a practice to provide safe, high-quality care, treatment, and services. The scoring of EP compliance determines a practice's overall compliance with a standard. EPs are evaluated on the following scale:

0 Insufficient compliance
1 Partial compliance
2 Satisfactory compliance
NA Not applicable

You will find a **measure of success** icon—Ⓜ—next to some EPs. Measures of success (MOS) need to be developed for certain EPs when a standard is judged to be out of compliance through the on-site survey. An MOS is defined as a quantifiable measure, usually related to an audit, that can be used to determine whether an action has been effective and is being sustained.*

HR

Using the Self-Assessment Grid to Assess Your Compliance

Once you are familiar with the parts of this chapter, you can begin to assess your compliance with its requirements. A self-assessment grid (otherwise known as a scoring grid) has been provided in the margins for your convenience. If you would like to assess your practice's performance, mark your scores for the EPs on the scoring grid by following the simple steps described below. **Note:** *You are **not** required to complete this scoring grid. It is provided simply to help you assess your own performance.*

Two components are scored for each EP: (1) compliance with the requirement itself **and** (2) compliance with the track record† for that requirement. Scoring has been simplified from the past edition of the manual, and track record achievements (which have always been part of the scoring) have been appropriately modified.

---

* For more information about Measures of Success, *see* "The New Joint Commission Accreditation Process" chapter in this manual.

† **Track record** The amount of time that a practice has been in compliance with a standard, element of performance, or other requirement.

Note: *Some standards and EPs do not apply to a particular type of practice; these standards and EPs are marked "not applicable" and the related text is not included. Your practice is not expected to comply with standards and EPs marked "not applicable."*

In addition, some standards and EPs that do apply to practices may not apply to the specific care, treatment, and services that your individual practice provides. Although these standards and EPs are included in the manual, you are not expected to comply with them. If you are unsure about the standards or EPs that apply to your practice, please contact the Joint Commission's Standards Interpretation Group at 630/792-5900.

Step 1: Score Your Compliance with Each Element of Performance

Before you can determine your compliance with the standards, you must score your compliance with each EP. First look at the EP scoring criterion category listed immediately preceding the scoring scale in the margin next to the EP. There are three scoring criterion categories: A, B, and C (described below). Please note that for each EP scoring criterion category, your practice must meet the performance requirement itself and the track record achievements (*see* below).

Category A

These EPs relate to the presence or absence of the requirement(s) and are scored either yes (2) or no (0); however, score 1 for partial compliance is also possible based on track record achievements (*see* below).

If an A EP has multiple components designated by bullets, your practice must be compliant with all the bullets to receive a score of 2. If your practice does not meet one or more requirements in the bullets, you will receive a score of 0.

Category B

Category B EPs are scored in two steps:

1. As with category A EPs, category B EPs relate to the presence or absence of the requirement(s). If your practice *does not meet* the requirement(s), the EP is scored 0; there is no need to assess your compliance with the principles of good process design (*see* below).
2. If your practice *does meet* the requirement(s), but there is concern about the quality or comprehensiveness of the effort, then and only then should you assess the qualitative aspect of the EP. That is, review the applicable principles of good process design and ask how the principles were applied in the situation under discussion. Good process design has the following characteristics:
   - Is consistent with your practice's mission, values, and goals
   - Meets the needs of patients
   - Reflects the use of currently accepted practices (doing the right thing, using resources responsibly, using practice guidelines)
   - Incorporates current safety information and knowledge such as sentinel event data and National Patient Safety Goals
   - Incorporates relevant performance improvement results

This two-part evaluation applies to both simple and bulleted B EPs. First, the EPs are assessed to determine if the requirements are present. If the EP has multiple components designated by bullets, as with the category A EPs, your practice must meet the requirements in *all* the bulleted items to get a score of 2. If your practice meets *none* of the requirements in the bullets, it receives a score of 0. If your practice meets *at least one, but not all,* of the bulleted requirements, it will receive a score of 1 for the EPs.

Use the following rules to determine your EP score:

- Your EP score is 0 if your practice does not meet the requirement(s); you *do not* need to assess your compliance with the preceding applicable principles of good process design
- Your EP score is 1 if your practice does meet the requirement(s), but considered only *some* of the preceding applicable principles of good process design

- Your EP score is 2 if your practice does meet the requirement(s) *and* considered *all* the preceding principles of good process design

Category C

C EPs are scored 0, 1, or 2 based on the number of times your practice does not meet the EP. These EPs are frequency based and require totaling the number of occurrences (that is, results of performance or nonperformance) related to a particular EP. Each situation discovered by a surveyor(s) will be counted as a separate occurrence.

Note: *Multiple events of the same type related to a single patient and single practitioner/staff member are counted as* one occurrence only.

Use the following rules to determine your EP score:
- Your EP score is 2 if you find one or fewer occurrences of noncompliance with the EP
- Your EP score is 1 if you find two occurrences of noncompliance with the EP
- Your EP score is 0 if you find three or more occurrences of noncompliance with the EP

If an EP in the C category has multiple requirements designated by bullets, the following scoring guidelines apply:
- If there are fewer than 2 findings in all bullets, the EP is scored 2
- If there are three or more findings in all bullets, the EP is scored 0
- In all other combinations of findings, the EP is scored 1

Track Record Achievements

In addition to meeting the requirement(s) in each EP, regardless of category, your practice must also meet the following track record achievements:

Score	Initial Survey	Full Survey
2	4 months or more	12 months or more
1	2 to 3 months	6 to 11 months
0	Fewer than 2 months	Fewer than 6 months

Sample Sizes

If during an on-site survey, your practice has been found to be not compliant with one or more standards, you must demonstrate Evidence of Standards Compliance (ESC) for each standard that is not compliant. The ESC must address compliance at the EP level; when an EP within a noncompliant standard requires an MOS, your practice must demonstrate achievement with the MOS when completing the ESC.

Note: *Not every EP requires an MOS. EPs that do require an MOS are clearly marked in this chapter Practices are required to demonstrate achievement with an MOS* only *for EPs within a noncompliant standard that require an MOS. Practices* do not *need to demonstrate achievement with an MOS for any EP within a compliant standard.*

When demonstrating achievement with an MOS during the ESC process, your practice is **required** to use the following sample sizes, which were established because of their statistical significance, their relative simplicity in application, and their sensitivity to a practice's population size:
- For a population size of fewer than 30 cases,* sample 100% of available cases
- For a population size of 30 to 100 cases, sample 30 cases
- For a population size of 101 to 500 cases, sample 50 cases
- For a population size greater than 500 cases, sample 70 cases

When demonstrating an ESC (mandatory use), use the following percentages to determine your EP score: 90% through 100% of your sample size is in compliance = score 2; 80% through 89% of your sample size is in compliance = score 1; less than 80% of your sample size is in compliance = score 0.

* "Case" refers to a single instance in which a situation related to a survey finding occurs. For example, if a survey finding was related to **pain assessment,** then a "case" would be any patient record. If a survey finding was related to **pain management,** a "case" would be any patient record for patients receiving pain management.

HR

In addition, the following information should govern your practice's selection of samples:

- The appropriate sample size should be determined by the specific population related to the survey findings.
- The sampling approach should involve either systematic random sampling (for example, your practice selects every second or third case for review) or simple random sampling (for example, your practice uses a series of random numbers generated by a computer to identify the cases to be reviewed).
- When submitting a clarifying ESC, if your practice selects records as part of its sample, the records should be from a period of no more than three months before the last date of the survey.
- Assessment of MOS compliance is conducted for a four-month period following the date of ESC approval. Your practice should select records as a part of your sample following the date of ESC approval and use the required sample sizes. MOS percentage compliance rates are derived from the average of all four months.

Step 2: Use Your EP Scores to Gauge Your Compliance with the Standards

Now that you have evaluated and scored each EP for a particular standard, use these simple rules to determine your compliance with the standard itself:

- Your practice is not in compliance (that is, "not compliant") with the standard if any EP is scored 0
- Otherwise, your practice is in compliance with a standard if 65% or more of its EPs are scored 2

Scoring Grid
0 Insufficient compliance
1 Partial compliance
2 Satisfactory compliance
NA Not applicable

Standards, Rationales, Elements of Performance, and Scoring

Planning

Standard HR.1.10

The practice provides an adequate number and mix of staff and licensed independent practitioners consistent with the practice's staffing plan.

❏ Compliant
❏ Not Compliant

Rationale for HR.1.10

A practice's ability to meet patients' needs with safe and effective care depends in part on attracting and retaining adequate numbers and types of qualified, competent staff.

Element of Performance for HR.1.10

1. The practice has an adequate number and mix of staff to meet the care, treatment, and service needs of the patients. **B** 0 | 1 | 2 | NA

Standard HR.1.20

The practice has a process to ensure that a person's qualifications are consistent with his or her job responsibilities.

❏ Compliant
❏ Not Compliant

Elements of Performance for HR.1.20

1. Through 17. Not applicable

18. Individuals who do not possess a license, registration, or certification do not provide or have not provided care, treatment, and services in the practice that would, under applicable law or regulation, require such a license, registration, or certification. **A** 0 | 1 | 2 | NA

19. Individuals who do not possess a license, registration, or certification do not provide or have not provided care, treatment, and services in the practice that would, under applicable law or regulation, require such a license, registration, or certification and that would have placed the practice's patients at risk for a serious adverse outcome. **A** 0 | 1 | 2 | NA

20. Through 42. Not applicable

43. Defined job qualifications, responsibilities, and expectations are based on the practice's scope of services; patient needs; staff education, training, and licensure; and the practice's and patient's expectations. **B** 0 | 1 | 2 | NA

44. Performance expectations are periodically reviewed and updated when necessary. **B** 0 | 1 | 2 | NA

Standard HR.1.30

Not applicable

Scoring Grid
0 Insufficient compliance
1 Partial compliance
2 Satisfactory compliance
NA Not applicable

Orientation, Training, and Education

❑ Compliant
❑ Not Compliant

Standard HR.2.10

Orientation provides initial job training and information.

Rationale for HR.2.10

Staff orientation promotes safe and effective job performance.

Elements of Performance for HR.2.10

As appropriate, each staff member, licensed independent practitioner, and student is oriented to the following:

C | 0 | 1 | 2 | NA | Ⓜ 1. The practice's mission and goals

C | 0 | 1 | 2 | NA | Ⓜ 2. Practicewide policies and procedures (including safety and infection control) and relevant unit, setting, or program-specific policies and procedures

C | 0 | 1 | 2 | NA | Ⓜ 3. Specific job duties and responsibilities related to safety and infection control

4. Not applicable

❑ Compliant
❑ Not Compliant

Standard HR.2.20

Staff members, licensed independent practitioners, students and volunteers, as appropriate, can describe or demonstrate their roles and responsibilities, based on specific job duties or responsibilities, relative to safety.

Elements of Performance for HR.2.20

Staff members, licensed independent practitioners, students, and volunteers, as appropriate, can describe or demonstrate the following:

C | 0 | 1 | 2 | NA | Ⓜ 1. Risks within the practice's environment

C | 0 | 1 | 2 | NA | Ⓜ 2. Actions to eliminate, minimize, or report risks

C | 0 | 1 | 2 | NA | Ⓜ 3. Procedures to follow in the event of an incident

C | 0 | 1 | 2 | NA | Ⓜ 4. Reporting processes for common problems, failures, and user errors

HR

❑ Compliant
❑ Not Compliant

Standard HR.2.30

Ongoing education, including in-services, training, and other activities, maintains and improves competence.

Rationale for HR.2.30

When developing recruitment, retention, development, and continuing education processes for all staff, the leaders consider the following factors:

- The practice's goals and values
- The case mix of patients and the degree and complexity of care they require
- Technology used in patient care, treatment, and services
- Identified learning needs

Elements of Performance for HR.2.30

The following occurs for staff, students, and volunteers who work in the same capacity as staff providing care, treatment, and services:

Scoring Grid
0 Insufficient compliance
1 Partial compliance
2 Satisfactory compliance
NA Not applicable

1. Training occurs when job responsibilities or duties change — B 0 1 2 NA

Ⓜ 2. Participation in ongoing in-services, training, or other activities occurs to increase staff, student, or volunteer knowledge of work-related issues — C 0 1 2 NA

Assessing Competence

Standard HR.3.10

Competence to perform job responsibilities is assessed, demonstrated, and maintained.

❑ Compliant
❑ Not Compliant

Elements of Performance for HR.3.10

1. Through 7. Not applicable

Ⓜ 8. The practice assesses and documents each person's ability to carry out assigned responsibilities safely, competently, and in a timely manner upon completion of orientation. — C 0 1 2 NA

9. Through 33. Not applicable

Ⓜ 34. Each staff member's competence to perform job duties is periodically assessed. — B 0 1 2 NA

35. The competence assessment evaluates the following: — B 0 1 2 NA
   - The staff member's ability to provide care, treatment, service, and support for the procedures performed by the practice
   - Responsibilities related to new procedures, techniques, technology, and equipment
   - Age-specific competencies required to care for the population served by the practice

Ⓜ 36. All individuals responsible for helping to provide services are competent and appropriately supervised. — C 0 1 2 NA

Standard HR.3.20 Through HR.3.60

Not applicable

Credentialing and Assignment of Clinical Responsibilities* of Licensed Independent Practitioners

Credentialing and Privileging

Introduction

The office setting is increasingly being used for invasive and surgical services. Surgeons, other licensed independent practitioners, and other clinical staff work collaboratively to provide sedation, anesthesia, and invasive and surgical care. The appropriateness of the physical setting and the qualifications and number of surgeons and licensed independent practitioners necessary to deliver quality care are determined by the complexity of the services offered. Ongoing evaluation of practitioner and staff competence (both employed and contracted) establishes a basis for providing safe, effective care in the office setting.

* Authorization granted by the practice to a practitioner to provide specific care, treatment, and services within well-defined limits based on the following factors, as applicable: license, education, training, experience, competence, health status, and judgment.

Scoring Grid
0 Insufficient compliance
1 Partial compliance
2 Satisfactory compliance
NA Not applicable

The credentialing and self-assessment processes in this chapter emphasize demonstration of qualifications and competence to perform the invasive and surgical procedures and sedation and anesthesia services offered at a particular office site. The section sets forth processes applicable to the office setting whereby the surgeons and the licensed independent practitioners identify the specific surgical or invasive procedures or anesthesia services to be offered; document the capabilities required for performance of the procedures or services; and establish current competence to perform the procedures or services by using and documenting evidenced-based criteria. In most small office practices, this is a self-credentialing process. In some office practices, a governance or administrative structure (in which a surgeon and/or qualified licensed independent practitioner credentials other individuals in the practice) may exist to support these processes.

The credentialing and self-assessment process described in this chapter applies to surgeons and licensed independent practitioners, including those providing services under a contract. A licensed independent practitioner is any individual permitted by law and by the practice to provide care, treatment, and services, without direction or supervision, within the scope of the individual's license.

❑ Compliant
❑ Not Compliant

Standard HR.4.10

There is a process for ensuring the competence of all practitioners permitted by law and the practice to practice independently.

Element of Performance for HR.4.10

1. Through 10. Not applicable

A | 0 | 1 | 2 | NA

11. The following occur at the time of hire:
    - Current licensure, including all actions against the license, is verified with the primary source and documented.
    - Relevant training and experience are verified from the primary source.
    - Current competence is verified from a knowledgeable source.
    - The applicant's ability to perform the clinical privileges* requested is evaluated.

12. Through 21. Not applicable

B | 0 | 1 | 2 | NA

22. The practice is responsible for reviewing the competence assessment process every two years or whenever the practice's scope changes or new procedures are introduced.

HR

B | 0 | 1 | 2 | NA

23. Policies and procedures address the following:
    - The individuals subject to them
    - Lines of administrative authority and oversight
    - The scope of the office-based surgery practice, including all invasive and surgical procedures and services offered
    - Standards of practice, clinical pathways, clinical practice guidelines, or protocols followed by the practice (the standards of practice and so forth may be incorporated by reference)
    - A process to verify individual surgeon and licensed independent practitioner credentials
    - The criteria employed by the practice to determine individual surgeon and licensed independent practitioner competence to perform a specific procedure, sedation, or anesthesia service
    - The mechanisms for ongoing evaluation of an individual surgeon's or licensed independent practitioner's competence to perform a specific procedure or service

* The Americans with Disabilities Act (ADA) bars certain discrimination based on physical or mental impairment. To prevent such discrimination, the act prohibits or mandates various activities. Health care practices need to determine the applicability of the ADA to their licensed independent practitioners. If applicable, the practice should examine its privileging or credentialing procedures as to how and when it ascertains and confirms an applicant's health status. For example, the act may prohibit inquiry as to an applicant's physical or mental health status before making an offer of membership and privileges, but may not prohibit such inquiry after an offer is extended (without specific reference to health matters) to perform the specific privileges requested. Thus, the inquiry may be made and confirmed as a component of the application process. The Joint Commission cannot provide legal advice to practices. However, the Joint Commission has and will absolutely construe this standard in such a manner as to be consistent with practice efforts to comply with the ADA.

Scoring Grid
0 Insufficient compliance
1 Partial compliance
2 Satisfactory compliance
NA Not applicable

- Surgeon and licensed independent practitioner involvement in developing performance expectations and conducting competence assessments of clinical and office staff subject to job descriptions

Ⓜ 24. Each surgeon's and licensed independent practitioner's credentials file contains sufficient documentation to show that the criteria have been verified and evaluated. — **C** 0 | 1 | 2 | NA

25. The credentials verification and assessment processes are periodically reviewed for effectiveness. — **B** 0 | 1 | 2 | NA

The practice obtains the following information and includes it in the credentials file:

26. Evidence of a current, unrestricted Drug Enforcement Administration registration and any history of revocation — **A** 0 | 1 | 2 | NA

27. Board certification, current recertification, or eligibility — **A** 0 | 1 | 2 | NA

Standard HR.4.20

Individuals permitted by law and the practice to practice independently are granted clinical privileges.

❑ Compliant
❑ Not Compliant

Elements of Performance for HR.4.20

1. Criteria for determining the licensed independent practitioner's clinical privileges are specified in writing. — **B** 0 | 1 | 2 | NA

Ⓜ 2. Clinical privileges for licensed independent practitioners are granted according to practice policy and based on the licensed independent practitioner's current credentials and competence, as well as the population(s) served and the types of care, treatment, and services provided in the practice. — **C** 0 | 1 | 2 | NA

Standards HR.4.30 Through HR.4.50

Not applicable

Standard HR.4.60

Individual surgeons' and licensed independent practitioners' credentials information that is subject to change is reverified at least every two years and reevaluated in the event of a change in services, an unexpected adverse outcome, or a sentinel event.

❑ Compliant
❑ Not Compliant

HR

Rationale for HR.4.60

Certain credentials information, such as the location and dates of completed medical education, residency, and internship, remain constant and do not need to be reverified. Other credentials information, such as active licensure to practice in a particular state, can change over time.

Elements of Performance for HR.4.60

1. No more than two years may elapse between verification and reverification of individual surgeons' and licensed independent practitioners' credentials information that is subject to change. — **A** 0 | 1 | 2 | NA

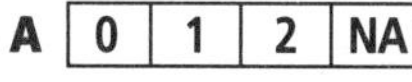

2. If there is a change in the surgical, invasive, sedation, or anesthesia procedures, services, or techniques offered, or if an unexpected or adverse outcome or sentinel event occurs, the practice reviews its credentialing and self-assessment processes and information to ensure that clinical qualifications and skill are appropriate to the procedure or service involved. — **B** 0 | 1 | 2 | NA

HR

Management of Information

Overview

The goal of information management in an office-based surgery practice is to obtain, manage, and use information to improve patient outcomes and practice performance. Effective management of information should do the following:

- Ensure timely and easy access to necessary clinical and procedural information
- Maintain accuracy of clinical, administrative, and procedural information
- Balance the requirements of security and ease of access
- Use aggregate and comparative data to identify and pursue opportunities for improvement

While efficiency might be improved by computerization and other technologies, the principles of good information management apply to all methods, whether paper based or electronic. These standards are designed to be equally compatible with noncomputerized systems and evolving technologies.

Glossary Terms

These key terms have specific Joint Commission definitions. Please access the Glossary found near the end of your manual for the Joint Commission definition and appropriate use.

accountability
analyzing
auditability
authentication
capture
confidentiality
data
electronic health information
integrity
interactive text
interoperability
knowledge-based information
nonrepudiation
privacy
processing
protected health information
report generation
retrievability
structured text
timeliness
transmission

Standards

The following is a list of all standards for this function. They are presented here for your convenience without footnotes or other explanatory text. If you have a question about a term used here, please check the Glossary.

Note: *A revised standard numbering system is being used with the reformatted standards. This revised numbering system allows for more flexibility to add standards while maintaining the current label for each standard.*

Information Management Planning

IM.1.10 Not applicable

Confidentiality and Security

IM.2.10 Information privacy and confidentiality are maintained.

IM.2.20 Information security, including data integrity, is maintained.

Patient-Specific Information

IM.6.10 The practice has a complete and accurate medical record for every individual assessed, cared for, treated, or served.

IM.6.20 Records contain patient-specific information, as appropriate to the care, treatment, and services provided.

IM.6.30 The medical record thoroughly documents operative or other high-risk procedures and the use of moderate or deep sedation or anesthesia.

IM.6.40 Not applicable

IM.6.50 Designated qualified personnel accept and transcribe verbal orders from authorized individuals.

IM.6.60 The practice can provide access to all relevant information from a patient's record when needed for use in patient care, treatment, and services.

Understanding the Parts of This Chapter

To help you navigate this reformatted standards chapter, it may be helpful to think of its parts this way:

- The **standard** is the "goal."
- The **rationale** explains why it's important to achieve this goal.
- The **elements of performance** identify the step(s) needed to achieve this goal.

These parts are defined as follows.

Standard A statement that defines the performance expectations and/or structures or processes that must be in place in order for a practice to provide safe, high-quality care, treatment, and services. An practice is either "compliant" or "not compliant" with a standard as reflected by the check boxes in the margin by the standard:

❑ Compliant
❑ Not Compliant

Accreditation decisions are based on simple counts of the standards that are determined to be "not compliant."

Rationale A statement that provides background, justification, or additional information about a standard. A standard's rationale is not scored. In some instances, the rationale for a standard is self-evident. Therefore, not every standard has a written rationale.

Elements of performance (EPs) The specific performance expectations and/or structures or processes that must be in place in order for a practice to provide safe, high-quality care, treatment, and services. The scoring of EP compliance determines a practice's overall compliance with a standard. EPs are evaluated on the following scale:

0 Insufficient compliance
1 Partial compliance
2 Satisfactory compliance
NA Not applicable

You will find a **measure of success** icon—Ⓜ—next to some EPs. Measures of success (MOS) need to be developed for certain EPs when a standard is judged to be out of compliance through the on-site survey. An MOS is defined as a quantifiable measure, usually related to an audit, that can be used to determine whether an action has been effective and is being sustained.*

Using the Self-Assessment Grid to Assess Your Compliance

Once you are familiar with the parts of this chapter, you can begin to assess your compliance with its requirements. A self-assessment grid (otherwise known as a scoring grid) has been provided in the margins for your convenience. If you would like to assess your practice's performance, mark your scores for the EPs on the scoring grid by following the simple steps described below. **Note:** *You are **not** required to complete this scoring grid. It is provided simply to help you assess your own performance.*

Two components are scored for each EP: (1) compliance with the requirement itself **and** (2) compliance with the track record† for that requirement. Scoring has been simplified from the past edition of the manual, and track record achievements (which have always been part of the scoring) have been appropriately modified.

---

* For more information about Measures of Success, *see* "The New Joint Commission Accreditation Process" chapter in this manual.

† **Track record** The amount of time that a practice has been in compliance with a standard, element of performance, or other requirement.

Note: *Some standards and EPs do not apply to a particular type of practice; these standards and EPs are marked "not applicable" and the related text is not included. Your practice is not expected to comply with standards and EPs marked "not applicable."*

In addition, some standards and EPs that do apply to practices may not apply to the specific care, treatment, and services that your individual practice provides. Although these standards and EPs are included in the manual, you are not expected to comply with them. If you are unsure about the standards or EPs that apply to your practice, please contact the Joint Commission's Standards Interpretation Group at 630/792-5900.

Step 1: Score Your Compliance with Each Element of Performance

Before you can determine your compliance with the standards, you must score your compliance with each EP. First look at the EP scoring criterion category listed immediately preceding the scoring scale in the margin next to the EP. There are three scoring criterion categories: A, B, and C (described below). Please note that for each EP scoring criterion category, your practice must meet the performance requirement itself and the track record achievements (*see* below).

Category A

These EPs relate to the presence or absence of the requirement(s) and are scored either yes (2) or no (0); however, score 1 for partial compliance is also possible based on track record achievements (*see* below).

If an A EP has multiple components designated by bullets, your practice must be compliant with all the bullets to receive a score of 2. If your practice does not meet one or more requirements in the bullets, you will receive a score of 0.

Category B

Category B EPs are scored in two steps:

1. As with category A EPs, category B EPs relate to the presence or absence of the requirement(s). If your practice *does not meet* the requirement(s), the EP is scored 0; there is no need to assess your compliance with the principles of good process design (*see* below).
2. If your practice *does meet* the requirement(s), but there is concern about the quality or comprehensiveness of the effort, then and only then should you assess the qualitative aspect of the EP. That is, review the applicable principles of good process design and ask how the principles were applied in the situation under discussion. Good process design has the following characteristics:
   - Is consistent with your practice's mission, values, and goals
   - Meets the needs of patients
   - Reflects the use of currently accepted practices (doing the right thing, using resources responsibly, using practice guidelines)
   - Incorporates current safety information and knowledge such as sentinel event data and National Patient Safety Goals
   - Incorporates relevant performance improvement results

This two-part evaluation applies to both simple and bulleted B EPs. First, the EPs are assessed to determine if the requirements are present. If the EP has multiple components designated by bullets, as with the category A EPs, your practice must meet the requirements in *all* the bulleted items to get a score of 2. If your practice meets *none* of the requirements in the bullets, it receives a score of 0. If your practice meets *at least one, but not all,* of the bulleted requirements, it will receive a score of 1 for the EPs.

Use the following rules to determine your EP score:

- Your EP score is 0 if your practice does not meet the requirement(s); you *do not* need to assess your compliance with the preceding applicable principles of good process design
- Your EP score is 1 if your practice does meet the requirement(s), but considered only *some* of the preceding applicable principles of good process design

IM

- Your EP score is 2 if your practice does meet the requirement(s) *and* considered *all* the preceding principles of good process design

Category C

C EPs are scored 0, 1, or 2 based on the number of times your practice does not meet the EP. These EPs are frequency based and require totaling the number of occurrences (that is, results of performance or nonperformance) related to a particular EP. Each situation discovered by a surveyor(s) will be counted as a separate occurrence.

Note: *Multiple events of the same type related to a single patient and single practitioner/staff member are counted as* one occurrence only.

Use the following rules to determine your EP score:

- Your EP score is 2 if you find one or fewer occurrences of noncompliance with the EP
- Your EP score is 1 if you find two occurrences of noncompliance with the EP
- Your EP score is 0 if you find three or more occurrences of noncompliance with the EP

If an EP in the C category has multiple requirements designated by bullets, the following scoring guidelines apply:

- If there are fewer than 2 findings in all bullets, the EP is scored 2
- If there are three or more findings in all bullets, the EP is scored 0
- In all other combinations of findings, the EP is scored 1

Track Record Achievements

In addition to meeting the requirement(s) in each EP, regardless of category, your practice must also meet the following track record achievements:

Score	Initial Survey	Full Survey
2	4 months or more	12 months or more
1	2 to 3 months	6 to 11 months
0	Fewer than 2 months	Fewer than 6 months

Sample Sizes

If during an on-site survey, your practice has been found to be not compliant with one or more standards, you must demonstrate Evidence of Standards Compliance (ESC) for each standard that is not compliant. The ESC must address compliance at the EP level; when an EP within a noncompliant standard requires an MOS, your practice must demonstrate achievement with the MOS when completing the ESC.

Note: *Not every EP requires an MOS. EPs that do require an MOS are clearly marked in this chapter Practices are required to demonstrate achievement with an MOS* only *for EPs within a noncompliant standard that require an MOS. Practices* do not *need to demonstrate achievement with an MOS for any EP within a compliant standard.*

When demonstrating achievement with an MOS during the ESC process, your practice is **required** to use the following sample sizes, which were established because of their statistical significance, their relative simplicity in application, and their sensitivity to a practice's population size:

- For a population size of fewer than 30 cases,* sample 100% of available cases
- For a population size of 30 to 100 cases, sample 30 cases
- For a population size of 101 to 500 cases, sample 50 cases
- For a population size greater than 500 cases, sample 70 cases

When demonstrating an ESC (mandatory use), use the following percentages to determine your EP score: 90% through 100% of your sample size is in compliance = score 2; 80% through 89% of your sample size is in compliance = score 1; less than 80% of your sample size is in compliance = score 0.

---

* "Case" refers to a single instance in which a situation related to a survey finding occurs. For example, if a survey finding was related to **pain assessment,** then a "case" would be any patient record. If a survey finding was related to **pain management,** a "case" would be any patient record for patients receiving pain management.

IM

In addition, the following information should govern your practice's selection of samples:

- The appropriate sample size should be determined by the specific population related to the survey findings
- The sampling approach should involve either systematic random sampling (for example, your practice selects every second or third case for review) or simple random sampling (for example, your practice uses a series of random numbers generated by a computer to identify the cases to be reviewed)
- When submitting clarifying ESC, if your practice selects records as part of its sample, the records should be from a period of no more than three months before the last date of the survey
- Assessment of MOS compliance is conducted for a four-month period following the date of ESC approval. Your practice should select records as a part of your sample following the date of ESC approval and use the required sample sizes. MOS percentage compliance rates are derived from the average of all four months.

Step 2: Use Your EP Scores to Gauge Your Compliance with the Standards

Now that you have evaluated and scored each EP for a particular standard, use these simple rules to determine your compliance with the standard itself:

- Your practice is not in compliance (that is, "not compliant") with the standard if any EP is scored 0
- Otherwise, your practice is in compliance with a standard if 65% or more of its EPs are scored 2

Scoring Grid
0 Insufficient compliance
1 Partial compliance
2 Satisfactory compliance
NA Not applicable

Standards, Rationales, Elements of Performance, and Scoring

Information Management Planning

Standard IM.1.10

Not applicable

Confidentiality and Security

Standard IM.2.10

Information privacy* and confidentiality† are maintained.

❑ Compliant
❑ Not Compliant

Element of Performance for IM.2.10

1. The practice has developed a process based on and consistent with applicable law that addresses the privacy and confidentiality of information.

   B | 0 | 1 | 2 | NA |

Standard IM.2.20

Information security, including data integrity,‡ is maintained.

❑ Compliant
❑ Not Compliant

Rationale for IM.2.20

Policies and procedures address security procedures to ensure that only authorized personnel gain access to data and information. These policies can range from access to the paper chart to the various security levels and distribution of passwords in an electronic system. The basic premise of the policies is to provide the appropriate level of security and protection for sensitive patient, employee, and other information, while facilitating access to data by those who have a legitimate need. The capture, storage, and retrieval processes for data and information are designed to provide for timely access without compromising the data and information's security and integrity.

Elements of Performance for IM.2.20

1. The practice has developed a process based on and consistent with applicable law that addresses information security, including data integrity.

   B | 0 | 1 | 2 | NA |

2. Through 5. Not applicable

6. The practice develops and implements controls to safeguard data and information, including the patient record, against loss, destruction, and tampering. Controls include the following:
   - Policies regarding when the removal of records is permitted
   - Data and information protection against unauthorized intrusion, corruption, or damage
   - Prevention of falsification of data and information

   B | 0 | 1 | 2 | NA |

* **Privacy** An individual's right to limit the disclosure of personal information.

† **Confidentiality** The safekeeping of data/information so as to restrict access to individuals who have need, reason, and permission for such access.

‡ **Data integrity** In the context of data security, data integrity means the protection of data from accidental or unauthorized intentional change.

IM

- Guidelines to prevent the loss and destruction of records
- Guidelines for destroying copies of records
- Protection of records in a manner that minimizes the possibility of damage from fire and water

Standards IM.2.30 Through IM.5.10

Not applicable

Patient-Specific Information

❑ Compliant
❑ Not Compliant

Standard IM.6.10

The practice has a complete and accurate medical record for every individual assessed or treated.

Elements of Performance for IM.6.10

A [0 | 1 | 2 | NA] 1. Only authorized individuals make entries in the medical record.

A [0 | 1 | 2 | NA] 2. The practice defines which entries made by nonindependent practitioners require countersigning consistent with law and regulation.

3. Not applicable

C [0 | 1 | 2 | NA] Ⓜ 4. Every medical record entry* is dated, the author identified and, when necessary according to law or regulation and practice policy, is authenticated.

C [0 | 1 | 2 | NA] Ⓜ 5. At a minimum, the following are authenticated either by written signature, electronic signature, or computer key or rubber stamp:†
- The history and physical examination
- Operative report
- Follow-up or discharge

C [0 | 1 | 2 | NA] Ⓜ 6. The medical record contains sufficient information to identify the patient; support the diagnosis/condition; justify the care, treatment, and services; document the course and results of care, treatment, and services; and promote continuity of care among providers.

7. Not applicable

8. Not applicable

A [0 | 1 | 2 | NA] 9. The practice defines a complete record and the time frame within which the record must be completed.

10. Through 13. Not applicable

B [0 | 1 | 2 | NA] 14. The retention time of medical record information is determined by the practice based on law and regulation and on its use for patient care, treatment, and services; legal; research; and operational purposes, as well as educational activities.

15. Through 26. Not applicable

---

* Signatures do not have to be dated if they occur in real time of the entry. For paper-based records, counter signatures entered for purposes of authentication after transcription or for verbal orders are dated when required by state or federal law and regulation and practice policy. For electronic records, electronic signatures will be date-stamped.

† Authentication can be shown by written signatures or initials, rubber-stamp signatures, or computer key. Authorized users of signature stamps or computer keys sign a statement assuring that they alone will use the stamp or key.

Scoring Grid
0 Insufficient compliance
1 Partial compliance
2 Satisfactory compliance
NA Not applicable

27. Medical records (electronic or hard copy) are periodically reviewed to determine whether they are completed on a timely basis and whether if all required data are present, accurate, authenticated, and legible. **B** | 0 | 1 | 2 | NA |

Standard IM.6.20

Records contain patient-specific information, as appropriate, to the care, treatment, and services provided.

❏ Compliant
❏ Not Compliant

Elements of Performance for IM.6.20

1. Not applicable
2. Not applicable
3. Not applicable

Ⓜ 4. When appropriate, summaries of treatment and other documents provided by the practice are forwarded to other care providers.

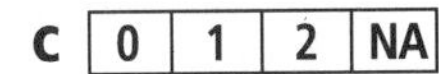

5. Through 22. Not applicable

Ⓜ 23. Each medical record contains, as applicable, the following clinical information: **C** | 0 | 1 | 2 | NA |
- Documentation and findings of assessments*
- Conclusions or impressions drawn from medical history and physical examination
- The diagnosis, diagnostic impression, or conditions
- All relevant diagnostic and therapeutic tests and results obtained during the course of care, treatment, and services
- History of all operative and other invasive procedures, including placement of any implants appropriate to the procedure being done
- Consultation† reports
- Allergies to foods and medicines
- Every dose of medication administered while on site, including the strength, dose, or rate of administration, administration devices used, access site or route, known drug allergies, adverse drug reactions, and patient's response to medication
- All relevant diagnoses/conditions established during the course of care, treatment, and services

Ⓜ 24. Each medical record contains, as applicable, the following demographic information:
- The patient's name, gender, address, phone number, date of birth, height and weight, and the name and phone number of any legally authorized representative

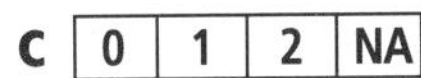

Ⓜ 25. Each medical record contains, as applicable, the following information: **C** | 0 | 1 | 2 | NA |
- Evidence of known advance directives
- Evidence of informed consent when required by practice policy
- Referrals or communications made to external or internal care providers and community agencies
- When appropriate, other pertinent documents to promote continuity of care, treatment, and services
- Documentation of clinical research interventions that is distinct from entries related to regular patient care

IM

* *See* the "Provision of Care, Treatment, and Services" (PC) chapter in this manual.

† **Consultation** 1. Provision of professional advice or services. 2. For the purposes of Joint Commission accreditation, advice given to staff of surveyed practices relating to compliance with standards that are the subject of the review. 3. A review of an individual's problem by a second practitioner, such as a physician or other health care provider, and the rendering of an opinion and advice to the referring practitioner. In most instances, the review involves the independent examination of the individual by the consultant. The opinion and advice are not usually binding on the referring individual.

Scoring Grid
0 Insufficient compliance
1 Partial compliance
2 Satisfactory compliance
NA Not applicable

- Records of communication with the patient regarding care, treatment, and services, for example, telephone calls or e-mail, if applicable
- Patient-generated information (for example, assessment tools the patient completes before the visit)

C 0 1 2 NA — Ⓜ 26. Clinical summaries of treatment received elsewhere are included in the medical record, and may include the following:
- Follow-up instruction
- Postoperative reports from surgery
- Therapy progress notes from visiting nurses or specialty consultants
- Progress reports from intermediate nursing facilities

❑ Compliant
❑ Not Compliant

Standard IM.6.30*

The medical record thoroughly documents operative or other high-risk procedures[†] and the use of moderate or deep sedation or anesthesia.

Elements of Performance for IM.6.30

C 0 1 2 NA — Ⓜ 1. A provisional diagnosis is recorded before the operative procedure by the licensed independent practitioner responsible for the patient.

C 0 1 2 NA — Ⓜ 2. Operative reports dictated or written immediately[‡] after a procedure record the name of the primary surgeon and assistants, findings, procedures performed and description of the procedure, estimated blood loss, as indicated, specimens removed, and postoperative diagnosis.

C 0 1 2 NA — Ⓜ 3. An operative progress note is entered in the medical record immediately after the procedure.

C 0 1 2 NA — Ⓜ 4. The completed operative or other high-risk procedure report is authenticated by the surgeon, physician, or dentist and made available in the medical record as soon as possible after the procedure.

C 0 1 2 NA — Ⓜ 5. Postoperative documentation records the patient's vital signs and level of consciousness; medications (including intravenous fluids, blood, and blood components administered, if applicable); and any unusual events or complications, including blood transfusion reactions and the management of those events.

C 0 1 2 NA — Ⓜ 6. Postoperative documentation records the patient's discharge from the postsedation or postanesthesia care phase by the responsible licensed independent practitioner or according to discharge criteria.

C 0 1 2 NA — Ⓜ 7. The use of approved discharge criteria to determine the patient's readiness for discharge is documented in the medical record.

C 0 1 2 NA — Ⓜ 8. Postoperative documentation records the name of the licensed independent practitioner responsible for discharge.

Standard IM.6.40

Not applicable

---

* **Note:** Also see *the "Provision of Care, Treatment, and Services" (PC) chapter, standards PC.13.30 and PC.13.40.*

† **Operative and other high-risk procedures** Procedures including operative, other invasive, and noninvasive procedures that place the patient at risk. The focus is on procedures and therefore is not meant to include use of medications that place patients at risk.

‡ Immediately after a procedure is defined as *upon completion of the operation or procedure, before the patient is transferred to the next level of care.* This is to ensure that pertinent information is available to the next caregiver. In addition, if the surgeon accompanies the patient from the operating room to the next unit or area of care, the operative note or progress note can be written in that unit or area of care.

Scoring Grid

- **0** Insufficient compliance
- **1** Partial compliance
- **2** Satisfactory compliance
- **NA** Not applicable

Standard IM.6.50

Designated qualified personnel accept and transcribe verbal orders from authorized individuals.

❑ Compliant
❑ Not Compliant

Elements of Performance for IM.6.50

1. Qualified personnel are identified, as defined by practice policy and, as appropriate, in accordance with state and federal law, and authorized to receive and record verbal orders. — **A** | 0 | 1 | 2 | NA |
2. Ⓜ Each verbal order is dated and identifies the names of the individuals who gave and received it, and the record indicates who implemented it. — **C** | 0 | 1 | 2 | NA |
3. When required by state or federal law and regulation, verbal orders are authenticated within the specified time frame. — **A** | 0 | 1 | 2 | NA |
4. Implement a process for taking verbal or telephone orders or receiving critical test results that require a verification read-back of the complete order or test result by the person receiving the order or test result. — **A** | 0 | 1 | 2 | NA |

Standard IM.6.60

The practice can provide access to all relevant information from a patient's record when needed for use in patient care, treatment, and services.

❑ Compliant
❑ Not Compliant

Rationale for IM.6.60

To facilitate continuity of care, providers have access to information about all previous care, treatment, and services provided to a patient by the practice.

Elements of Performance for IM.6.60

1. There is a manual or automated mechanism to track the location of all components of the medical record. — **B** | 0 | 1 | 2 | NA |
2. The practice uses a system to assemble required information or make available a summary of information relative to patient care, treatment, and services when the patient is seen. — **B** | 0 | 1 | 2 | NA |

IM

Crosswalks of Previous Standards to New Standards

Crosswalk of Previous Standards for Office-Based Surgery Practices to the New "Practice Ethics, and Patient Rights and Responsibilities" Standards for Office-Based Surgery Practices

This crosswalk is designed to show where the previous standards requirements appear in the reformatted "Practice Ethics, and Patient Rights and Responsibilities" (RI) standards for the second edition of the manual. The left column, "Previous Standards," lists consecutively each standard that was effective in the first edition. The right column, New Standards, indicates the RI standards, with revised numbers, which become effective January 1, 2005.

Previous Standards	New Standards
RI.1 Patients' cultural, psychosocial, spiritual, and personal values are respected.	**RI.2.10** The practice respects the rights of patients. **RI.2.30** Patients are involved in decisions about care, treatment, and services provided. **RI.2.70** Patients have the right to refuse care, treatment, and services in accordance with law and regulation. **RI.3.10** Patients are given information about their responsibilities while receiving care, treatment, and services.
RI.1 Informed consent is obtained.	**RI.1.20** The practice addresses conflicts of interest. **RI.2.40** Informed consent is obtained. **RI.2.60** Patients receive adequate information about the person(s) responsible for the delivery of their care, treatment, and services.
RI.1.1.1 During the initial consultation period, the patient receives written materials that disclose the current licensure, relevant education, training, and experience of the surgeon who will perform the procedure.	**RI.2.60** Patients receive adequate information about the person(s) responsible for the delivery of their care, treatment, and services.
RI.1.2 Patients involved in investigational studies and clinical trials participate in care decisions throughout the care process.	**RI.2.30** Patients are involved in decisions about care, treatment, and services provided. **RI.2.180** The practice protects research subjects and respects their rights during research, investigation, and clinical trials involving human subjects.
RI.1.3 Patients are involved in resolving conflicts about care decisions.	**RI.2.30** Patients are involved in decisions about care, treatment, and services provided.
RI.1.4 The practice demonstrates respect for privacy. **RI.1.5** The practice demonstrates respect for communication. **RI.1.6** The practice demonstrates respect for resolution of complaints.	**RI.2.100** The practice respects the patient's right to and need for effective communication. **RI.2.120** The practice addresses the resolution of complaints from patients and their families. **RI.2.130** The practice respects the needs of patients for confidentiality, privacy, and security.

Previous Standards	New Standards
RI.2 A code of ethical business and professional behavior addresses billing and marketing practices; relationships with other health care providers, educational institutions, and payers; and concern for the cost of care. **RI.2.1** A code of ethical business and professional behavior addresses protection of the integrity of clinical decision making, regardless of how the practice compensates or shares financial risk with its leaders, managers, surgeons, licensed independent practitioners, and clinical staff.	**RI.1.10** The practice follows ethical behavior in its care, treatment, services, and business practices. **RI.1.20** The practice addresses conflicts of interest. **RI.1.30** The practice follows ethical behavior in its care, treatment, services, and business practices.

Crosswalk of Previous "Surgical and Invasive Procedures, Sedation, Anesthesia, and Recovery" and "Education" Standards for Office-Based Surgery Practices to the New "Provision of Care, Treatment, and Services" Standards for Office-Based Surgery Practices

This crosswalk is designed to show where the previous standards requirements appear in the reformatted "Provision of Care, Treatment, and Services" (PC) standards for the second edition of the manual. The left column, Previous Standards, lists consecutively each standard that was effective in the first edition. The right column, New Standards, indicates the updated standards, with revised numbers, which become effective January 1, 2005.

Previous Standards	New Standards
PC.1 An initial medical assessment of each patient's physical and psychological status and health history is conducted.	**PC.2.130** Initial assessments are performed as defined by the practice.
PC.1.2 Diagnostic testing necessary for determining the patient's health care needs is performed. **PC.1.3** Results of previous diagnostic testing are considered in patient assessment.	**PC.3.230** Diagnostic testing necessary for determining the patient's health care needs is performed.
PC.1.4 Each patient's need for follow-up care is assessed.	**PC.15.20** The transfer or discharge of a patient is based on the patient's assessed needs and the practice's capabilities.
PC.1.5 A presedation or preanesthesia clinical assessment is conducted for each patient for whom moderate or deep sedation or anesthesia is planned to determine whether the patient is an appropriate candidate for moderate or deep sedation or anesthesia.	**PC.13.20** Operative or other procedures and/or the administration of moderate or deep sedation or anesthesia are planned.
PC.1.6 Based on the presedation or preanesthesia assessment, the surgeon gives final approval of whether the patient is an appropriate candidate for moderate or deep sedation or anesthesia.	**PC.13.20** Operative or other procedures and/or the administration of moderate or deep sedation or anesthesia are planned.
PC.1.7 As appropriate, patients' dietary needs are met.	**PC.7.10** The practice has a process for preparing and/or distributing food and nutrition products as appropriate.
PC.2 The planned procedure is appropriate to the patient's needs and severity of disease, condition, impairment, or disability.	**PC.4.10** Development of a plan for care, treatment, and services is individualized and appropriate to the patient's needs, strengths, limitations, and goals.
PC.3 The surgeon defines the scope of appropriate clinical assessment for all surgical and invasive procedures. **PC.3.1** Determining the appropriateness of a procedure for each patient is based, in part, on a review of the patient's history, physical status, and diagnostic data and an assessment of the procedure's risks and benefits.	**PC.13.10** Licensed independent practitioners define the scope of assessment for operative or other procedures and/or the administration of moderate or deep sedation or anesthesia.
PC.3.2 A surgeon performs the surgical or invasive procedure.	**PC.13.20** Operative or other procedures and/or the administration of moderate or deep sedation or anesthesia are planned.

Previous Standards	New Standards
PC.4 Each patient is reevaluated clinically immediately before moderate and deep sedation use and before anesthesia induction.	**PC.13.20** Operative or other procedures and/or the administration of moderate or deep sedation or anesthesia are planned.
PC.5 While patients are undergoing procedures and until discharged from the setting, there are at least two staff members on-site at all times to help in the event of a patient emergency.	**PC.9.20** The practice responds to life-threatening emergencies according to practice policy and procedure.
PC.6 The practice takes action to prevent or reduce the risk of nosocomial infection in patients, staff, and visitors. **PC.6.1** The practice takes action to control outbreaks of nosocomial infections when they are identified.	**IC.1.10 Through IC.9.10** (Please see IC-1 through IC-12 for standards)
PC.7 As appropriate, the practice has procedures for obtaining blood and blood components.	**PC.9.10** Blood and blood components are administered safely.
PC.8 Qualified clinical staff provides moderate or deep sedation and anesthesia.	**PC.13.20** Operative or other procedures and/or the administration of moderate or deep sedation or anesthesia are planned. **PC.13.30** Patients are monitored during the procedure and/or administration of moderate or deep sedation or anesthesia.
PC.8.1 Each patient's moderate or deep sedation and anesthesia care is planned.	**PC.4.10** Development of a plan for care, treatment, and services is individualized and appropriate to the patient's needs, strengths, limitations, and goals. **PC.13.20** Operative or other procedures and/or the administration of moderate or deep sedation or anesthesia are planned.
PC.8.2 Sedation and anesthesia options and risks are discussed with the patient and, as appropriate family or legal guardian, before administration.	**RI.2.40** Informed consent is obtained.
PC.8.3 Each patient's physiological status is monitored during sedation or anesthesia administration.	**PC.13.30** Patients are monitored during the procedure and/or administration of moderate or deep sedation or anesthesia.
PC.8.4 The licensed independent practitioner responsible for the sedation or anesthesia service discharges the patient from the postsedation or postanesthesia recovery phase.	**PC.13.40** Patients are monitored immediately after the procedure and/or administration of moderate or deep sedation or anesthesia.
PC.8.4.1 The patient is discharged from the setting by the surgeon responsible for the patient.	**PC.13.40** Patients are monitored immediately after the procedure and/or administration of moderate or deep sedation or anesthesia.
PC.8.5 Patients who have received moderate to deep sedation or anesthesia are discharged in the company of a responsible, designated adult.	**PC.13.40** Patients are monitored immediately after the procedure and/or administration of moderate or deep sedation or anesthesia.

Previous Standards	New Standards
PC.9 Surgical and anesthesia services and care are provided under clinical protocols or guidelines approved by the practice.	**LD.5.50** Clinical practice guidelines are used in designing or improving processes that evaluate and treat specific diagnoses, conditions, and/or symptoms. **LD.5.60** The leaders identify criteria for selecting and implementing clinical practice guidelines. **LD.5.70** Appropriate leaders, practitioners, and health care professionals in the practice review and approve clinical practice guidelines selected for implementation. **LD.5.80** The leaders evaluate the outcomes related to clinical practice guidelines and refine the guidelines to improve processes.
PC.9.1 Qualified clinical staff members are available to help provide invasive, surgical, sedation, and anesthesia services.	**HR.3.10** Competence to perform job responsibilities is assessed, demonstrated, and maintained.
PC.9.2 Each patient's physical, physiological, mental, and functional status is monitored throughout the postprocedure period by qualified clinical staff.	**PC.9.20** The practice responds to life-threatening emergencies according to practice policy and procedure. **PC.13.40** Patients are discharged from the recovery area and the practice by a qualified licensed independent practitioner or according to rigorously applied criteria approved by the clinical leaders.
PC.10 An established procedure(s) governs patient consultations and referrals or transfers to another level of care, health professional, or setting.	**PC.15.10** A process addresses the needs for continuing care, treatment, and services after transfer.
PC.10.1 Appropriate patient care and clinical information are exchanged when patients are referred, transferred, or discharged.	**PC.15.30** When patients are transferred or discharged, appropriate information related to the care, treatment, and services provided is exchanged with other service providers.
PC.10.2 Patients are reassessed at specified points to determine their responses to care.	**PC.13.40** Patients are monitored immediately after the procedure and/or administration of moderate or deep sedation or anesthesia. **IM.6.20** Records contain patient-specific information, as appropriate to the care, treatment, and services provided.
PC.11 Criteria are used to identify possible victims of abuse or neglect.	**PC.3.10** Patients who might be victims of abuse, neglect, or exploitation are assessed.
PC.11.1 Victims of alleged or suspected abuse or neglect are assessed with the consent of the patient, parent, or legal guardian, or as otherwise provided by law. **PC.11.2** Notification and release of information are provided to the proper authorities, as required by law. **PC.11.3** Victims of abuse are referred to private or public agencies that provide or arrange for evaluation and care.	**RI.2.40** Informed consent is obtained. **PC.3.10** Patients who might be victims of abuse, neglect, or exploitation are assessed. **LD.1.30** The practice complies with applicable law and regulation.

Previous Standards	New Standards
PF.1 The patient receives education specific to his or her assessed needs, abilities, learning preferences, and readiness to learn as appropriate to the care, treatment, and services provided by the practice. **PF.1.1** The patient receives education on the procedure and related options. **PF.1.2** The patient receives education on sedation, anesthesia, and related options. **PF.1.3** The patient receives education on the duration of the procedure and recovery. **PF.1.4** The patient receives education on signs and symptoms (including their duration) that he or she might anticipate following discharge. **PF.1.5** The patient receives education on preoperative preparations he or she must undertake. **PF.1.6** The patient receives education on the need to have a responsible adult escort postdischarge, postdischarge care instructions, and the appropriate contact for questions following discharge.	**PC.6.10** The patient receives education and training specific to the patient's needs and as appropriate to the care, treatment, and services provided. **PC.6.30** The patient receives education and training specific to the patient's abilities as appropriate to the care, treatment, and services provided by the practice.
PF.2 Patients are educated about pain and managing pain.	**PC.6.10** The patient receives education and training specific to the patient's needs and as appropriate to the care, treatment, and services provided.
PF.3 Patients are educated about habilitation or rehabilitation techniques to help them be more functionally independent, as appropriate.	**PC.6.10** The patient receives education and training specific to the patient's needs and as appropriate to the care, treatment, and services provided.
PF.4 Education includes information about the patient's responsibilities in his or her care.	**RI.2.30** Patients are involved in decisions about care, treatment, and services provided. **RI.3.10** Patients are given information about their responsibilities while receiving care, treatment, and services.

Crosswalk of Previous "Clinical Support Services" Standards for Office-Based Surgery Practices to the New "Medication Management" Standards for Office-Based Surgery Practices

This crosswalk is designed to show where the previous standards requirements appear in the reformatted "Medication Management" (MM) standards for the second edition of the manual. The left column, Previous Standards, lists consecutively each standard that was effective in the first edition. The right column, New Standards, indicates the updated standards, with revised numbers, which become effective January 1, 2005.

Previous Standards	New Standards
SU.1 Prescribing and ordering medications follow established procedures.	**MM.5.30** Prescribing and ordering medications follow established procedures.
SU.1.1 Preparing, dispensing, and recalling medication(s) adheres to law, regulation, licensure, and professional standards of practice.	**MM.4.70** Medications dispensed by the practice are retrieved when recalled or discontinued by the manufacturer or the Food and Drug Administration for safety reasons. **MM.4.30** Medications are appropriately labeled.
SU.1.2 When preparing and dispensing a medication(s) for a patient, important patient medication information is considered.	**MM.1.10** Patient-specific information is readily accessible to those involved in the medication management system.
SU.1.3 The practice has emergency medication systems.	**MM.2.30** Emergency medications and/or supplies, if any, are consistently available, controlled, and secure in the practice's patient care areas.
SU.1.4 Prescriptions or orders are verified and patients are identified before medication is administered.	**PC.5.10** The practice provides care, treatment, and services for each patient according to the plan for care, treatment, and services. **MM.4.10** All prescriptions or medication orders are reviewed for appropriateness. **MM.5.10** Medications are safely and accurately administered. **MM.2.20** Medications are properly and safely stored throughout the practice. **MM.4.20** Medications are prepared safely. **MM.4.30** Medications are appropriately labeled. **MM.4.40** Medications are dispensed safely. **MM.7.40** Investigational medications are safely controlled and administered. **MM.8.10** The practice evaluates its medication management system.
SU.2 Pathology and clinical laboratory services and consultation are readily available to meet patients' needs.	**PC.2.130** Initial assessments are performed as defined by the practice. **LD.3.50** Services provided by consultation, contractual arrangements, or other agreements are provided safely and effectively.

CW

Previous Standards	New Standards
SU.2.1 While the patient is under the practice's care, all laboratory testing is done in the practice's laboratories or approved reference laboratories. **SU.2.2** The practice identifies acceptable reference or contract laboratory services. **SU.2.3** Reference and contract laboratory services meet applicable federal standards for clinical laboratories.	**LD.3.50** Services provided by consultation, contractual arrangements, or other agreements are provided safely and effectively.
SU.2.4 The practice defines the extent to which the test results are used in an individual's treatment (definitive or used only as a screen).	**PC.16.10** The practice defines the context in which quantitative waived test results are used in patient care, treatment, and services.
SU.2.5 The practice identifies the staff responsible for performing and supervising waived testing.	**PC.16.20** The practice identifies the staff responsible for performing and supervising waived testing.
SU.2.6 Staff members performing tests have adequate, specific training and orientation to perform the tests and demonstrate satisfactory levels of competence in the testing performed.	**PC.16.30** Staff performing tests have adequate, specific training and orientation to perform the tests and demonstrate satisfactory levels of competence.
SU.2.7 Procedures governing specific testing-related processes are current and readily available.	**PC.16.40** Approved policies and procedures for specific testing-related processes are current and readily available.
SU.2.8 Quality control checks are conducted on each procedure as identified by the practice. **SU.2.8.1** At a minimum, manufacturers' instructions are followed.	**PC.16.50** Quality control checks, as defined by the practice, are conducted on each procedure.
SU.2.9 Appropriate quality control and test records are maintained.	**PC.16.60** Appropriate quality control and test records are maintained.

Crosswalk of Previous "Staff Development, Training, and Competence" and "Credentialing and Self-Assessment" Standards for Office-Based Surgery Practices to the New "Management of Human Resources" Standards for Office-Based Surgery Practices

This crosswalk is designed to show where the previous standards requirements appear in the reformatted "Management of Human Resources" (HR) standards for the second edition of the manual. The left column, Previous Standards, lists consecutively each standard that was effective in the first edition. The right column, New Standards, indicates the updated HR standards, with revised numbers, which become effective January 1, 2005.

Previous Standards	New Standards
HR.1 The practice develops processes for recruiting, retaining, developing, and continuing the education of all staff.	**HR.1.10** The practice provides an adequate number and mix of staff consistent with the practice's staffing plan. **HR.2.30** Ongoing education, including in-services, training, and other activities, maintains and improves competence.
HR.2 Qualifications, job descriptions, and performance expectations are defined for all staff.	**HR.1.20** The practice has a process to ensure that a person's qualifications are consistent with his or her job responsibilities.
HR.3 New staff orientation provides initial job training and information and assesses capability to perform job responsibilities.	**HR.2.10** Orientation provides initial job training and information.
HR.4 Ongoing education and training are provided to maintain and improve staff competence.	**HR.2.30** Ongoing education, including in-services, training, and other activities, maintains and improves competence. **HR.3.10** Competence to perform job responsibilities is assessed, demonstrated, and maintained.
HR.5 Staff members' abilities to fulfill expectations of their job descriptions are periodically assessed.	**HR.2.20** Staff members, licensed independent practitioners, students, and volunteers, as appropriate, can describe or demonstrate their roles and responsibilities, based on specific job duties or responsibilities, relative to safety. **HR.3.10** Competence to perform job responsibilities is assessed, demonstrated, and maintained.
CS.1 The office-based surgery practice establishes policies and procedures that guide the practice in assessing individual surgeon and licensed independent practitioner qualifications and competence to perform the surgical or invasive procedures and anesthesia services offered in the office setting.	**HR.4.10** There is a process for ensuring the competence of all practitioners permitted by law and the practice to practice independently. **HR.4.20** Individuals permitted by law and the practice to practice independently are granted clinical privileges.

Previous Standards	New Standards
CS.2 The practice establishes a process to determine and document an individual surgeon's and licensed independent practitioner's qualifications and competence to perform a specific surgical or invasive procedure and sedation or anesthesia service. **CS.2.1** When verifying and documenting an individual surgeon's or licensed independent practitioner's credentials to perform a specific invasive or surgical procedure and sedation or anesthesia service, the practice obtains the following information from the primary source and includes it in the individual surgeon's or licensed independent practitioner's credentials file: a. Current licensure or certification b. Relevant education c. Relevant training d. Relevant experience **CS.2.2** When verifying and documenting an individual surgeon's or licensed independent practitioner's credentials to perform a specific invasive or surgical procedure and sedation or anesthesia service, the practice obtains the following information (from the primary source when possible) and includes it in the individual surgeon's or licensed independent practitioner's credentials file: a. Continuing medical/dental education in the area of current practice b. Evidence of a current, unrestricted Drug Enforcement Administration registration and any history of revocation c. Board certification, current recertification, or eligibility. **CS.2.3** When verifying and documenting an individual surgeon's or licensed independent practitioner's credentials to perform a specific surgical or invasive procedure and sedation or anesthesia service, the practice includes the following information, if applicable, in the surgeon's or licensed independent practitioner's credentials file: a. Results of a clinical record review by a same-specialty practitioner b. Peer recommendations addressing the type and number of procedures or services performed as the surgeon or licensed independent practitioner's of record; c. The skill demonstrated in performing the procedure or service d. Information on resulting clinical outcomes **CS.2.4** Practitioner-specific outcomes data are reviewed in the practice's credentialing process and included in the individual surgeon's and licensed independent practitioner's credentials file. **CS.3** Individual surgeons' and licensed independent practitioners' credentials information that is subject to change is reverified at least every two years.	**HR.4.10** There is a process for ensuring the competence of all practitioners permitted by law and the practice to practice independently. **HR.4.20** Individuals permitted by law and the practice to practice independently are granted clinical privileges. **HR.4.60** Individual surgeons' and licensed independent practitioners' credentials information that is subject to change is reverified at least every two years and reevaluated in the event of a change in services, an unexpected adverse outcome, or a sentinel event.

Previous Standards	New Standards
CS.3.1 Individual surgeons' and licensed independent practitioners' credentials information is reevaluated any time there is a change in the surgical, invasive, sedation, or anesthesia procedures, services, or techniques offered, or there is an unexpected adverse outcome or sentinel event.	**HR.4.60** Individual surgeons' and licensed independent practitioners' credentials information that is subject to change is reverified at least every two years and reevaluated in the event of a change in services, an unexpected adverse outcome, or a sentinel event.
CS.4 The individual surgeon and licensed independent practitioner engage in ongoing review of clinical outcomes.	**PI.1.10** The practice collects data about its performance.

Crosswalk of Previous "Management of the Environment of Care" Standards for Office-Based Surgery Practices to the New "Management of the Environment of Care" Standards for Office-Based Surgery Practices

This crosswalk is designed to show where the previous standards requirements appear in the reformatted "Management of the Environment of Care" (EC) standards for the second edition of the manual. The left column, Previous Standards, lists consecutively each standard that was effective in the first edition. The right column, New Standards, indicates the updated standards, with revised numbers, which become effective January 1, 2005.

Previous Standards	New Standards
EC.1 The practice plans for a safe environment that is accessible, effective, efficient, and consistent with its goals and values, services, law, and regulation.	**EC.1.10** The practice manages safety risks. **EC.1.20** The practice maintains a safe environment.
EC.1.1 The practice provides for staff safety.	**EC.1.25** The practice provides for staff safety.
EC.1.1.1 The practice develops and implements a smoking policy.	**EC.1.30** The practice develops and implements a policy to prohibit smoking except in specified circumstances.
EC.2.1 The practice provides for a secure environment.	**EC.2.10** The practice identifies and manages its security risks.
EC.2.2 The practice safely manages hazardous materials and wastes.	**EC.3.10** The practice manages its hazardous materials and waste risks.
EC.2.3 The practice plans for and manages emergencies.	**EC.4.10** The practice addresses emergency management.
EC.2.4 The practice implements fire prevention processes.	**EC.5.10** The practice manages fire safety risks.
EC.2.5 The practice provides for the safe and effective use of medical equipment.	**EC.6.10** The practice manages medical equipment risks. **HR.2.10** Orientation provides initial job training and information.
EC.2.6 The practice provides for effective and safe utility systems.	**EC.7.10** The practice manages its utility risks. **HR.2.10** Orientation provides initial job training and information.
EC.2.6.1 The practice provides a reliable emergency power source as required.	**EC.7.20** The practice provides an emergency electrical power source.
EC.2.7 Staff members have been oriented to and educated about the environment of care and have the knowledge and skills to perform their responsibilities in the environment of care.	**HR.2.10** Orientation provides initial job training and information. **HR.2.20** Staff members, licensed independent practitioners, students, and volunteers, as appropriate, can describe or demonstrate their roles and responsibilities, based on specific job duties or responsibilities, relative to safety.
EC.2.8.2 Fire drills are conducted regularly.	**EC.5.30** The practice conducts fire drills regularly.
EC.2.9 Operational components of the environment are maintained, tested, and inspected. **EC.2.9.1** Safety elements of the environment of care are maintained, tested, and inspected.	**EC.1.20** The practice maintains a safe environment.

CW

Previous Standards	New Standards
EC.2.9.2 Fire safety elements in the environment of care are maintained, tested, and inspected.	**EC.5.40** The practice maintains fire-safety equipment and building features.
EC.2.9.3 Medical equipment is maintained, tested, and inspected.	**EC.6.20** Medical equipment is maintained, tested, and inspected.
EC.2.9.4 Utility systems are maintained, tested, and inspected.	**EC.7.30** The practice maintains, tests, and inspects its utility systems.
EC.2.9.4.1 Emergency power systems are maintained, tested, and inspected.	**EC.7.40** The practice maintains, tests, and inspects its emergency power systems.
EC.3 Building(s) and grounds are suitable to services provided and patients served.	**LD.3.80** The leaders provide for adequate space, equipment, and other resources. **PC.13.20** Operative or other procedures and/or the administration of moderate or deep sedation or anesthesia are planned. **EC.1.10** The practice manages safety risks. **EC.8.10** The practice establishes and maintains an appropriate environment. **EC.7.20** The practice provides an emergency electrical power source.
EC.3.2 Newly constructed and existing environments of care are designed and maintained to comply with the *Life Safety Code*®*	**EC.5.20** Newly constructed and existing environments of care are designed and maintained to comply with the *Life Safety Code*®

* *Life Safety Code*® is a registered trademark of the National Fire Protection Association, Quincy, MA.

CW

Crosswalk of Previous "Planning and Directing Practice Services" Standards for Office-Based Surgery Practices to the New "Practice Leadership" Standards for Office-Based Surgery Practices

This crosswalk is designed to show where the previous standards requirements appear in the reformatted "Practice Leadership" (LD) standards for the second edition of the manual. The left column, Previous Standards, lists consecutively each standard that was effective in the first edition. The right column, New Standards, indicates the updated standards, with revised numbers, which become effective January 1, 2005.

Previous Standards	New Standards
LD.1 Planning addresses patient care and practice functions.	**PC.1.10** The practice accepts for care, treatment, and services only those patients whose identified care, treatment, and service needs it can meet. **LD.1.30** The practice complies with applicable law and regulation. **LD.2.50** The leaders develop and monitor an annual operating budget and, as appropriate, a long-term capital expenditure plan. **LD.3.10** The leaders engage in both short-term and long-term planning. **LD.3.20** Patients with comparable needs receive the same standard of care, treatment, and services throughout the practice. **LD.3.60** Communication is effective throughout the practice. **LD.3.70** The leaders define the required qualifications and competence of those staff who provide care, treatment, and services and recommend a sufficient number of qualified and competent staff to provide care, treatment, and services. **LD.3.80** The leaders provide for adequate space, equipment, and other resources.
LD.1.1 Care is available in a timely manner to meet patient needs. **LD.1.2** The practice leaders approve sources of patient service outside the practice.	**PC.5.60** The practice coordinates the care, treatment, and services provided to a patient as part of the plan for care, treatment, and services and consistent with the practice's scope of care, treatment, and services. **LD.3.50** Services provided by consultation, contractual arrangements, or other agreements are provided safely and effectively.
LD.1.3 The practice's scope of services is defined in writing and approved by the practice leaders.	**LD.1.20** Governance responsibilities are defined in writing, as applicable. **LD.3.90** The leaders develop and implement policies and procedures for care, treatment, and services.
LD.1.4 The practice leaders provide for uniform performance of patient care processes throughout the practice.	**LD.3.20** Patients with comparable needs receive the same standard of care, treatment, and services throughout the practice.
LD.1.5 Clinical practice guidelines are used in designing or improving processes that evaluate and treat specific diagnoses, conditions, or symptoms, as appropriate.	**LD.5.50** Clinical practice guidelines are used in designing or improving processes that evaluate and treat specific diagnoses, conditions, and/or symptoms.

CW

Previous Standards	New Standards
LD.2 The practice leaders are responsible for developing, implementing, and maintaining procedures that guide and support the provision of care. **LD.2.1** The practice leaders are responsible for providing an adequate number of qualified, competent staff. **LD.2.2** The practice leaders are responsible for determining the qualifications and competence of patient care staff members who are not surgeons or licensed independent practitioners.	**LD.2.20** The practice has effective leadership. **LD.3.70** The leaders define the required qualifications and competence of those staff who provide care, treatment, and services and recommend a sufficient number of qualified and competent staff to provide care, treatment, and services. **LD.3.90** The leaders develop and implement policies and procedures for care, treatment, and services. **HR.1.20** The practice has a process to ensure that a person's qualifications are consistent with his or her job responsibilities.
LD.3 The practice leaders ensure that processes and activities that most affect patient outcomes are continually and systematically assessed and improved.	**LD.4.10** The leaders set expectations, plan, and manage processes to measure, assess, and improve the practice's management, clinical, and support activities. **LD.4.50** The leaders set performance improvement priorities and identify how the practice adjusts priorities in response to unusual or urgent events.
LD.3.1 The practice leaders ensure that the processes for identifying and managing sentinel events are defined and implemented.	**PI.2.30** Processes for identifying and managing sentinel events are defined and implemented. **PI.3.10** Information from data analysis is used to make changes that improve performance and patient safety and reduce the risk of sentinel events.
LD.3.2 The practice leaders assign adequate resources, including staff, to performance improvement activities.	**LD.4.60** The leaders allocate adequate resources for measuring, assessing, and improving the practice's performance and improving patient safety.
	LD.4.20 New or modified services or processes are designed well.
	LD.4.40 The leaders ensure that an integrated patient safety program is implemented throughout the practice.

CW

Crosswalk of Previous "Management of Information" Standards for Office-Based Surgery Practices to the New "Management of Information" Standards for Office-Based Surgery Practices

This crosswalk is designed to show where the previous standards requirements appear in the reformatted "Management of Information" (IM) standards for the second edition of the manual. The left column, Previous Standards, lists consecutively each standard that was effective in the first edition. The right column, New Standards, indicates the updated IM standards, with revised numbers, which become effective January 1, 2005.

Previous Standards	New Standards
IM.1 The practice determines appropriate levels of security and confidentiality for data and information. **IM.1.1** Collection, storage, and retrieval systems are designed to allow timely and easy use of data and information without compromising their security and confidentiality. **IM.1.2** Records and information are protected against loss, destruction, tampering, and unauthorized access or use.	**IM.2.10** Information privacy and confidentiality are maintained. **IM.2.20** Information security, including data integrity, is maintained.
IM.2 Medical records are periodically reviewed for completeness, accuracy, and timely completion of all information, and action is taken as necessary to improve.	**IM.6.10** The practice has a complete and accurate medical record for every individual assessed or treated.
IM.3 The practice determines the retention time of medical record information based on law and regulation and on its use for patient care, legal, research, and educational activities.	**IM.6.10** The practice has a complete and accurate medical record for every individual assessed or treated.
IM.4 The practice initiates and maintains a medical record for every individual assessed or treated. **IM.4.1** Only authorized staff makes entries in medical records. **IM.4.2** The medical record contains sufficient information to identify the patient, support the diagnosis, justify the procedure, document the course and results, and promote continuity of care among health care providers.	**IM.6.10** The practice has a complete and accurate medical record for every individual assessed or treated. **IM.6.20** Records contain patient-specific information, as appropriate, to the care, treatment, and services provided. **IM.6.60** The practice can provide access to all relevant information from a patient's record when needed for use in patient care, treatment, and services.

Previous Standards	New Standards
IM.4.3 The surgeon responsible for the patient records a preoperative diagnosis before surgery. **IM.4.4** Operative reports dictated or written immediately after surgery record the name of the surgeon who performed the procedure, the licensed independent practitioner responsible for sedation or anesthesia services, assisting clinical staff, findings, technical procedures used, specimens removed, and postoperative diagnosis. **IM.4.5** The surgeon who performed the procedure authenticates the completed operative report, and it is filed in the medical record as soon as possible. **IM.4.6** When there is a delay in filing the operative report, an operative progress note is entered in the medical record immediately after surgery. **IM.4.7** Postoperative documentation records the patient's vital signs and level of consciousness; medications (including intravenous fluids), blood, and blood components administered; and any unusual events or postoperative complications, including blood transfusion reactions and the management of those events. **IM.4.8** Postoperative documentation records the patient's discharge from the postanesthesia care area by the responsible licensed independent practitioner. **IM.4.9** Discharge criteria are approved by the appropriate surgeon(s) on staff and rigorously applied to determine the patient's readiness for discharge from the setting. **IM.4.10** Postoperative documentation records the name of the surgeon responsible for discharge from the setting.	**IM.6.30** The medical record thoroughly documents operative or other procedures and the use of moderate or deep sedation or anesthesia.
IM.4.11 Medical record data and information are managed in a timely manner.	**IM.6.10** The practice has a complete and accurate medical record for every individual assessed or treated.
IM.4.12 Verbal orders of authorized practitioners are accepted and transcribed by designated, qualified staff.	**IM.6.50** Designated, qualified personnel accept and transcribe verbal orders from authorized individuals.
IM.4.13 Every medical record entry is dated, its author is identified, and (when necessary) it is authenticated.	**IM.6.10** The practice has a complete and accurate medical record for every individual assessed or treated.
IM.4.14 The practice can quickly assemble and have accessible all relevant information from a patient's record when needed for use in patient care.	**IM.6.60** The practice can provide access to all relevant information from a patient's record when needed for use in patient care, treatment, and services.

Crosswalk of Previous "Improving Practice Performance" Standards for Office-Based Surgery Practices to the New "Improving Practice Performance" Standards for Office-Based Surgery Practices

This crosswalk is designed to show where the previous standards requirements appear in the reformatted "Improving Practice Performance" (PI) standards for the second edition of the manual. The left column, Previous Standards, lists consecutively each standard that was effective in the first edition. The right column, New Standards, indicates the updated standards, with revised numbers, which become effective January 1, 2005.

Previous Standards	New Standards
PI.1 The practice collects data to monitor its performance.	**PI.1.10** The practice collects data to monitor its performance. **LD.4.50** The leaders set performance improvement priorities and identify how the practice adjusts priorities in response to unusual or urgent events.
PI.1.1 The practice collects data to monitor the performance of processes that involve risks or might result in sentinel events.	**PI.1.10** The practice collects data to monitor its performance. **PI.3.10** Information from data analysis is used to make changes that improve performance and patient safety and reduce the risk of sentinel events. **LD.4.50** The leaders set performance improvement priorities and identify how the practice adjusts priorities in response to unusual or urgent events.
PI.1.1.1 The practice collects data to monitor clinical outcomes.	**PI.1.10** The practice collects data to monitor its performance.
PI.1.2 The practice collects data to monitor improvements in performance.	**PI.1.10** The practice collects data to monitor its performance. **LD.4.50** The leaders set performance improvement priorities and identify how the practice adjusts priorities in response to unusual or urgent events.
PI.2 Data are systematically aggregated and analyzed on an ongoing basis.	**PI.2.10** Data are systematically aggregated and analyzed.
PI.2.2 Undesirable patterns or trends in performance and sentinel events are intensively analyzed.	**PI.2.20** Undesirable patterns or trends in performance are analyzed. **PI.2.30** Processes for identifying and managing sentinel events are defined and implemented.
PI.3 Improved performance is achieved and sustained.	**PI.1.10** The practice collects data to monitor its performance. **PI.2.30** Processes for identifying and managing sentinel events are defined and implemented. **PI.3.10** Information from data analysis is used to make changes that improve performance and patient safety and reduce the risk of sentinel events. **LD.4.60** The leaders allocate adequate resources for measuring, assessing, and improving the practice's performance and improving patient safety.

Previous Standards	New Standards
	PI.3.20 An ongoing, proactive program for identifying and reducing unanticipated adverse events and safety risks to patients is defined and implemented.

CW

Appendix A: *2005–2006 Comprehensive Accreditation Manual for Ambulatory Care* Crosswalk to the *Accreditation Manual for Office-Based Surgery Practices, Second Edition*

2005–2006 Comprehensive Accreditation Manual for Ambulatory Care	*Accreditation Manual for Office-Based Surgery Practices, Second Edition*
Ethics, Rights, and Responsibilities	
Organization Ethics	**Practice Ethics**
RI.1.10	RI.1.10
RI.1.20	RI.1.20
RI.1.30	RI.1.30
RI.1.40	
Individual Rights	**Patient Rights**
RI.2.10	RI.2.10
RI.2.20	
RI.2.30	RI.2.30
RI.2.40	RI.2.40
RI.2.50	
RI.2.60	RI.2.60
RI.2.70	RI.2.70
RI.2.80	
RI.2.90	RI.2.90
RI.2.100	RI.2.100
RI.2.120	RI.2.120
RI.2.130	RI.2.130
RI.2.150	
RI.2.160	
RI.2.180	RI.2.180
Individual Responsibilities	**Individual Responsibilities**
RI.3.10	RI.3.10

Provision of Care, Treatment, and Services	
Entry to Care, Treatment, and Services	**Entry to Care, Treatment, and Services**
PC.1.10	PC.1.10
Assessment	**Assessment**
PC.2.20	
PC.2.120	

AXA

2005–2006 Comprehensive Accreditation Manual for Ambulatory Care	*Accreditation Manual for Office-Based Surgery Practices, Second Edition*
Provision of Care, Treatment, and Services *(continued)*	
PC.2.130	PC.2.130
PC.2.150	
Additional Standard for Victims of Abuse	**Additional Standard for Victims of Abuse**
PC.3.10	PC.3.10
Diagnostic Services	**Diagnostic Services**
PC.3.230	PC.3.230
Planning Care, Treatment, and Services	**Planning Care, Treatment, and Services**
PC.4.10	PC.4.10
Providing Care, Treatment, and Services	**Providing Care, Treatment, and Services**
PC.5.10	PC.5.10
PC.5.50	
PC.5.60	PC.5.60
Education	**Education**
PC.6.10	PC.6.10
PC.6.30	PC.6.30
Nutritional Care	**Nutritional Care**
PC.7.10	PC.7.10
Pain	**Pain**
PC.8.10	PC.8.10
Specific Procedures	**Specific Procedures**
Administering Blood and Blood Components	*Administering Blood and Blood Components*
PC.9.10	PC.9.10
Responding to Life-Threatening Emergencies	*Responding to Life-Threatening Emergencies*
PC.9.20	PC.9.20
Restraint and Seclusion	*Restraint and Seclusion*
PC.11.70	
PC.11.100	
Operative or Other High-Risk Procedures and/or the Administration of Moderate or Deep Sedation or Anesthesia	*Operative or Other High-Risk Procedures and/or the Administration of Moderate or Deep Sedation or Anesthesia*
PC.13.10	PC.13.10
PC.13.20	PC.13.20
PC.13.30	PC.13.30
PC.13.40	PC.13.40
Discharge or Transfer	**Discharge or Transfer from the Practice**
PC.15.10	PC.15.10
PC.15.20	PC.15.20

2005–2006 Comprehensive Accreditation Manual for Ambulatory Care	*Accreditation Manual for Office-Based Surgery Practices, Second Edition*
Provision of Care, Treatment, and Services *(continued)*	
PC.15.30	PC.15.30
Waived Testing	**Waived Testing**
PC.16.10	PC.16.10
PC.16.20	PC.16.20
PC.16.30	PC.16.30
PC.16.40	PC.16.40
PC.16.50	PC.16.50
PC.16.60	PC.16.60
Medication Management	
Patient-Specific Information	**Patient-Specific Information**
MM.1.10	MM.1.10
Selection and Procurement	
MM.2.10	
Storage	**Storage**
MM.2.20	MM.2.20
MM.2.30	MM.2.30
MM.2.40	
Ordering and Transcribing	
MM.3.20	
Preparing and Dispensing	**Preparing and Dispensing**
MM.4.10	MM.4.10
MM.4.20	MM.4.20
MM.4.30	MM.4.30
MM.4.40	MM.4.40
MM.4.50	
MM.4.60	
MM.4.70	MM.4.70
MM.4.80	
Administering	**Administering**
MM.5.10	MM.5.10
MM.5.30	
Monitoring	
MM.6.10	
MM.6.20	
High-Risk Medications	**High-Risk Medications**
MM.7.10	MM.7.10

2005–2006 Comprehensive Accreditation Manual for Ambulatory Care	*Accreditation Manual for Office-Based Surgery Practices, Second Edition*
Medication Management *(continued)*	
MM.7.40	MM.7.40
Evaluation	**Evaluation**
MM.8.10	MM.8.10
Surveillance, Prevention, and Control of Infection	
IC.1.10	IC.1.10
IC.2.10	IC.1.120
IC.3.10	IC.1.30
IC.4.10	IC.4.10
IC.5.10	IC.5.10
IC.6.10	IC.7.10
IC.6.20	IC.8.10
IC.7.10	IC.9.10
IC.8.10	
IC.9.10	
Improving Organization/Practice Performance	
Data Collection	**Data Collection**
Monitoring Performance Through Data Collection	*Monitoring Performance Through Data Collection*
PI.1.10	PI.1.10
Aggregation and Analysis	**Aggregation and Analysis**
Aggregating and Analyzing Data to Support Performance Improvement	*Aggregating and Analyzing Data to Support Performance Improvement*
PI.2.10	PI.2.10
PI.2.20	PI.2.20
PI.2.30	PI.2.30
Performance Improvement	**Performance Improvement**
PI.3.10	PI.3.10
PI.3.20	PI.3.20
Leadership/Practice Leadership	
LD.1.10	
LD.1.20	LD.1.20
LD.1.30	LD.1.30
LD.2.10	
LD.2.20	LD.2.20
LD.2.50	LD.2.50
LD.3.10	LD.3.10

2005–2006 Comprehensive Accreditation Manual for Ambulatory Care	*Accreditation Manual for Office-Based Surgery Practices, Second Edition*
Leadership *(continued)*	
LD.3.20	LD.3.20
LD.3.50	LD.3.50
LD.3.60	LD.3.60
LD.3.70	LD.3.70
LD.3.80	LD.3.80
LD.3.90	LD.3.90
LD.3.120	
LD.4.10	LD.4.10
LD.4.20	LD.4.20
LD.4.40	LD.4.40
LD.4.50	LD.4.50
LD.4.60	LD.4.60
LD.4.70	
LD.5.50	LD.5.50
LD.5.60	LD.5.60
LD.5.70	LD.5.70
LD.5.80	LD.5.80

Management of the Environment of Care	
Planning and Implementation Activities	**Planning and Implementation Activities**
EC.1.10	EC.1.10
EC.1.20	EC.1.20
EC.1.25	
EC.1.30	EC.1.30
EC.2.10	EC.2.10
EC.3.10	EC.3.10
EC.4.10	EC.4.10
EC.4.20	EC.4.20
EC.5.10	EC.5.10
EC.5.20	EC.5.20
EC.5.30	EC.5.30
EC.5.40	EC.5.40
EC.5.50	
EC.6.10	EC.6.10
EC.6.20	EC.6.20
EC.7.10	EC.7.10
EC.7.20	EC.7.20

2005–2006 Comprehensive Accreditation Manual for Ambulatory Care	*Accreditation Manual for Office-Based Surgery Practices, Second Edition*
Management of the Environment of Care *(continued)*	
EC.7.30	EC.7.30
EC.7.40	EC.7.40
EC.7.50	
EC.8.10	EC.8.10
EC.8.30	
Measuring and Improving Activities	
EC.9.10	
EC.9.20	
EC.9.30	

Management of Human Resources	
Planning	**Planning**
HR.1.10	HR.1.10
HR.1.20	HR.1.20
Orientation, Training, and Education	**Orientation, Training, and Education**
HR.2.10	HR.2.10
HR.2.20	HR.2.20
HR.2.30	HR.2.30
Assessing Competence	**Assessing Competence**
HR.3.10	HR.3.10
HR.3.20	
Credentialing and Privileging	**Credentialing and Privileging**
HR.4.10	HR.4.10
HR.4.20	HR.4.20
HR.4.30	
HR.4.40	
HR.4.50	
HR.4.60	HR.4.60

Management of Information	
Information Management Planning	**Information Management Planning**
IM.1.10	
Confidentiality and Security	**Confidentiality and Security**
IM.2.10	IM.2.10
IM.2.20	IM.2.20
IM.2.30	
IM.6.10	
IM.6.20	

AXA

2005–2006 Comprehensive Accreditation Manual for Ambulatory Care	*Accreditation Manual for Office-Based Surgery Practices, Second Edition*
Management of Information *(continued)*	
IM.6.30	
IM.6.50	
IM.6.60	
Information Management Processes	
IM.3.10	
Information-Based Decision Making	
IM.4.10	
Knowledge-Based Information	
IM.5.10	
Patient-Specific Information	
IM.6.10	IM.6.10
IM.6.20	IM.6.20
IM.6.30	IM.6.30
IM.6.40	
IM.6.50	IM.6.50
IM.6.60	IM.6.60

AXA

Appendix B: Required Written Policies and Documentation

The following list provides examples of documentation to have readily accessible during the different elements of a survey. One document can address several requirements. You may find it useful to use this document as a checklist when preparing for survey.

While documentation is important, the primary emphasis of the survey is on how the practice carries out the functions described in the manual. The surveyors may use a combination of data sources, including interviews with leaders of the organization, staff, patients, and patient family members, visits to patient care settings; and review of documentation to arrive at an assessment of the organization's compliance with a standard.

For unannounced Medicare deemed-status surveys, the surveyors may request to review documentation while staff are informed of their arrival and gathered for the opening conference.

Note: *This is not an exhaustive list, nor should you create documentation that is not relevant for your organization. This list is meant to be a guide in preparing for a survey. To assist in identifying the correct materials for review, the list identifies issues in which the surveyors have an interest, as a result of the standards' requirements. The names and format of specific documents may vary from organization to organization.*

Standard	A	B	Description of Documentation Required	Examples of Typical Data Sources
Accreditation Participation Requirements (APR)				
APR 1		X	Official records and reports of all public or publicly recognized licensing, examining, reviewing, or planning bodies.	
APR 2		X	Copies of correspondence with the Joint Commission indicating changes in ownership, control, location, capacity, category of services offered, and any mergers or acquisitions.	
APR 4		X	Notice of Public Information Interview (PII).	Joint Commission form
APR 5		X	Copies of written requests to participate in PIIs that the organization received.	
APR 7		X	Providing accurate representation of accreditation status.	Marketing aterials if any
Practice Ethics, and Patient Rights and Responsibilities (RI)				
RI.1.10		X	Business practices	Marketing materials
RI.1.20		X	Conflicts of interest	Patient's rights document
RI.1.30	X		Decisions based on patient care, treatment, and services	

A = Required Written Policy/Procedures
B = Required Written Documentation *(e.g. in the patient's chart, handout, policy, procedure, etc.)*

AXB

Standard	A	B	Description of Documentation Required	Examples of Typical Data Sources
RI.2.10		X	Policies addressing patient rights	Patient's rights document
RI.2.30		X	Patient participation in the decisions of care, treatment, and services provided	
RI.2.40	X		Policies addressing informed consent	Patient's rights document
RI.2.40		X	Informed consent documented	Chart
RI.2.60		X	Information regarding person responsible for care, treatment, and services	Organization Form
RI.2.70		X	Patient's rights to refuse care, treatment, and services	Patient's rights document
RI.2.100		X	Policy addressing patient's rights to effective communication	Patient's Rights Document
RI.2.120		X	Policy addressing the need for patient complaint resolution process	Patient's rights document
RI.2.180		X	Consent forms related to patient participation in research, investigation, or clinical trials	Chart
RI.3.10		X	Policy that defines the mechanism for communicating the responsibilities of patients	Organization Form
Provision of Care, Treatment, and Services (PC)				
PC.1.10	X		Written process that defines patient eligibility	
PC.2.130		X	Collecting information appropriate to patient's health status	Chart
PC.3.10		X	List of community agencies that serve abuse victims	
PC.3.230		X	Necessary diagnostic testing for determining patient's health care needs	Chart
PC.6.10		X	Procedures for providing patient with education and training specific to the patient's needs in the care, treatment, and services provided	Chart Organization materials
PC.8.10		X	Pain assessment and treatment	Chart
PC.9.10	X		Procedures for how to obtain blood components or blood products	
PC.13.20		X	Assessment information recorded	Chart
PC.13.30		X	Operative procedures and/or the administration of moderate or deep sedation or anesthesia are documented in the patients' record.	Chart

A = Required Written Policy/Procedures
B = Required Written Documentation *(e.g. in the patient's chart, handout, policy, procedure, etc.)*

AXB

Standard	A	B	Description of Documentation Required	Examples of Typical Data Sources
PC.13.40		X	Monitoring patients after the procedure and/or administration of moderate or deep sedation or anesthesia	Chart
PC.15.20		X	Written discharge instructions	Chart Organization form
PC.16.10	X		Written procedure to define the use of waived test results in patient care, treatment, and services	
PC.16.30		X	Documentation showing current competence for staff who perform waived testing	HR file
PC.16.40	X		Policies and procedures for waived testing	
PC.16.50	X		Written quality control plan for waived testing	
PC.16.60		X	Quality control test results and test results	Log book/chart
Medication Management (MM)				
MM.4.30	X		Policy addressing medication labeling	
MM.4.30		X	Medication labels	
MM.5.10	X		Policies addressing medication administration	
MM.7.40	X		Procedures for the use of investigational medications	
Surveillance, Prevention, and Control of Infection (IC)				
IC.1.10	X		Written IC Plan	
IC.2.10		X	Infection Surveillance data	
IC.4.10		X	Infection Control Interventions	
IC.5.10		X	Evaluating the effectiveness of IC intervention	
IC.9.10		X	Allocating adequate resources for the IC program	
Improving Practice Performance (PI)				
PI.1.10		X	Required Performance data	
PI.2.10		X	Analysis and related display of data	
PI.2.30		X	Documentation of a risk-reduction strategy to reduce the risks of sentinel events	
Practice Leadership (LD)				
LD.1.20	X		Definition of governance responsibilities	
LD.2.50		X	Operating budget and long-term capital expenditure plan, as appropriate	
LD.3.10		X	Vision, mission, and goal statements	
LD.3.50		X	Definition of the nature and scope of any services provided by consultation, contractual arrangements, or other agreements	Contracts

A = **Required Written Policy/Procedures**
B = **Required Written Documentation** *(e.g. in the patient's chart, handout, policy, procedure, etc.)*

Standard	A	B	Description of Documentation Required	Examples of Typical Data Sources
LD.3.90	X		Policies that guide and support patient care, treatment, and services	
LD.4.20		X	Designing new or modified services of processes—testing and analysis	Meeting minutes
LD.4.40		X	Reports on the organization's patient safety program	
LD.5.50		X	Clinical practice guidelines	
Management of the Environment of Care (EC)				
EC.1.20		X	Maintaining a safe environment	Minutes, notes, organization forms
EC.1.30	X		Policy addressing smoking	
EC.4.10		X	Written emergency management plan	
EC.4.20		X	Performing drills to test emergency management plan	
EC.5.10		X	Written fire safety management plan	
EC.5.20		X	Statement of Conditions or equivalency when required	Statement of Conditions
EC.5.30		X	Evaluating the effectiveness of fire-response training	
EC.5.40		X	Documentation of testing of fire safety equipment and building features	
EC.6.10		X	Written medical equipment management plan	
EC.6.20		X	Inventory of medical equipment management and documentation of safety and performance testing as specified	
EC.7.10		X	Written utility management plan	
EC.7.30		X	Inventory of operating components of the utility management system	
EC.7.40		X	Maintaining and testing emergency electrical power system	
EC.8.10	X		Maintaining an appropriate environment for the patient's care, treatment, and services	
Management of Human Resources (HR)				
HR.1.20		X	Defined job qualifications	
HR.2.10		X	Documentation of each person's competency upon completion of orientation	
HR.3.10		X	Assessing and maintaining staff members' job competence	
HR.4.10		X	Credentialing information as specified	

A = Required Written Policy/Procedures
B = Required Written Documentation *(e.g. in the patient's chart, handout, policy, procedure, etc.)*

Standard	A	B	Description of Documentation Required	Examples of Typical Data Sources
HR.4.20		X	Criteria for determining licensed independent practitioners' clinical privileges	
HR.4.60		X	Reverification of credentialing information	
Management of Information (IM)				
IM.6.10 Through 6.30		X	Medical records—documentation as specified	Chart
IM.6.50	X		Policy designating who is authorized to receive and record verbal orders	

A = Required Written Policy/Procedures
B = Required Written Documentation *(e.g. in the patient's chart, handout, policy, procedure, etc.)*

Glossary

abuse Intentional maltreatment of an individual that may cause injury, either physical or psychological. *See also* neglect.

mental abuse Includes humiliation, harassment, and threats of punishment or deprivation.

physical abuse Includes hitting, slapping, pinching, or kicking. Also includes controlling behavior through corporal punishment.

sexual abuse Includes sexual harassment, sexual coercion, and sexual assault.

accountability *See* information management.

accreditation Determination by the Joint Commission's accrediting body that an eligible health care practice complies with applicable Joint Commission standards. *See also* accreditation decisions.

accreditation cycle A period of accreditation at the conclusion of which, accreditation expires unless a full survey is performed.

accreditation decisions Categories of accreditation that a practice can achieve based on a Joint Commission full survey. These decision categories are:

Accredited The organization is in compliance with all standards at the time of the on-site survey or has successfully addressed all requirements for improvement (*see* definition), in an Evidence of Standards Compliance (*see* definition), within 90 days following the survey (45 days beginning July 1, 2005).

Provisional Accreditation The organization fails to successfully address all requirements for improvement in an Evidence of Standards Compliance within 90 days following the survey (45 days beginning July 1, 2005).

Conditional Accreditation The organization is not in substantial compliance with the standards, as usually evidenced by a count of the number of standards identified as not compliant at the time of survey which is between two and three standard deviations above the mean number of noncompliant standards for organizations in that accreditation program. The organization must remedy identified problem areas through preparation and submission of a plan of correction and subsequently undergo an on-site, follow-up survey.

Preliminary Denial of Accreditation There is justification to deny accreditation to the organization, as usually evidenced by a count of the number of noncompliant standards at the time of survey that is at least three standard deviations above the mean number of noncompliant standards for organizations in that accreditation program. The decision is subject to appeal prior to the determination to deny accreditation; the appeal process may also result in a decision other than Denial of Accreditation.

Denial of Accreditation The organization has been denied accreditation. All review and appeal opportunities have been exhausted.

Preliminary Accreditation The organization demonstrates compliance with selected standards in the first of two surveys conducted under the Early Survey Policy Option 1 (*see* Early Survey Policy).

accreditation process A continuous process whereby health care organizations are required to demonstrate to the Joint Commission that they are providing safe, high-quality care, as determined by compliance with Joint Commission standards, National Patient Safety Goals recommendations, and performance measurement requirements. Key components of this process are an on-site evaluation of a practice by Joint Commission surveyors, a Periodic Performance Review, and quarterly submission of performance measurement data to the Joint Commission, as applicable.

Accreditation Report A report of a practice's survey findings; the report includes practice strengths, requirements for improvement (*see* definition), and supplemental findings (*see* definition), as appropriate.

accreditation survey findings Findings from an on-site evaluation conducted by Joint Commission's surveyors that results in a practice's accreditation decision.

administration **1.** The fiscal and general management of a practice, as distinct from the direct provision of services. **2.** *See* medication management, administration.

admitting Acceptance of a patient to the health care setting or service.

admitting privileges Authority issued to admit individuals to an office-based surgery practice. Individuals with admitting privileges may practice only within the scope of the clinical privileges granted by the practice's governing body.

advance directive A document or documentation allowing a person to give directions about future medical care or to designate another person(s) to make medical decisions if the individual loses decision-making capacity. Advance directives may include living wills, durable powers of attorney, do-not-resuscitate (DNR) orders, right to die, or similar documents listed in the Patient Self-Determination Act, which express the patient's preferences.

advanced practice nurse A registered nurse who has gained additional knowledge and skills through successful completion of an organized program of nursing education that prepares nurses for advanced practice roles and has been certified by the Board of Nursing to engage in the practice of advanced practice nursing.

adverse drug event A patient injury resulting from a medication, either because of a pharmacological reaction to a normal dose, or because of a preventable adverse reaction to a drug resulting from an error.

adverse drug reaction (ADR) Unintended, undesirable, or unexpected effects of prescribed medications or of medication errors that require discontinuing a medication or modifying the dose; require initial or prolonged hospitalization; result in disability; require treatment with a prescription medication; result in cognitive deterioration or impairment; are life threatening; result in death; or result in congenital anomalies.

advocate A person who represents the rights and interests of another individual as though they were the person's own, to realize the rights to which the individual is entitled, obtain needed services, and remove barriers to meeting the individual's needs. *See also* surrogate decision maker.

ambulatory health care All types of health services provided to individuals on an outpatient basis. Ambulatory care services are provided in many settings ranging from freestanding ambulatory surgical facilities to cardiac catheterization centers.

ambulatory health care occupancy *See* occupancy.

analyzing *See* information management.

anesthesia and sedation The administration to an individual, in any setting, for any purpose, by any route, of medication to induce a partial or total loss of sensation for the purpose of conducting an operative or other procedure. Definitions of four levels of sedation and anesthesia include the following:

minimal sedation (anxiolysis) A drug-induced state during which patients respond normally to verbal commands. Although cognitive function and coordination might be impaired, ventilatory and cardiovascular functions are unaffected.

moderate sedation/analgesia (conscious sedation) A drug-induced depression of consciousness during which patients respond purposefully to verbal commands, either alone or accompanied by light tactile stimulation. Reflex withdrawal from a painful stimulus is not considered a purposeful response. No interventions are required to maintain a patent airway, and spontaneous ventilation is adequate. Cardiovascular function is usually maintained.

deep sedation/analgesia A drug-induced depression of consciousness during which patients cannot be easily aroused, but respond purposefully following repeated or painful stimulation. The ability to independently maintain ventilatory function might be impaired. Patients might require assistance in maintaining a patent airway and spontaneous ventilation might be inadequate. Cardiovascular function is usually maintained.

anesthesia Consists of general anesthesia and spinal or major regional anesthesia. It does not include local anesthesia. General anesthesia is a drug-induced loss of consciousness during which patients are not arousable, even by painful stimulation. The ability to independently maintain ventilatory function is often impaired. Patients often require assistance in maintaining a patent airway, and positive pressure ventilation might be required because of depressed spontaneous ventilation or drug-induced depression of neuromuscular function. Cardiovascular function might be impaired.

anesthetic gases Any gas delivered through the respiratory system as a component of general anesthesia or sedation. This may include inhalation anesthetics distributed in liquid form that when vaporized produce an anesthetic gas (for example, isoflurane, sevoflurane) or nonliquid compressed gases (for example, nitrous oxide). Oxygen is not included in this definition.

anesthetizing location Any area used for the administration of anesthetic agents.

appeal proces The process afforded to a practice that receives a Preliminary Denial of Accreditation (*see* accreditation decisions), which includes the practice having a right to make a presentation to a Review Hearing Panel (*see* definition) before the Accreditation Committee takes final action to deny accreditation.

assessment **1.** For purposes of patient assessment, the process established by a practice for obtaining appropriate and necessary information about each individual seeking entry into a health care setting or service. The information is used to match an individual's need with the appropriate setting, care level, and intervention. **2.** For purposes of performance improvement, the systematic collection and review of patient-specific data.

auditability *See* information management.

authenticate To verify that an entry is complete, accurate, and final.

authentication *See* information management.

best practices Clinical, scientific, or professional practices that are recognized by a majority of professionals in a particular field. These practices are typically evidence based and consensus driven.

biologicals Medicines made from living organisms and their products, including serums, vaccines, antigens, and antitoxins.

blood component A fraction of separated whole blood, for example, red blood cells, plasma, platelets, and granulocytes.

blood derivative A pooled blood product, such as albumin, gamma globulin, or Rh immune globulin, whose use is considered significantly lower in risk than that of blood or blood components.

blood transfusion services Services relating to transfusing and infusing individuals with blood, blood components, or blood derivatives.

blood usage measurement An activity that entails measuring, assessing, and improving the ordering, distributing, handling, dispensing, administering, and monitoring of blood and blood components.

business occupancy *See* occupancy.

bylaws A governance framework that establishes the roles and responsibilities of a body and its members.

capture *See* information management.

care plan A written plan, based on data gathered during assessment, that identifies care needs, describes the strategy for providing services to meet those needs, documents treatment goals and objectives, outlines the criteria for terminating specified interventions, and documents the progress in meeting goals and objectives. The format of the plan in some practices may be guided by patient-specific policies and procedures, protocols, practice guidelines, clinical paths, care maps, or a combination thereof. The care plan may include care, treatment, habilitation, and rehabilitation.

care planning (or planning of care) Individualized planning and provision of services that addresses the needs, safety, and well-being of a patient. The plan, which formulates strategies, goals, and objectives, may include narratives, policies and procedures, protocols, practice guidelines, clinical paths, care maps, or a combination of these.

CLIA '88 The Clinical Laboratory Improvement Amendments of 1988.

clinical privileges Authorization granted by the appropriate authority (for example, the governing body) to a practitioner to provide specific care, treatment, or services in a practice within well-defined limits, based on the following factors, as applicable: license, education, training, experience, competence, health status, and judgment.

clinical record *See* record.

clinical/service groups (CSGs) Groups of patients in distinct, clinical populations for which data are collected. Tracer patients are selected according to CSGs.

community The individuals, families, groups, agencies, facilities, or institutions within the geographic area served by a health care organization.

competence or competency A determination of an individual's skills, knowledge, and capability to meet defined expectations.

compliance with a standard (*see* definition) Meeting the requirements of a standard through compliance with its element(s) of performance.

component A health care delivery entity (for example, service, program, related entity) that meets survey eligibility criteria under one of the the Joint Commission accreditation programs. Multiple components comprise a complex organization.

confidentiality An individual's right, within the law, to personal and informational privacy, including his or her health care records. *See also* information management.

consultation **1.** Provision of professional advice or services. **2.** For purposes of Joint Commission accreditation, advice that is given to staff members of surveyed practices relating to compliance with standards that are the subject of the survey.

consultation report **1.** A written opinion by a consultant that reflects, when appropriate, an examination of the individual and the individual's medical record(s). **2.** Information given verbally by a consultant to a care provider that reflects, when appropriate, an examination of the individual. The individual's care provider usually documents those opinions in the clinical/case record.

continuing care Care provided over time; in various settings, programs, or services; spanning the illness-to-wellness continuum.

continuing education Education beyond initial professional preparation that is relevant to the type of care delivered in a practice, that provides current knowledge relevant to an individual's field of practice or service responsibilities, and that might be related to findings from performance-improvement activities.

continuity The degree to which the care of individuals is coordinated among practitioners, among practices, and over time.

contract A formal agreement for care, treatment, or services with any practice, agency, or individual that specifies the services, personnel, products, or space provided by, to, or on behalf of the practice and specifies the consideration to be expended in exchange. The agreement is approved by the governing body or comparable entity.

contracted services Services provided through a written agreement with another practice, agency, or individual. The agreement specifies the services or personnel to be provided on behalf of the applicant practice and the fees to provide these services or personnel.

control chart A graphic display of data in the order they occur with statistically determined upper and lower limits of expected common-cause variation. A control chart is used to identify special causes of variation, to monitor a process for maintenance, and to determine whether process changes have had the desired effect.

control limit In statistics, an expected limit of common-cause variation, sometimes referred to as either an upper or a lower limit. Variation beyond a control limit is evidence that special causes are affecting a process. Control limits are calculated from process data and are not to be confused with engineering specifications or tolerance limits. Control limits are typically plotted on a control chart.

coordination of care The process of coordinating care, treatment, or services provided by a health care organization, including referral to appropriate community resources and liaison with others (such as the individual's physician, other health care organizations, or community services involved in care, treatment, or services) to meet the ongoing identified needs of individuals, to ensure implementation of the plan of care, and to avoid unnecessary duplication of services.

credentialing The process of obtaining, verifying, and assessing the qualifications of a health care practitioner to provide patient care services in or for a health care organization.

credentials Documented evidence of licensure, education, training, experience, or other qualifications.

criteria 1. Expected level(s) of achievement, or specifications against which performance or quality can be compared. 2. For purposes of eligibility for a Joint Commission survey, the conditions necessary for health care organizations and networks to be surveyed for accreditation by the Joint Commission.

data *See* information management.

decentralized laboratory testing *See* point-of-care testing.

decentralized pharmaceutical services *See* pharmaceutical care and services.

deemed status Status conferred by the Centers for Medicare & Medicaid Services (CMS) on a health care provider when that provider is judged or determined to be in compliance with relevant Medicare Conditions of Participation because it has been accredited by a voluntary organization whose standards and survey process are determined by CMS to be equivalent to those of the Medicare program or other federal laws, such as the Clinical Laboratory Improvement Amendments of 1988 (CLIA '88).

delineation of clinical privileges The listing of the specific clinical privileges an organization's staff member is permitted to perform in the organization.

dental services Services provided by a dentist, or a qualified individual under the supervision of a dentist, to improve or maintain the health of an individual's teeth, oral cavity, and associated structures.

dentist An individual who has received the degree of either doctor of dental surgery or doctor of dental medicine and who is licensed to practice dentistry.

disaster *See* emergency.

disaster plan *See* emergency management plan.

discharge The point at which an individual's active involvement with an organization or program is terminated and the organization or program no longer maintains active responsibility for the care of the individual.

discharge planning A formalized process in a health care organization through which the need for a program of continuing and follow-up care is ascertained and, if warranted, initiated for each patient.

disinfection The use of a chemical procedure that eliminates virtually all recognized pathogenic microorganisms but not necessarily all microbial forms (e.g. bacterial endospores) on inanimate objects.

dispensing *See* medication management, pharmacy services.

drug *See* medication.

drug administration *See* medication management.

drug allergies A state of hypersensitivity induced by exposure to a particular drug antigen resulting in harmful immunologic reactions on subsequent drug exposures, such as a penicillin drug allergy. *See also* medication.

drug dispensing *See* medication management.

e-App The electronic version of an organization's application for accreditation.

Early Survey Policy A policy that provides two options to organizations undergoing their first Joint Commission survey. Under both options, the organization undergoes two surveys. Under the first option, the first survey is limited in scope and successful completion results in Preliminary Accreditation (*see* accreditation decisions). Under the second option, the first survey is a full survey, and successful completion can lead to the organization being Accredited (*see* accreditation decisions). The second survey in both options is required and addresses all standards and a 4-month track record of compliance with the standards.

effectiveness The degree to which care is provided in the correct manner, given the current state of knowledge, to achieve the desired or projected outcome(s) for the individual.

efficacy The degree to which the care of the individual has been shown to accomplish the desired or projected outcome(s).

efficiency The relationship between the outcomes (results of care) and the resources used to deliver care.

electronic health information *See* information management.

elements of performance (EPs) The specific performance expectations , structures or

GL

processes that must be in place for an organization to provide safe, high-quality care, treatment, and services.

emergency 1. An unexpected or sudden occasion, as in emergency surgery needed to prevent death or serious disability. 2. A natural or man-made event that significantly disrupts the environment of care (for example, damage to the organization's building(s) and grounds due to severe winds, storms, or earthquakes); that significantly disrupts care and treatment (for example, loss of utilities such as power, water, or telephones due to floods, civil disturbances, accidents, or emergencies in the organization or its community); or that results in sudden, significantly changed or increased demands for the organization's services (for example, bioterrorist attack, building collapse, or plane crash in the organization's community). Some emergencies are called *disasters* or *potential injury creating events* (PICEs).

emergency, life-threatening A situation (e.g., major trauma, neck injury) in which an individual might require resuscitation or other support to sustain life.

emergency, medical A situation (e.g., major trauma, neck injury) in which an individual might require resuscitation or other support to sustain life.

emergency management plan The organization's written document describing the process it would implement for managing the consequences of natural disasters or other emergencies that could disrupt the organization's ability to provide care, treatment, and services. The plan identifies specific procedures that describe mitigation, preparedness, response and recovery strategies, actions, and responsibilities. *See also* emergency, mitigation activities, preparedness activities.

endemic infection *See* infection, endemic infection.

entry The process by which an individual comes into a setting, including screening and/or assessment by the organization or the practitioner, to determine the capacity of the organization or practitioner to provide the care or services required to meet the individual's needs.

environmental tours Activities routinely used by the organization to determine the presence of unsafe conditions and whether the organization's current processes for managing environmental safety risks are being practiced correctly and are effective.

epidemic infection *See* infection, epidemic infection.

equipment management Activities selected and implemented by the organization to assess and control the clinical and physical risks of fixed and portable equipment used for diagnosis, treatment, monitoring, and care.

evidence-based guidelines Guidelines that have been scientifically developed based on current literature and are consensus driven. These are also referred to as National Guidelines or Professional Guidelines.

Evidence of Standards Compliance (ESC) report A report submitted by a surveyed organization within 45 days (90 days between January 1, 2004, and June 30, 2005) of its survey, which details the action(s) that it took to bring itself into compliance with a standard or clarifies why the organization believes that it was in compliance with the standard for which it received a requirement for improvement. An ESC report must address compliance at the element of performance (EP) level and include a measurement of success (MOS) (*see* definition) for all appropriate EP corrections.

exploitation Taking unjust advantage of another for one's own advantage or benefit.

failure modes and effect analysis *See* risk assessment, proactive.

family The person(s) who plays a significant role in an individual's life. This may include a person(s) not legally related to the individual. This person(s) is often referred to as a surrogate decision maker if authorized to make care decisions for the individual should he or she lose decision-making capacity. *See also* guardian; surrogate decision maker.

fire safety management Activities selected and implemented by the organization to assess and control the risks of fire, smoke, and other byproducts of combustion that could occur during the organization's provision of care, treatment, or services.

governance The individual(s), group, or agency that has ultimate authority and responsibility for establishing policy, maintaining quality of care, and providing for organization management and planning.

Other names for this group include the board, board of trustees, board of governors, and board of commissioners.

guardian A parent, trustee, conservator, committee, or other individual or agency empowered by law to act on behalf of or be responsible for an individual. *See also* family; surrogate decision maker.

hazard vulnerability analysis The identification of potential emergencies and the direct and indirect effects these emergencies might have on the health care organization's operations and the demand for its services.

hazardous condition Any set of circumstances (exclusive of the disease, disorder, or condition for which the patient is undergoing care, treatment, or services) defined by the organization that significantly increases the likelihood of a serious adverse outcome.

hazardous materials and waste Materials whose handling, use, and storage are guided or defined by local, state, or federal regulation (for example, the Occupational Safety and Health Administration's Regulations for Bloodborne Pathogens regarding the disposal of blood and blood-soaked items; the Nuclear Regulatory Commission's regulations for the handling and disposal of radioactive waste), hazardous vapors (for example, gluteraldehyde, ethylene oxide, nitrous oxide), and hazardous energy sources (for example, ionizing or nonionizing radiation, lasers, microwave, ultrasound). Although the Joint Commission considers infectious waste as falling into this category of materials, federal regulations do not define infectious or medical waste as hazardous waste.

hazardous materials and waste management Activities selected and implemented by the organization to assess and control occupational and environmental hazards of materials and waste that require special handling. *See also* hazardous materials and waste.

health care occupancy *See* occupancy.

high-complexity test A test that meets CLIA '88 requirements based on personnel with specialized scientific and technical knowledge, specialized training, and substantial experience to perform the test; possibly labile reagents and materials that might require special handling to ensure reliability and reagents and materials preparation that might include manual steps; operational steps in the testing process that require close monitoring or control and may require special specimen preparation, precise temperature control or timing of procedural steps, accurate pipetting, or extensive calculations; and calibration, quality control, and proficiency testing of materials that may not be available or may be labile. In these tests, troubleshooting is not automatic and requires decision-making and direct intervention to resolve most problems; maintenance requires special knowledge, skills, and abilities. Extensive independent interpretation and judgment are required to perform preanalytic, analytic, and postanalytic processes, and resolution of problems requires extensive interpretation and judgment.

human subject research The use of individuals in the systematic study, observation, or evaluation of factors on preventing, assessing, treating, and understanding an illness. The term applies to all behavioral and medical experimental research that involves human beings as experimental subjects.

indicator A measure used to determine, over time, an organization's performance of functions, processes, and outcomes.

infection The transmission of a pathogenic microorganism to a host, with subsequent invasion and multiplication, with or without resulting symptoms of

- **endemic infection** The usual level or presence of an agent or disease in a defined population during a defined period.
- **epidemic infection** A higher than expected level of infection by a common agent in a defined population during a defined period.
- **health care–acquired infection** An infection acquired while receiving care or services in the health care organization.

infection control program Organized system of services designed to meet the needs of the organization or individual in relation to the surveillance, prevention, and control of infection.

information management Terms applicable to information management functions:

- **accountability** All information is attributable to its source (person or device).
- **analyzing** The process that interprets data and transforms it into information.

GL

auditability The capability to do a methodical examination and verification of all information activities such as entering and accessing.

authentication The validation of correctness for both the information itself and the person who is the author or user of the information.

capture The process of recording representations of human thought, perceptions, or actions, as well as device-generated data or information that is gathered and/or computed about a patient as part of a health care encounter or about other matters in a health care organization.

confidentiality The safekeeping of data/information so as to restrict access to individuals who have need, reason, and permission for such access.

data Uninterpreted observations or facts.

electronic health information A computerized format of the health care information in paper records that is used for the same range of purposes as paper records, namely to familiarize readers with the patient's status; to document care, treatment, and services; to plan for discharge; to document the need for care, treatment, and services; to assess the quality of care, treatment, and services; to determine reimbursement rates; to justify reimbursement claims; to pursue clinical or epidemiological research; and to measure outcomes of the care, treatment, and service process.

integrity In the context of data security, data integrity means the protection of data from accidental or unauthorized intentional change.

interactive text A more complex version of structured text, as it interactively prompts and provides feedback to the person using it. Typically, it uses a higher level of computer intelligence that interacts with the person who records information.

interoperability Enables authorized users to capture, share, and report information from any system, whether paper based or electronic based.

knowledge-based information A collection of stored facts, models, and information that can be used for designing and redesigning processes and for problem solving. In the context of the manual, knowledge-based information is found in the clinical, scientific, and management literature.

nonrepudiation The inability to dispute a document's content or authorship.

privacy An individual's right to limit the disclosure of personal information.

processing The manipulation of data and information by editing and updating.

protected health information Health information that contains information such that an individual person can be identified as the subject of that information.

report generation The process of analyzing, organizing, and presenting recorded information for authentication and inclusion in the patient's health care record or in financial or business records.

retrievability The capability of efficiently finding relevant information.

security The protection of data from intentional or unintentional destruction, modification, or disclosure.

structured text A process that requires authors to put specific information into specific fields with passive guidance by the information system. In paper-based systems, a form encourages a practitioner to fill in fields or boxes. Electronic systems use the same principle for templates or macros, which are guides used to create standardized information documentation. The purpose is to produce data of more consistent quality, make information more usable for decision support, make information more complete and more easily retrievable, and save documentation time.

timeliness The time between the occurrence of an event and the availability of data about the event. Timeliness is related to the use of the data.

transmission The sending of data and information from one location to another.

informed consent Agreement or permission accompanied by full notice about what is being consented to. A patient must be apprised of the nature, risks, and alternatives of a medical procedure or treatment before the physician or other health care professional begins any such course. After receiving this information, the patient then either consents to or refuses such a procedure or treatment.

initial survey An accreditation survey of a health care organization not previously accredited by the Joint Commission, or an accreditation survey of an organization performed without reference to any prior survey findings.

integrity *See* information management.

interactive text *See* information management.

interdisciplinary Communication; discussion; planning; evaluation; and care, treatment, and service activities that occur formally and informally between and among team members who are representatives of multiple disciplines.

interim life safety measures (ILSM) A series of 11 administrative actions intended to temporarily compensate for significant hazards posed by existing National Fire Protection Association 101® 2000 *Life Safety Code*® (*LSC*)* deficiencies or construction activities. See also *Life Safety Code*®; fire safety management.

interoperability *See* information management.

intravenous (IV) admixture The preparation of pharmaceutical product that requires the measured addition of a medication to a 50ml or greater bag or bottle of IV fluid (e.g., IV, IM, IT, SC, etc.). It does not include the drawing-up of medications into a syringe for immediate use (i.e., reconstitution) or the assembly and activation of an IV system that does not involve the measurement of the additive.

invasive procedure A procedure involving puncture or incision of the skin, or insertion of an instrument or foreign material into the body.

investigational medication A medication or placebo used as part of a research protocol or clinical trial.

Joint Commission on Accreditation of Healthcare Organizations An independent, not-for-profit organization dedicated to improving the quality of care in organized health care settings. Founded in 1951, its members represent the American College of Physicians-American Society of Internal Medicine, the American College of Surgeons, the American Dental Association, the American Hospital Association, the American Medical Association, the public, and the nursing profession. The Joint Commission engages in issues and activities concerning the advancement of health care safety and quality, including public policy initiatives, standards development, and accreditation and certification programs.

knowledge-based information *See* information management.

laboratory *See* pathology and clinical laboratory services.

leader An individual who sets expectations, develops plans, and implements procedures to assess and improve the quality of the organization's governance, management, clinical, and support functions and processes. Leaders include, when applicable to the organization's structure, the owners, members of the governing body, the chief executive officer, director of nursing, medical director, and other senior managers, and the leaders of the licensed independent practitioners.

licensed independent practitioner Any individual permitted by law and by the organization to provide care and services, without direction or supervision, within the scope of the individual's license.

licensure A legal right that is granted by a government agency in compliance with a statute governing an occupation (such as medicine, nursing, psychiatry, or clinical social work) or the operation of an activity (such as in a long term care or residential treatment center).

***Life Safety Code*® (*LSC*)** A set of standards for the construction and operation of buildings, intended to provide a reasonable degree of safety to life during fires; prepared, published, and periodically revised by the National Fire Protection Association and adopted by the Joint Commission to evaluate health care organizations under its life-safety management program. *See also* interim life safety measures; fire safety management; occupancy.

life support equipment Any device used for the purpose of sustaining life and whose failure to perform its primary function, when used according to manufacturer's instructions

* *Life Safety Code*® is a registered trademark of the National Fire Protection Association, Quincy, MA.

and clinical protocol, leads to patient death in the absence of immediate intervention (examples include ventilators, anesthesia machines, and heart-lung bypass machines).

loss of protective reflexes An inability to handle secretions without aspiration or to maintain a patent airway independently.

measure of success (MOS) A numerical or quantifiable measure usually related to an audit that determines whether an action was effective and sustained due four months after Evidence of Standards Compliance (*See* definition) approval.

measurement The systematic process of data collection, repeated over time or at a single point in time.

medical equipment Fixed and portable equipment used for the diagnosis, treatment, monitoring, and direct care of individuals. *See also* equipment management.

medical history A component of the medical record consisting of an account of an individual's history, obtained whenever possible from the individual, and including at least the following information: chief complaint, details of the present illness or care needs, relevant history, and relevant inventory by body systems.

medical record *See* record.

medical record review The process of measuring, assessing, and improving the quality of medical record documentation, that is, the degree to which medical record documentation is accurate, complete, and performed in a timely manner. This process is carried out with the cooperation of relevant departments or services.

medication Any prescription medications; sample medications; herbal remedies; vitamins; nutriceuticals; over-the-counter drugs; vaccines; diagnostic and contrast agents used on or administered to persons to diagnose, treat, or prevent disease or other abnormal conditions; radioactive medications; respiratory therapy treatments; parenteral nutrition; blood derivatives; intravenous solutions (plain, with electrolytes and/or drugs); and any product designated by the Food and Drug Administration (FDA) as a drug. This definition of medication does not include enteral nutrition solutions (which are considered food products), oxygen, and other medical gases.

medication error Any preventable event that might cause inappropriate medication use or jeopardize patient safety. *See also* adverse drug reaction; sentinel event.

medication history A delineation of the drugs used by an individual (both past and present), including prescribed and unprescribed drugs and alcohol, along with any unusual reactions to those drugs. *See* medication.

medication management The process an organization uses to provide medication therapy to individuals served by the organization. The steps in the medication management process include:

> **selection** Safe and appropriate selection of medications available for prescribing, storage, and/or use in the organization.
>
> **procurement** The task of obtaining selected medications from a source outside the organization. It does not include obtaining a medication from the organization's own pharmacy, which is considered part of the ordering and dispensing processes.
>
> **storage** The task of appropriately maintaining a supply of medications on the organization's premises.
>
> **prescribing or ordering** Synonymous terms for when a licensed independent practitioner transmits a legal order or prescription to the organization directing the preparing, dispensing, and administering of a specific medication to a specific patient. It does not include requisitions for medication supplies.
>
> **transcribing** The process by which an order from a licensed independent practitioner is documented either in writing or electronically.
>
> **preparing** The compounding, manipulation, or other activity needed to get a medication ready for administration exactly as ordered by the licensed independent practitioner.
>
> **dispensing** Providing, furnishing, or otherwise making available a supply of medications to the individual for whom it was ordered or their representative by a licensed pharmacy according to a specific prescription or medication order, or by a licensed independent practitioner authorized by law

to dispense. Dispensing does not involve providing an individual a dose of medication previously dispensed by the pharmacy.

administration The provision of a prescribed and prepared dose of an identified medication to the individual for whom it was ordered to achieve its pharmacological effect. This includes directly introducing the medication into or onto the individual's body.

self-administration Independent use by a patient of a medication, including medications that may be held by the organization for independent use by the patient.

monitoring The ongoing evaluation of an individual to whom a medication was administered, to ascertain the effectiveness and efficacy of the medication therapy and prevent the occurrence of any serious adverse outcomes.

medication-management measurement The measurement, assessment, and improvement of the prescribing or ordering, preparing and dispensing, administering, and monitoring of medications.

mental abuse *See* abuse.

mission statement A written expression that sets forth the purpose of an organization or one of its components. The generation of a mission statement usually precedes the formation of goals and objectives.

mitigation activities Those activities an organization undertakes in attempting to lessen the severity and impact of a potential emergency. *See also* emergency.

moderate-complexity test A test that meets CLIA '88 requirements based on knowledge required to perform the test; minimal training and limited experience required to perform the test; reagents and materials that are generally stable and reliable and reagents and materials that are prepackaged, premeasured, or require no special handling, precautions, or storage conditions; operational steps that are either automatically executed or are easily controlled; and stable and readily available calibration, quality control, and proficiency testing materials. Test system troubleshooting is automatic or self-correcting, or is clearly described or requires minimal judgment. Equipment maintenance provided by the manufacturer is seldom needed, or can easily be performed. Minimal interpretation and judgment are required to perform preanalytic, analytic, and postanalytic processes and resolution of problems requires limited independent interpretation and judgment.

multidisciplinary team A group of clinical staff members composed of representatives of a range of professions, disciplines, or service areas.

near miss Used to describe any process variation that did not affect an outcome, but for which a recurrence carries a significant chance of a serious adverse outcome. Such a near miss falls within the scope of the definition of a sentinel event, but outside the scope of those sentinel events that are subject to review by the Joint Commission under its Sentinel Event Policy.

neglect The absence of minimal services or resources to meet basic needs. Neglect includes withholding or inadequately providing food and hydration (without physician, patient, or surrogate approval), clothing, medical care, and good hygiene. It may also include placing the individual in unsafe or unsupervised conditions. *See also* abuse.

nonrepudiation *See* information management.

nursing The health profession dealing with nursing care and services as (1) defined by the Code of Ethics for Nurses with Interpretive Statements, Nursing's Social Policy Statement, Nurses' Bill of Rights, Scope and Standards of Nursing Practice of the American Nurses Association and specialty nursing organizations; and (2) defined by relevant state, commonwealth, or territory nurse practice acts and other applicable laws and regulations.

nursing care Professional processes of assessment, diagnosis, planning, implementation, and evaluation based on the art and science of nursing to promote health, its recovery, or a peaceful and dignified death. This includes, but is not limited to, assisting individuals, families, communities, and/or populations in understanding health needs and carrying out therapeutic plans and activities.

nursing staff Personnel within a health care organization who are accountable for providing and assisting in the provision of nursing care. Such personnel must include registered nurses (RNs), and may include others such as advanced practice registered nurses (APRNs), licensed practical or vocational nurses (LPNs/LVNs), and nursing assistants or other designated unlicensed assistive personnel.

nutriceuticals Nutritional supplements formulated in a pharmaceutical dosage form and used with the intention of deriving medical or health benefits, including preventing and treating disease. Such products may range from isolated nutrients, dietary supplements, and diets to genetically engineered "designer" foods, herbal products, and processed foods such as cereals, soups, and beverages.

nutrition assessment A comprehensive process for defining an individual's nutrition and hydration status using medical, nutrition, and medication intake histories, physical examination, anthropomorphic measurements, and laboratory data.

nutrition care Interventions and counseling to promote appropriate nutrition and fluid intake, based on nutrition and hydration assessment and information about food, other sources of nutrients, and meal preparation consistent with the individual's cultural background and socioeconomic status. Nutrition therapy, a component of medical treatment, includes enteral and parenteral nutrition.

occupancy The purpose for which a building or portion there of is used or intended to be used.

> **ambulatory health care occupancy** An occupancy used to provide services or treatment to four or more patients at the same time that either (1) renders them incapable of providing their own means of self-preservation in an emergency or (2) provides outpatient surgical treatment requiring general anesthesia.
>
> **business occupancy** An occupancy used to provide outpatient care, treatment, or services that does not meet the criteria in the ambulatory health care occupancy definition (for example, three or fewer patients at the same time who are either rendered incapable of self-preservation in an emergency or are undergoing general anesthesia).
>
> **health care occupancy** An occupancy used for purposes such as medical or other treatment or care of persons suffering from physical or mental illness, disease or infirmity; and for the care of infants, convalescents, or infirm aged persons. Health care occupancies provide sleeping facilities for four or more occupants and are occupied by persons who are mostly incapable of self-preservation because of age, physical or mental disability, or because of security measures not under the occupant's control. Health care occupancies include hospitals, nursing homes, and limited care facilities.

office-based surgery Operative or invasive procedures that are performed in an office setting.

operative and other high-risk procedures Surgical or other procedures that put the patient at risk of death or disability. This does not include use of medications that place patients at risk.

oral and maxillofacial surgeon An individual who has successfully completed a postgraduate program in oral and maxillofacial surgery accredited by a nationally recognized accrediting body approved by the United States Department of Education. As determined by the medical staff, the individual is also currently competent to perform a complete history and physical examination in order to assess the medical, surgical, and anesthetic risks of the proposed operative and other procedure(s).

pathology and clinical laboratory services The services that provide information on diagnosis, prevention, or treatment of disease or the assessment of health, through the examination of the structural and functional changes in tissues and organs of the body that cause or are caused by disease. It also includes the biological, microbiological, serological, chemical, immunohematological, hematological, or other examination of materials derived from the human body.

patient An individual who receives care or services. For hospice providers, the patient and family are considered a single unit of care. Synonyms used by various health care fields include client, resident, customer, patient and family unit, consumer, and health care consumer.

patient tracer The process of evaluating a patient's total care experience within a health care organization.

performance improvement (PI) The continuous study and adaptation of an office-based surgery practice's functions and processes to increase the probability of achieving desired outcomes and to better meet the needs of individuals and other users of services.

pharmaceutical care and services Services provided directly or through written contract with another organization that include procuring, preparing, dispensing, and/or distributing pharmaceutical products and the ongoing monitoring of the recipient to identify, prevent, and resolve medication-related problems.

pharmaceutical equivalence The degree to which two formulations of the same medication are identical in strength, concentration, and dosage form.

pharmacy A licensed location where drugs are stored and dispensed.

pharmacy services The provision of pharmaceutical care and services involving the preparation and dispensing of medications, and medication-related devices and supplies by a licensed pharmacy, with or without the provision of clinical or consultant pharmacist services.

physical abuse *See* abuse.

physical restraint *See* restraint.

physician A doctor of medicine or doctor of osteopathy who, by virtue of education, training, and demonstrated competence, is granted clinical privileges by a practice to perform a specific diagnostic or therapeutic procedure(s) and who is fully licensed to practice medicine.

physician assistant An individual who practices medicine with supervision by licensed physicians, providing patients with services ranging from primary medicine to specialized surgical care. The scope of practice is determined by state law, the supervising physician's delegation of responsibilities, the individual's education and experience, and the specialty and setting in which the individual works.

physician licensure The process by which a legal jurisdiction, such as a state, grants permission to a physician to practice medicine after finding that he or she has met acceptable qualification standards. Licensure also involves ongoing regulation of physicians by the legal jurisdiction, including the authority to revoke or otherwise restrict a physician's license to practice.

plan A detailed method, formulated beforehand, that identifies needs, lists strategies to meet those needs, and sets goals and objectives. The format of a plan may include narratives, policies and procedures, protocols, practice guidelines, clinical paths, care maps, or a combination of these.

plan for improvement For purposes of Joint Commission accreditation, a practice's written statement that details the procedures to be taken and time frames to correct existing *Life Safety Code*® (LSC) deficiencies. *See also* Statement of Conditions™; interim life safety measures; *Life Safety Code*®.

plan of action A plan detailing the action(s) that a practice will take to come into compliance with a Joint Commission standard. A plan of action must be completed for each element of performance (EP) (*see* definition) associated with a not compliant standard. A measure of success (MOS) (*see* definition) must also be included in the plan of action as indicated in the accreditation manual.

podiatrist An individual who has received the degree of doctor of podiatry medicine and who is licensed to practice podiatry.

point-of-care testing (POCT) Analytical testing performed at sites outside the traditional laboratory environment, usually at or near where care is delivered to individuals. Testing may range from simple waived procedures, such as fecal occult blood, to more sophisticated chemical analyzers. The testing may be under the control of the main laboratory, the direction of another specialized laboratory (such as for arterial blood gas), or under the nursing service. Testing may be categorized as waived, moderate, or high complexity under CLIA '88. Also called alternate site testing, decentralized laboratory testing, and distributed site testing.

policies and procedures The formal, approved description of how a governance, management, or clinical care process is defined, organized, and carried out.

practice, office-based surgery An organization comprised of four or fewer surgeons (physician, dentist, or podiatrist) who perform operative or invasive procedures requiring the administration of local anesthesia, minimal sedation, conscious sedation, or general anesthesia. The practice must be surgeon owned or operated (e.g., a professional services corporation, private physician office, small group practice).

practice guidelines Tools that describe processes found by clinical trials or by consensus opinion of experts to be the most effective in evaluating and/or treating a patient who has a specific symptom, condition, or diagnosis, or describe a specific procedure. Synonyms include practice parameter, protocol, preferred practice pattern, and guideline.

practice's strengths Areas in which a practice's performance is exemplary, as evidenced by the implementation of innovative approaches to meeting Joint Commission standards. A practice will not be cited for having a strength if the practice has a related noncompliantstandard and/or partially compliant element of performance (EP).

practitioner Any individual who is qualified to practice a health care profession (for example, a physician or nurse) and is engaged in the provision of care, treatment, and services. Practitioners are often required to be licensed as defined by law.

Preliminary Denial of Accreditation *See* accreditation decisions.

preparedness activities Those activities a practice undertakes to build capacity and identify resources that can be used if an emergency occurs. *See also* emergency.

prescribing or ordering *See* medication management.

primary source The original source of a specific credential that can verify the accuracy of a qualification reported by an individual health care practitioner. Examples include medical school, graduate medical education program, and state medical board.

priority focus areas (PFAs) Processes, systems, or structures in a health care organization that significantly impact the quality and safety of care. The PFAs are:

- Assessment and care/services
- Communication
- Credentialed practitioners
- Equipment use
- Infection control
- Information management
- Medication management
- Organizational structure
- Orientation and training
- Patient safety
- Physical environment
- Quality improvement expertise and activity
- Rights and ethics
- Staffing

primary priority focus area Every standard is linked to one or more priority focus areas (PFAs). When a surveyor has findings under a standard, s/he determines which of the linked PFAs is most related to the specific finding—this becomes the *primary* PFAs. For example, a finding under standard HR.1.10 may be assigned a primary priority focus area of Staffing. The organization's accreditation report is organized by PFA.

secondary priority focus areas The additional priority focus areas (PFAs) that are also related to a specific finding, in addition to the primary PFA. For example, a finding under standard HR.1.10 may be assigned a secondary PFA of Orientation and Training. The organization's accreditation report also lists the secondary PFAs.

Priority Focus Process (PFP) The process for standardizing the priorities for sampling during a practice's survey based on information collected about the practice prior to survey. The process also helps to focus the survey on areas that are critical to that practice's patient safety and quality of care processes. Examples of such information may include, but not be limited to, data from the practice's e-App (*see* definition), complaint and sentinel event information, and previous survey results.

Priority Focus Tool (PFT) An automated tool that supports the Priority Focus Process (PFP) through the use of algorithms, or sets of rules, to transform an office-based surgery practice's data into information that guides the survey process.

privacy *See* information management.

privileging The process whereby a specific scope and content of patient care services (that is, clinical privileges) are authorized for a health care practitioner by an office-based surgery practice, based on evaluation of the individual's credentials and performance. *See* licensed independent practitioner.

processing *See* information management.

program An organized system of services designed to address the needs of the practice or individual.

protected health information *See* information management.

provisional accreditation *See* accreditation decisions.

Public Information Policy A Joint Commission policy governing the disclosure of specific information about the performance of an office-based surgery practice or network, as well as accreditation-related information that remains confidential. This policy covers the Joint Commission's Quality Reports, information publicly disclosed on request, complaint information, aggregate performance data, data released to government agencies, and the Joint Commission's right to clarify information an accredited practice releases about its accreditation status.

qualified individual An individual or staff member who is qualified to provide care, treatment, or services by virtue of the following: education, training, experience, competence, registration, certification,applicable licensure, or law or regulation. Examples of qualified individuals can include: activities coordinator, administrator, audiologist, child psychiatrist, clinical chaplain, creative arts therapist, dietetic services supervisor, dietitian, registered dietitian, health information administrator, health information technician, licensed practical nurse (LPN), medical radiation physician, medical technologist, music therapist, occupational therapist, occupational therapy assistant, physiatrist, physical therapist assistant, physical therapist, psychiatric nurse, psychologist, radiologic technologist, recreational therapist, recreational therapist assistant or technician, respiratory care technician, respiratory therapist, respiratory therapy technician, social work assistant, social worker, and speech-language pathologist.

qualified individual, infection control An individual who is qualified to participate in one or all of the mechanisms outlined in the standards by virtue of one or more of the following: education, training, certification or licensure, or experience. Certification by the Certification Board for Infection Control is often a requirement for infection control practitioners.

quality control A process that consists of measuring performance, comparing performance against goals, and acting on the differences when performance falls short of defined goals.

quality of care The degree to which health services for individuals and populations increase the likelihood of desired health outcomes and are consistent with current professional knowledge. Dimensions of performance include the following: patient perspective issues; safety of the care environment; and accessibility, appropriateness, continuity, effectiveness, efficacy, efficiency, and timeliness of care.

Quality Report A report that is available to the public that provides information about a practice's accreditation decision and the effective date for the decision, any special quality awards the practice received, the accreditation services included in the practice's accreditation award, any disease-specific care certification(s) and the effective date of each certification received by the practice, and the implementation of National Patient Safety Goals by the practice.

rationale for a standard Background, justification, or additional information about a standard. A rationale is not scored. Not every standard has a rationale.

reassessment Ongoing data collection, which begins on initial assessment, comparing the most recent data with the data collected at earlier assessments.

record **1.** The account compiled by physicians and other health care professionals of a variety of patient health information, such as assessment findings, treatment details, and progress notes. **2.** (data source) Data obtained from the records or documentation maintained on a patient in any health care setting (for example, hospital, home care, long term care, practitioner office). Includes automated and paper medical record systems.

referral The sending of an individual (1) from one clinician to another clinician or specialist, (2) from one setting or service to another, or (3) by one physician (the referring physician) to another physician(s) or other resource, either for consultation or care.

registered nurse An individual who is qualified by an approved postsecondary program or baccalaureate or higher degree in nursing and licensed by the state, commonwealth, or territory to practice professional nursing.

report generation *See* information management.

reprocessing All operations performed to render a contaminated reusable or single-use device patient ready. The steps may include cleaning and disinfection/sterilization. The manufacturer of reusable devices and single-use devices that are marketed as nonsterile should provide validated reprocessing instructions in the labeling.

requirement for improvement A survey finding cited in a practice's Accreditation Report that must be addressed in the organization's Evidence of Standards Compliance (ESC).

restraint Any method (chemical or physical) of restricting a patient's freedom of movement, including seclusion, physical activity, or normal access to his or her body that (1) is not a usual and customary part of a medical diagnostic or treatment procedure to which the patient or his or her legal representative has consented; (2) is not indicated to treat the patient's medical condition or symptoms; or (3) does not promote the patient's independent functioning.

chemical restraint The inappropriate use of a sedating psychotropic drug to manage or control behavior.

physical restraint Any method of physically restricting a person's freedom of movement, physical activity, or normal access to his or her body.

retrievability *See* information management.

Review Hearing Panel A panel of three individuals, including one member of the the Joint Commission Accreditation Committee, who hear a presentation on the facts of a case by a practice in Preliminary Denial of Accreditation, should the organization desire such a presentation.

risk assessment, proactive An assessment that examines a process in detail including sequencing of events; assesses actual and potential risk, failure, or points of vulnerability; and, through a logical process, prioritizes areas for improvement based on the actual or potential patient care impact (criticality).

risk-management activities Clinical and administrative activities that practices undertake to identify, evaluate, and reduce the risk of injury to patients, staff, and visitors and the risk of loss to the practice itself.

root cause analysis A process for identifying the basic or causal factor(s) that underlie variation in performance, including the occurrence or possible occurrence of a sentinel event.

run chart A display of data in which data points are plotted as they occur over time (for example, observed weights over time) to detect trends or other patterns and variation occurring over time. Run charts, as opposed to tabular frequency displays, are capable of time-order analytic studies.

safety The degree to which the risk of an intervention (for example, use of a drug or a procedure) and risk in the care environment are reduced for a patient and other persons, including health care practitioners.

safety management Activities selected and implemented by the practice to assess and control the impact of environmental risk, and to improve general environmental safety.

scope of care, treatment, and services The activities performed by governance, managerial, clinical, or support staff.

secure In locked containers, in a locked room, or under constant surveillance.

security *See* information management.

security management A component of a practice's management of the environment of care program that maintains and improves the general security of the care environment.

sentinel event An unexpected occurrence involving death or serious physical or psychological injury, or the risk thereof. Serious injury specifically includes lolimb or function. The phrase *or the risk thereof* includes any process variation for which a recurrence carries a significant chance of a serious adverse outcome.

sexual abuse *See* abuse.

Shared Visions–New Pathways® An initiative to progressively sharpen the focus of the accreditation process on care systems critical to the safety and quality of patient care.

staff Individuals, such as employees, contractors, or temporary agency personnel, who provide services in a practice.

staffing effectiveness The number, competence, and skill mix of staff as related to the provision of needed services.

standard A statement that defines the performance expectations, structures, or processes that must be in place for a practice to provide safe and high-quality care, treatment, and services.

Statement of Conditions™ (SOC) A proactive document that helps a practice do a critical self-assessment of its current level of compliance and describe how to resolve any *Life Safety Code®* (*LSC*) deficiencies. The SOC was created to be a "living, ongoing" management tool that should be used in a management process that continually identifies, assesses, and resolves *LSC* deficiencies.

sterilization The use of a physical or chemical procedure to destroy all microbial life, including highly resistant bacterial endospores.

structured text *See* information management.

supplemental finding A recommendation that is not required to be addressed in a practice's Evidence of Standards Compliance report (*see* definition), but should be addressed by the practice internally. A supplemental finding is also factored into a practice's priority focus process at its next survey.

surrogate decision maker Someone appointed to act on behalf of another. Surrogates make decisions only when an individual is without capacity or has given permission to involve others. *See also* advocate; family.

survey A key component in the accreditation process, whereby a surveyor(s) conducts an on-site evaluation of a practice's compliance with Joint Commission standards.

full survey A survey that assesses a practice's compliance with all applicable Joint Commission standards.

initial survey A survey of an office-based surgery practice not previously accredited by the Joint Commission, or a survey of a practice performed without reference to any prior survey findings.

surveyor For purposes of Joint Commission accreditation, a physician, nurse, administrator, laboratorian, or any other health care professional who meets the Joint Commission's surveyor selection criteria, evaluates standards compliance, and provides education and consultation regarding standards compliance to surveyed practices or networks.

system A set of interrelated parts that work together toward a common goal.

system tracer A session during the on-site survey devoted to evaluating high-priority safety and quality-of-care issues on a systemwide basis throughout a practice. Examples of such issues may include infection control, medication management, and the use of data.

systems analysis The evaluation of how well an office-based surgery practice's systems function.

threshold for Conditional Accreditation At least two, but not more than three, standard deviations above the mean number of not compliant standards; the threshold for Conditional Accreditation is one rule for receiving Conditional Accreditation.

threshold for Preliminary Denial of Accreditation At least three standard deviations above the mean number of not compliant standards; the threshold for Preliminary Denial of Accreditation is one rule for receiving Preliminary Denial of Accreditation.

timeliness *See* information management.

tracer methodology A process surveyors use during the on-site survey to analyze a practice's systems, with particular attention to identified priority focus areas, by following individual patients through the practice's health care process in the sequence experienced by the patients. Depending on the health care setting, this might require surveyors to visit multiple care units, departments, or areas within a practice or a single care unit to trace the care rendered to a patient.

transfer The formal shifting of responsibility for the care of an individual (1) from one care unit to another, (2) from one clinical service to another, (3) from one licensed independent practitioner to another, or (4) from one practice to another.

transfer agreement A written understanding that provides for the reciprocal transfer of individuals between health care organizations.

transmission *See* information management.

utilities management Activities selected and implemented by a practice to assess and control the risks of utility systems of buildings that support the provision of care, treatment, or services. Included are those activities that ensure the operational reliability of such systems and those activities for responding to a failure of such systems.

utility systems Building systems for life support; surveillance, prevention, and control of infection; environment support; and equipment support. May include electrical distribution; emergency power; vertical and horizontal transport; heating, ventilating, and air conditioning; plumbing, boiler, and steam; piped gases; vacuum systems; or communication systems including data-exchange systems.

waived testing Tests that meet the Clinical Laboratory Improvement Amendments of 1988 (CLIA '88) requirements for waived tests; are cleared by the Food and Drug Administration for home use; employ methodologies that are so simple and accurate as to render the likelihood of erroneous results negligible; or pose no risk of harm to the patient if the test is performed incorrectly. *See also* CLIA '88.

Index

This index is designed to help the user find items quickly and efficiently. The majority of entries are referenced to specific standards. The standards numbers are listed in parentheses before the page number references. For example, if you are looking for information on monitoring medications, you would look up "medication management" in this index. Under this heading you would find the sub-heading "administering" and be directed to standards MM.5.10 and MM.5.30 on page MM-12.

IX

IX

IX

IX

S

T

U

Joint Commission Resources Educational Products

The following is a list of publications from Joint Commission Resources that might be of interest to office-based surgery practices. These publications are intended to help you improve the quality of care and services your practice provides as well as to help you prepare for a Joint Commission survey. If you would like to receive a free Joint Commission Resources publications catalog or order one of the publications listed here, please call Joint Commission Resources' Customer Service toll free at 877/223-6866.

Patient Safety Resources

The Physician's Promise: Protecting Patients from Harm

The only book on sentinel events and error prevention written specifically for physicians, *The Physician's Promise* helps physicians learn how to:

- Become more involved in preventing and analyzing sentinel events without taking time away from patient care activities
- Identify the system failures that can cause sentinel events and near misses
- Standardize care protocols and improve communication of care plans to other staff
- Use technology to streamline care practices and reduce the potential for error
- Understand strategies that can prevent sentinel events from occurring within the system
- Use Joint Commission standards to further their own patient safety goals.

The Physician's Promise approaches the patient safety initiative from the unique perspective of physicians and addresses issues important to physicians, such as workload, time constraints, communication issues, and how to contribute to improving the systems in which their patients receive care.
2003. 170 pages.
ISBN: 0-86688-798-9
Price: $55 **Order Code: PPPH-02BDK**

Front Line of Defense: The Role of Nurses in Preventing Sentinel Events

Written especially for nurses in all disciplines and health care settings, *Front Line of Defense* devotes chapters to nine categories of sentinel events. Each chapter is full of examples of sentinel events and near misses within a variety of health care settings to help you identify the following:

- Possible root causes of sentinel events
- The nurse's role in the systems that can lead to sentinel events
- Strategies nurses can use to prevent sentinel events from occurring

Help create a safer, more efficient environment. Use these error prevention techniques to empower yourself and become a stronger advocate for those in your care!
2001. 153 pages.
ISBN: 0-86688-727-X
Price: $50 **Order Code: NSE-01BDK**

Root Cause Analysis in Health Care: Tools and Techniques, Second Edition

This new edition includes the following information:

- An increased focus on multiple and interrelated root causes
- Lessons learned from root cause analysis (RCA) use in health care
- Updated terms and definitions
- Tips from surveyors who conduct reviews of sentinel events and RCAs
- Updated versions of the Joint Commission's Sentinel Event Policy, Minimum Scope of Root Cause Analysis Table, and Framework for a Root Cause Analysis Action Plan

This new book updates the Joint Commission's framework for conducting an *RCA* on adverse events, near misses, and unexpected outcomes.

Root Cause Analysis in Health Care helps organizations do the following:

- Establish which problems call for *RCA*
- Conduct a thorough and credible *RCA*
- Interpret analysis results
- Analyze and implement an action plan for improvement
- Integrate *RCA* with other programs
- Use *RCA* proactively to prevent failures before they happen

2003. 214 pages.
ISBN: 0-86688-781-4
Price: $60 Order Code: RCA-200BDK

Failure Mode and Effects Analysis in Health Care: Proactive Risk Reduction

This book is designed to help health care organizations meet the Joint Commission's new proactive identification and management of potential risks requirement. Proactive approaches to patient safety have the obvious advantage of preventing adverse occurrences, rather than simply reacting when they occur.

Failure mode and effects analysis (FMEA) is a systematic way of examining a process prospectively for possible ways in which failure can occur.

Special features of *Failure Mode and Effects Analysis in Health Care* include the following:

- The first book written specifically about FMEA for health care
- Real examples of FMEAs conducted by health care organizations
- A step-by-step guide through the process in a logical manner
- Clear, helpful process summaries, tips, and keyword definitions

2002. 160 pages.
ISBN: 0-86688-758-X
Price: $60 Order Code: FMEA-01BDK

Sentinel Events: Evaluating Cause and Planning Improvement, Second Edition

Serious and undesirable events in health care organizations should trigger analysis and response to minimize the risk of recurrence. *Sentinel Events: Evaluating Cause and Planning Improvement* describes the types of errors and sentinel events that have been reported in health care organizations, how organizations can respond to these events, how sentinel events are investigated through root cause analysis, and the Joint Commission's policy on sentinel events.

Sentinel Events shows how to perform the following tasks:

- Respond immediately to a sentinel event
- Gather the right people for an event investigation
- Conduct a root cause analysis to uncover the system-based causes for an event
- Set priorities for improvement
- Design and implement those improvements
- Prevent sentinel events before the first occurrence through risk-reduction strategies

Several case studies and examples demonstrate successful event investigation and improvement efforts in health care organizations. Foreword by Troy Brennan, MD, JD.
1998. 175 pages.
ISBN: 0-86688-554-4
Price: $50 Order Code: SE-101BDK

Lessons in Patient Safety

Edited by Lorri Zipperer, MA, and Susan Cushman, MPH

This publication offers easy access to information about patient safety, including the study and experience of those in health care and other industries who help provide a road map for those who want to change systems and make them safer.

"In a relatively short time, any health professional or manager can become grounded in the basic concepts and learn a great deal about how to redesign systems for safety." (From the Foreword by Lucian Leape, MD.)
2001. 134 pages.
Price: $42.50 Order Code: LIP-01BDK

NEW! *Meeting the Joint Commission's 2005 National Patient Safety Goals*

Get the patient safety information you need in one easy-to-use format. Learn how to meet the Joint Commission's 2005 National Patient Safety Goals with these useful explanations, strategies, and tips. This convenient CD-ROM product is a compilation of valuable articles, useful tips, and suggestions for meeting the Joint Commission's National Patient Safety Goals.

This electronic toolbox is a compilation of previously published articles from various JCR publications providing detailed information on the following:

- Improving the effectiveness of communication among caregivers
- Improving the safety of using high-alert medications
- Improving the safety of using infusion pumps
- Reducing the risk of health care–associated infections
- New goals on reducing surgical fires
- New goal on reconciling medications

The CD-ROM provides easy navigation of this information with a linked table of contents through Adobe Acrobat. No new software to buy or download!
Available January 2005.
Price: $60 Order Code: NPSCD-05BDK

NEW! *Patient Safety Posters, 2nd edition*

Enhance your patient safety program!

Use these colorful posters to communicate and reinforce the importance of patient safety to staff!

Communicating to staff about important care issues can be challenging. Health care organizations can keep essential patient safety issues in the minds of their staff by posting colorful, informative posters throughout their organization. Each poster contains key messages or tips on important safety issues including the following:

- Preventing falls
- Preventing medication errors
- Safe medication use
- Preventing surgical mistakes
- Communication
- Anesthesia safety
- Infection control
- Fire safety
- Recognizing abuse
- Assessment

Special Features: These color-fast posters are easy to read—and make safety tips easy to remember! A great how-to tool for information for all staff. Posters are suitable for display alone or framing and are shipped in a protective canister. Each poster is glossy, full color, fade resistant, and attention-getting, on heavy 18" x 24" paper.
2005.

Price: $95 for 10-pack of posters. Posters not sold separately, only in sets of all 10.
Order Code: JCPST-05BDK

NEW! *Hand Hygiene Posters*

Easy reminders for staff about the importance of hand hygiene in preventing infections!

Use these four new posters to communicate the importance of hand hygiene to your health care staff. Posters can be displayed in nursing stations and staff washrooms to encourage staff to clean their hands to help prevent the spread of infections and improve patient safety.

Each poster covers a different aspect of hand hygiene, including the following:

- The human and monetary costs of infections
- The recommended amount of time to clean hands
- How and when to clean hands

Order multiple sets to place prominently in your organization. Each poster is bold and brightly colored to attract staff attention, with clever messages and catchy graphics to get the point across to your busy staff. Posters are 8.5" x 11" and printed on durable, splash-resistant, laminated paper.

Price: $20 for set of all 4. Posters sold only in sets of 4.
Order Code: INVPST-04BDK

NEW! *Meeting the Joint Commission's Infection Control Requirements: A Priority Focus Area*

Meeting the Joint Commission's Infection Control Requirements: A Priority Focus Area illustrates the growing crisis in infection control across the spectrum of health care organizations and how compliance with the Joint Commission's infection control standards can provide a solid structure and foundation to tackle key infection control issues.

Coinciding with the release of the Joint Commission's new infection control standards and the new infection control–related National Patient Safety Goal, this book provides timely and helpful information on the standards and their elements of performance, provides examples of compliance for all types of health care organizations, and includes a comprehensive description of the newest National Patient Safety Goal related to the reduction of health care–associated infections. Also featured is a foreword written by Dr. Dennis O'Leary, President of the Joint Commission on Accreditation of Healthcare Organizations.
2004. 150 pages.
ISBN: 0-86688-857-8
Price: $70 **Order Code: MICS-01BDK**

Universal Protocol for Preventing Wrong Site, Wrong Procedure, Wrong Person Surgery: Brochure and Poster Products

Wrong site, wrong procedure, and wrong person surgery can be prevented. This universal protocol is intended to achieve that goal. It is based on the consensus of experts from the relevant clinical specialties and professional disciplines and is endorsed by more than 40 professional medical associations and organizations.

Purchase brochures that provide patients tips for preparing for surgery. Posters are available to provide guidance on preventing wrong site, wrong procedure, and wrong person surgery.

Brochure (Quantity of 100)
Price: $25.00 **Order Code: UPBR04BDK**

Poster (Quantity of 3)
Price: $10.00 **Order Code: UPPST04BDK**

Quality Improvement Resources

NEW! *Tracer Methodology: Tips and Strategies for Continuous Systems Improvement*

With its new accreditation process, Shared Visions–New Pathways®, the Joint Commission asks health care organizations to move beyond viewing the on-site survey as an activity to achieve a score to a continuous systems improvement approach where organizations are constantly improving the quality of care and patient safety. As a result, accreditation becomes the logical result of such continuous improvement efforts. An integral component of Shared Visions–New Pathways is the tracer methodology. By tracing areas of care within the organization with the use of tracers, surveyors pinpoint where organizations should be focusing to ensure continuous systems improvement.

Tracer Methodology: Tips and Strategies for Continuous Systems Improvement gives readers a comprehensive overview of tracer methodology and all the kinds of tracers (individual, systems) that can take place during an on-site survey. It also includes examples, from both organizations and surveyors, of health care setting–specific tracers. *Tracer Methodology: Tips and Strategies for Continuous Systems Improvement* provides readers with concrete tips on how to conduct their own mock tracers, identify and assess priority focus areas during mock tracers, and perform effective ongoing surveillance of their organization to ensure that their organization is continuously improving.
2004. Approximately 150 pages.
ISBN: 0-86688-898-5
Price: $65 Order Code: JTM-04BDK

NEW! *The Joint Commission Guide to Priority Focus Areas*

The Joint Commission has identified 14 broad categories of priority focus areas (PFAs) that are crucial to patient safety and quality of care. The Joint Commission's new accreditation process uses these PFAs as a guide to setting customized survey agendas for each organization undergoing accreditation.

The Joint Commission Guide to Priority Focus Areas is an all-in-one source for information. For each *PFA*, you'll find:

- Official Joint Commission definitions of the PFA and its related subprocesses
- The relevant Joint Commission requirements
- Common challenges faced by health care organizations
- Practical strategies for overcoming challenges
- Common instances of failures that can occur relative to the PFA and strategies to correct them
- Case studies of successful performance improvement initiatives for the PFA
- Concrete performance improvement suggestions that your organization can put into practice

This resource will be a valuable guide to your performance improvement initiatives as you move toward the goal of continuous standards compliance.
2004. 220 pages.
ISBN: 0-86688-841-1
Price: $70 Order Code: PFA-04BDK

NEW! *Shared Visions–New Pathways Essentials for Health Care*

Shared Visions–New Pathways Essentials is your guide to the Joint Commission's new accreditation process. You can use this new publication in conjunction with *Joint Commission Perspectives®* to help you get the most benefit from Shared Visions–New Pathways. This new resource includes the following:

- Information from the Shared Visions–New Pathways focus groups, pilot tests, and pilot surveys
- Clear explanations of all the elements of Shared Visions–New Pathways
- P.I.T. (Practical Information Time out) Stops that provide key information, quick definitions of key terms, and short lists throughout the text

You'll learn about the following components of Shared Visions–New Pathways:

- What it is
- What it is not
- What it means for health care organizations

2004. 148 pages.
ISBN: 0-86688-852-7
Price: $70 **Order Code: AE-04BDK**

Care Delivery and the Environment of Care: A Teamwork Approach

No health care discipline conducts its activities in isolation. With the increasing emphasis in health care on safety, emergency management, and sentinel events, the responsibilities of direct care staff and environment of care (*EC*) staff are beginning to overlap. Direct care staff and *EC* staff must work together to improve care delivery. *Care Delivery and the Environment of Care* gives you the following:

- Tips on implementing and supporting teamwork to bridge the gap between EC and direct care staff
- Tips on streamlining processes and procedures to avoid duplication of efforts and encourage cooperation between direct care staff and EC staff
- Examples of policies, procedures, forms, and checklists to help health care organizations improve processes

2003. 175 pages.
ISBN: 0-86688-759-8
Price: $55 **Order Code: ECCS-02BDK**

Putting Evidence to Work: Tools and Resources

Demands are coming from many quarters to integrate evidence into clinical practice. The chief difficulty is how to use existing evidence effectively. That requires health care organizations to create systems and programs for acquiring or assessing evidence, for anchoring practices in evidence, and for considering the needs of patients and the public.

Putting Evidence to Work helps you get started in the right direction, with the following information:

- Concepts, principles, and techniques of evidence-based practice (EBP)
- Information on where to find and how to use top sources and authorities
- Tools for appraising evidence
- Models and examples for starting or improving EBP programs
- Tools and templates for incorporating patients' values and shared decision making

2003. 162 pages.
ISBN: 0-86688-797-0
Price: $55 **Order Code: JCGE-02BDK**

NEW! *A Guide to JCAHO's Medication Management Standards*

A Guide to JCAHO's Medication Management Standards addresses compliance with the new and revised standards and serves as a guide on how to establish safe, high-quality, and effective medication management systems. The examples in the book illustrate setting-specific issues covering a wide range of patient populations.

A Guide to JCAHO's Medication Management Standards helps ambulatory care, behavioral health care, hospitals, home care, and long term care organizations meet the Joint Commission's medication management standards with the following:

- Explanations of key medication management standards and elements of performance
- Surveyor tips for complying with standards
- Compliance suggestions and other supplemental information that addresses a specific component of a particular goal
- Practical case studies that provide operational details to help organizations identify deficiencies and implement process improvements to improve care and address medication management standards

2004. 165 pages.
ISBN: 0-86688-856-X
Price: $70 Order Code: MMS-01BDK

Approaches to Pain Management: An Essential Guide for Clinical Leaders

In *Approaches to Pain Management: An Essential Guide for Clinical Leaders,* best-practice organizations tell the behind-the-scenes stories of how they developed and implemented pain management programs and made pain management an integral part of their care and services. This book is geared toward helping medical staff leaders, nursing leaders, and other clinicians and leaders in pain management initiatives evaluate and improve how they assess and manage pain across the continuum of care. It gives expert advice on how to meet the Joint Commission's pain assessment and management standards.

Approaches to Pain Management discusses how to perform the following tasks:

- Identify and use the best available resources for evidence-based pain management
- Address the challenges in pain management
- Commit the organization to pain management
- Establish an effective pain management program

It includes policies, procedures, protocols, and tools, such as a pain management policy, assessment forms and treatment guidelines, care plans, patient and family education materials, and staff education resources. Examples and tools come from seven inpatient, residential, and outpatient settings.
2003. 165 pages.
ISBN: 0-86688-800-4
Price: $55 Order Code: PMPP-02BDK

Essential Issues for Leaders: Emerging Challenges in Health Care

With the rapid rate of change in the industry, health care leaders in all types of organizations want and need to stay on top of today's most pertinent issues. This publication brings together the hot leadership topics identified and discussed by pre-eminent experts in the field. The chapters explore issues at the forefront of health care including the following:

- Cultivating a culture of safety and quality
- Ethics
- Confidentiality
- Evidence-based practice
- Integration of settings and services

Chapters include an introduction that sets the stage for the reader and provides important background information, as well as a summation that links the topic to accreditation and Joint Commission initiatives.
2001. 178 pages.
ISBN: 0-86688-702-4
Price: $55 Order Code: EIL-100BDK

Benchmarking in Health Care: Finding and Implementing Best Practices

Benchmarking is one of the most powerful tools available today for health care organizations to use to identify areas for improvement and to implement change.

Benchmarking in Health Care provides the following:

- A step-by-step guide to the different types of benchmarking and their application to health care
- Tips on finding and screening benchmarking partners
- Guidelines on collecting and analyzing benchmarking data
- Tips on avoiding common benchmarking mistakes

2000. 114 pages.
ISBN: 0-86688-675-3
Price: $50 Order Code: BM-100BDK

Ethical Issues and Patient Rights Across the Continuum of Care

Health care professionals encounter ethical issues almost daily, yet many are uncertain about how to recognize and address them. *Ethical Issues and Patient Rights* provides a comprehensive guide to understanding ethical tenets and decision making as well as meeting Joint Commission standards. Learn how to do the following:

- Understand the basic tenets of ethical decision making in the context of contemporary health care
- Design and implement a framework for clinical and organization ethics that meets Joint Commission standards
- Write clinical and organization policies and procedures to address ethical issues
- Develop a patient rights document and code of ethics
- Adopt a model for ethical inquiry and decision making
- Form and implement an ethics committee

Case studies address common ethical concerns in a variety of health care settings. Sample documents and policies address ethical issues including advance directives, withdrawal of life-sustaining care, patient rights, informed decision making, and organization ethics statements.
1998. 155 pages.
ISBN: 0-86688-591-9
Price: $45 Order Code: EI-100BDK

Clinical Improvement Action Guide, *edited by Eugene C. Nelson, DSc, MPH; Paul B. Batalden, MD; and Jeanne Ryer, MS*

The *Clinical Improvement Action Guide* offers a practical workbook that can be used by front-line clinical teams for rapidly improving quality, reducing costs, and getting better results. The *Clinical Improvement Action Guide* shows flexible methods to do the following:

- Develop specific clinical improvement aims and related measures of outcomes and costs
- Analyze the current delivery process and identify high-leverage changes
- Use benchmarking to identify best practices and best known results
- Plan and conduct rapid, sequential tests of change and measure the results against the original aim
- Sustain positive changes and deploy them to other parts of the organization

The book includes contributions by nationally recognized experts on health care quality: Eugene C. Nelson, DSc, MPH; Paul B. Batalden, MD; Jeanne Ryer, MS; Brent James, MD, MStat; Christina C. Mahoney, RN, MSN; Julie J. Mohr, MSPH; and Stephen K. Plume, MD; with a foreword by Donald M. Berwick, MD, MPH.
1998. 210 pages.
ISBN: 0-86688-553-6
Price: $45 Order Code: AG-100BDK

Using Performance Improvement Tools in Health Care Settings, Revised Edition

The tools and methods described in this book help ensure that performance improvement efforts are planned and systematic, based on reliable data and accurate analysis, and carried out with effective teamwork and communication. Almost all quality improvement projects go through the stages of planning, team formation, data collection, data analysis, and determining root causes of problems.

Through real-world case studies and examples, *Using Performance Improvement Tools* shows you how to choose the best tools for each stage. It includes a discussion on comparison and control charts that will help your organization understand ORYX® data. Ideal for quality improvement (QI) directors and staff, executives, and managers, *Using Performance Improvement Tools* is a survival guide for organizations that must demonstrate to payers, purchasers, and consumers that they provide high-quality, cost-effective care.
2000. 170 pages.
ISBN: 0-86688-689-3
Price: $50 Order Code: PI-401BDK

Topics in Clinical Care Improvement

Each monograph presents an overview of the topic, discusses standards requirements and survey issues, and provides strategies to address problems and improve performance. You'll find real-world examples and case studies of outstanding practices that profile a range of approaches to each topic.

There is one monograph for office-based surgery practices:

Anesthesia and Sedation

Developed to help organizations comply with the revised Joint Commission standards on anesthesia and conscious sedation, this monograph explains the changes to the standards, discusses the challenges and strategies for effective anesthesia and sedation, and provides case scenarios involving hospital and ambulatory care settings.
2001. 100 pages.
ISBN: 0-86688-696-6
Price: $24.95 Order Code: CC-1600BDK

NEW! *Assessing and Improving Staff Competence (CD-ROM)*

This product is an electronic compilation/toolbox of resources, strategies, and tips for assessing and improving staff competence in various types of health care organizations. It explains the Joint Commission's requirements in this area and offers suggestions and solutions for meeting these requirements based on the experiences of actual health care organizations. Many of the resources have been previously published elsewhere in JCR publications, but are now compiled for the first time in a user-friendly toolbox format.
2004. 60 pages.
ISBN: 0-86688-899-3
Price: $60 Order Code: AIC-CD01BDK

Staff Education Resources

NEW! *Educating Your Staff About JCAHO's New Accreditation Process*

As the Joint Commission's new accreditation process is implemented, health care leaders need to not only educate themselves on the new process, they will need to educate their staff. *Educating Your Staff About JCAHO's New Accreditation Process* is an essential tool for health care leaders to do just that. This book will provides health care leaders with the information they need to understand the new process, disseminate information, and involve key staff in activities that help the organization deliver safe, quality care.

Unique features of this book include the following:

- Explanations of the new accreditation process, broken out by component
- Tips on how to educate your staff about the process
- Practical examples of staff education
- Guidelines for conveying the information on the new process to staff
- Strategies for using the new accreditation process to promote safe, quality care

2004. 150 pages.
ISBN: 0-86688-854-3
Price: $75 Order Code: ESAP-01BDK

The Joint Commission Guide to Staff Education

The Joint Commission Guide to Staff Education gives you useful advice from experts in the field and examples from organizations that are breaking new ground in health care staff education.

The collaboration between the Joint Commission and the Health Care Education Association (HCEA) includes a collection of contributed essays from experts on today's key topics in health care education, such as the following:

- Recruiting and retaining employees
- Competency assessment
- Orientation, mentoring, preceptorship, and coaching
- Technological advances in learning media
- Ensuring appropriate budget, resources, and administrative support
- Documenting staff education

2002. 239 pages.
ISBN: 0-86688-725-3
Price: $55 Order Code: SEG-100BDK

A Pocket Guide to Using Performance Improvement Tools, Revised Edition

This convenient pocket guide summarizes major performance improvement tools. Clear and concise explanations make this booklet ideal for providing all levels of staff with easy access to these valuable tools.
2000. 48 pages.

Quantity	**Price**	**Order Code**
10-pack	**$25**	**PI-610BDK**
20-pack	**$45**	**PI-620BDK**

Patient Education

The Joint Commission Guide to Patient and Family Education

As the patient's role as part of the health care team continues to expand, patient and family education is key to safe and effective patient care. This book gives useful advice from experts in the field on patient and family education techniques. You will find real-world examples for today's education needs from many health care settings.

The Joint Commission Guide to Patient and Family Education provides methods of assessing patient learning needs and a summary of education techniques.

Hands-on examples included in the book feature the following:

- Examples on how to assess the effectiveness of education efforts
- Explanations of related Joint Commission requirements
- Documentation examples
- Examples for special patient populations, such as pediatric and geriatric patients
- Examples selected as good practices by the Health Care Education Association (HCEA)

2003. 154 pages.
ISBN 0-86688-815-2
Price: $65 Order Code: GPFE-01

Environment of Care Resources

The Joint Commission Guide to Managing the Statement of Conditions™

The Joint Commission Guide to Managing the Statement of Conditions is the authoritative guide to understanding and filling out this important document. *The Joint Commission Guide to Managing the Statement of Conditions* walks you through the Statement of Conditions (SOC) document, showing how to translate your building maintenance program activities into the required SOC information.

This publication includes the following:

- Easy-to-understand explanations of all the sections and components of the SOC
- Step-by-step guidelines for completing the SOC
- Explanation of occupancy-specific requirements of the core chapters of the *Life Safety Code*® (*LSC*)
- Explanation of the key differences between the 2000 *LSC* of the National Fire Protection Association and the 1987 edition
- Explanation of what surveyors may ask while reviewing SOC documents

- Tips for how surveyors use the SOC during survey
- Samples of completed portions of the SOC

Includes a special section explaining The Statement of Fire Safety for assisted living facilities.
2003. 168 pages.
ISBN: 0-86688-817-9
Order Code: NSC-01BDK   Price: $65

Guide to Emergency Management Planning in Health Care

Guide to Emergency Management Planning in Health Care helps health care organizations prepare to respond to most emergencies by examining their existing emergency management plans to identify areas for improvement within the four phases of preparedness: mitigation, preparedness, response, and recovery. In addition, this guide offers advice on developing a comprehensive, proactive, and practical emergency management plan; describes how to establish collaborative community relationships to respond to disasters; and strikes a balance between a generic and a specific approach to emergency management planning.

Guide to Emergency Management Planning in Health Care includes case studies, examples, and checklists from health care organizations, associations, and agencies highlighting effective emergency management plans. Chapters on dealing with the psychological impact resulting from disasters and working with the media are included to round out the content.
2002. 252 pages.
ISBN: 0-86688-755-5
Price: $60   Order Code: EMPHC-01BDK

Security Issues for Today's Health Care Organization

In today's tumultuous environment, safety and security are on everyone's minds—and in health care they are everyone's concern. From frontline security staff to nursing and pharmacy personnel, this publication demonstrates how security concerns all areas and levels within an organization to protect patients, residents and other care recipients.

This book discusses the key standards related to security in health care organizations and provides practical guidance on key topics including the following:

- Developing and implementing an up-to-date security plan
- Addressing setting-specific security concerns including infant abductions, workplace violence, drug theft, access control, resident wandering, and patient or resident suicide
- How terrorism and violence impact security and the workplace

2002. 130 pages.
ISBN: 0-86688-757-1
Price: $55   Order Code: SITHC-01BDK

Preventing Sentinel Events in the Environment of Care

What causes an environment of care sentinel event? How can errors be prevented? How is a root cause analysis conducted? *Preventing Sentinel Events* answers these questions and more by providing pertinent information on the occurrence of sentinel events. It includes examples of environment of care sentinel events, tips on how to avoid the occurrence of sentinel events, and examples of root cause analysis in the environment of care. Case studies include an infant abduction, a power and emergency generator failure and a defibrillator failure in a hospital setting, a patient suicide and fire in a behavioral health care setting, and a resident elopement in a long term care setting.
2000. 136 pages.
ISBN: 0-86688-646-1
Price: $50   Order Code: SEEC-50BDK

NEW! *Environment of Care Handbook, 2nd Edition*

Significant changes have been made over the past few years to the environment of care standards. To make sure you keep up with these important changes, we have introduced the new, updated

Environment of Care Handbook to give you the most up-to-date, state-of-the-art information about every area of the environment of care.

Learn about the following:
- Integrating performance monitoring into the environment of care
- Managing the information collection and evaluation system (ICES)
- New approaches to the seven environment of care management plans
- Environment of care standards in action with real-life examples in hospitals, long term care facilities, and ambulatory care settings

The Environment of Care Handbook is an indispensable guide for safety and facility managers in hospitals, long term care facilities, or ambulatory care settings, or for health care consultants.
2004. 146 pages.
ISBN: 0-86688-864-0
Price: $75 Order Code: EC-200BDK

NEW! *Infection Control Issues in the Environment of Care*

While the majority of health care–associated infections can be linked to clinical failures, a significant number of deaths have been linked to environmental failures, such as the presence of waterborne or airborne microbes. *Infection Control Issues in the Environment of Care* addresses infection control (*IC*) issues from the point of view of the environment of care (*EC*) professional for all health care settings.

Infection Control Issues in the Environment of Care does the following:
- Breaks down the IC issues into specific categories (personnel, equipment, utilities, building, construction, and performance measurement and improvement)
- Explores IC issues from an EC perspective
- Provides examples and tools on how to assess IC risks and address IC issues
- Includes advice on how EC professionals can work with IC professionals

2004. Approximately 150 pages.
ISBN: 0-86688-874-8
Price: $75 Order Code: ICEOC-01BDK

Newsletters

Joint Commission Resources Periodicals

To order any of these periodicals, or to request a FREE sample issue, click on InfoMart when you visit our Web site: http://www.jcrinc.com or call 800/346-0085, ext 558.

All JCR periodicals are online! The online versions provide the following benefits:
- **Speed**—You'll receive each issue directly, before it arrives in the mail.
- **Access**—Online issues have full-text access as well as hyperlinks to more information on the Joint Commission Web site and elsewhere.
- **Searchability**—You'll be able to search current issues and the archives of past issues.

You can subscribe to the print version only, the online version only, or the print and online versions together.

Joint Commission Perspectives®

Perspectives is the only official source of credible, timely, and complete information about Joint Commission standards changes, the Joint Commission's new accreditation process, sentinel events, ORYX®, and much more. *Perspectives* is the Joint Commission's official newsletter.

Rely on *Perspectives* every month to bring you updates to standards, the accreditation process, and policies. *Perspectives* includes the following:
- **Joint Commission Requirements**—This feature clearly highlights new or revised Joint Commission requirements, including standards changes, affecting your accreditation program.

- **News**—Learn everything you need to know about new Joint Commission initiatives and policy issues.
- **In Sight**—Monitor proposed changes to standards, survey processes, and key initiatives while they are in development.
- **The Fact on Fiction**—Get information correcting confusing and inaccurate communications about the Joint Commission published elsewhere and myths from the health care field.

Subscription term: 1 year - 12 issues

Call Customer Service for Canada, Mexico, and international rates.

To order, and for subscription rate information, call 800/346-0085, ext. 558, or visit InfoMart at http://www.jcrinc.com/infomart.

Joint Commission: The Source™

The how-to resource from Joint Commission Resources!

The Source is the authority on timely, complete, and correct information for complying with key Joint Commission initiatives, standards, and policies and procedures. It's the perfect companion to *Joint Commission Perspectives®* because it provides examples of how to comply with requirements published in *Perspectives*.

The Source provides health care organizations with expert, practical, how-to information, including sample forms, tools, and strategies for meeting Joint Commission requirements. Count on each issue of *The Source* to do the following:

- Help performance improvement directors learn to implement current and new Joint Commission standards and initiatives
- Target the most frequently cited standards and explain how to improve performance
- Provide practical information on how to maintain continuous standards compliance
- Keep health care organizations up-to-date about the Joint Commission's new accreditation process
- Present case studies that focus on hands-on lessons in meeting requirements
- Supply answers to the most frequently asked questions about Joint Commission requirements from health care professionals
- Spotlight surveyors' experiences in the field, providing guidance for meeting Joint Commission requirements

Turn to *The Source* to get clear, concise tips to help your organization strive toward continuous performance improvement.

Subscription term: 1 year - 12 issues

Call Customer Service for Canada, Mexico, and international rates.

To order, and for subscription rate information, call 800/346-0085, ext. 558, or visit InfoMart at http://www.jcrinc.com/infomart.

Joint Commission Perspectives on Patient Safety™

A monthly newsletter on important patient safety issues!

Perspectives on Patient Safety is the newsletter you'll want to keep at your fingertips every month. *Perspectives on Patient Safety* gives you information you can count on—straight from the source. You'll find the following in future issues:

- Practical, how-to information for implementing Joint Commission safety standards, National Patient Safety Goals, and safety-related components of the Joint Commission's new accreditation process
- Clear, concise explanations of Joint Commission safety standards requirements, with compliance tips for accreditation preparation
- Helpful discussions on how key safety changes can affect your continuous standards compliance efforts

- Practical tips for incorporating proactive risk assessment techniques into your performance improvement and error-prevention processes
- Strategies for preventing root causes of medication errors, falls, suicide, and other errors
- Useful advice to help risk managers and performance improvement coordinators incorporate safety improvement efforts into their daily practice

You'll also find case studies showing an organization's experience in preventing sentinel events and addressing safety. New features focus on improving specific aspects of the medication-use process and incorporating proactive risk assessment techniques into your improvement processes.

Subscription term: 1 year - 12 issues

Call Customer Service for Canada, Mexico, and International rates.

To order, and for subscription rate information, call 800/346-0085, ext. 558, or visit InfoMart at http://www.jcrinc.com/infomart.

Environment of Care® News

Environment of Care® News provides practical, accurate advice on Joint Commission EC standards, plus all the latest developments that affect EC.

Some new features in *Environment of Care® News* include the following:

- **EC & IC**—Address infection control from the EC point of view and help clinicians meet the new National Patient Safety Goal and the Joint Commission priority focus area (PFA)
- **Worker Safety**—Discover key links between OSHA and Joint Commission standards as you address ergonomic issues, workplace violence, biohazards, and more
- **Shared Visions–New Pathways® & EC**—How Shared Visions–New Pathways® impacts EC, PFAs of concern to EC, and more
- **Special Series**—Ongoing, in-depth coverage of the EC angle on patient flow, design and construction, and other emerging EC topics

Environment of Care® News also includes the following features you've come to depend on:

- **Standards News—**Late-breaking EC standards news
- **Q&A**—Expanded
- **Case Study**—Practical, hands-on examples of how organizations address EC compliance
- **Accreditation Session**—Tips, checklists, and ideas from Joint Commission surveyors and JCR consultants
- **Featured Form**— The best EC policies and procedures, management plans, and other forms
- **Nuts & Bolts**—Instructions, how-tos, and diagrams to help you tackle everyday EC problems

All designed and written for health care organizations across the board—hospital, ambulatory care, long term care, behavioral health care, home care, and laboratories.

You can choose how you want to receive your *Environment of Care® News* subscription: in print form, online, or both! Save on two- and three-year subscriptions! Update your existing print subscription to include the online newsletter for $20!

Subscription term: 1 year - 12 issues

Call Customer Service for Canada, Mexico, and international rates.

To order, and for subscription rate information, call 800/346-0085, ext. 558, or visit InfoMart at http://www.jcrinc.com/infomart.

Joint Commission Benchmark®

Joint Commission Benchmark®, a bi-monthly JCR periodical, has been redesigned with a new look and an expanded focus on critical performance measurement issues affecting health care organizations. *Benchmark®* now includes:

- A new expert **Editorial Advisory Board,** consisting of Joint Commission and other national performance measurement experts, providing new insight into important performance measurement issues.

- **Joint Commission Focus** provides an update on the latest Joint Commission performance measurement news, such as core measures.
- **PM Beat** focuses on national performance measurement news and trends
- **National Data Report** summarizes performance measures from nationally recognized organizations such as NQF, AHRQ, and CMS.

Benchmark also continues to provide how-to information on Joint Commission performance measurement requirements, including solutions and strategies to help health care organizations turn data into useful and actionable information. Expert advice on data collection and analysis issues continues to be addressed in the "Data Corner" feature. ORYX® experts continue to answer questions related to compliance with the Joint Commission's ORYX initiatives.

Subscription term: 1 year - 6 issues

Call Customer Service for Canada, Mexico, and international rates.

To order, and for subscription rate information, call 800/346-0085, ext. 558, or visit InfoMart at http://www.jcrinc.com/infomart.

The Joint Commission Journal on Quality and Safety™

The only monthly, peer-reviewed journal devoted to quality and safety in health care!

The Joint Commission Journal on Quality and Safety™ is the **trusted resource for health care professionals** who want practical, innovative ways to improve the quality and safety of care—all in step-by-step detail.

Rely on the *Journal* as your first resource in planning and testing improvements in care. Learn what works from leading health care experts and practitioners around the world. **Get information you can use** in your own health care organization.

Look at the following exciting new features in the *Journal*:

- **Authoritative, peer-reviewed articles from around the world** on the topics that you need to know about—short, easy to adapt, and very hands-on.
- **Sure-fire checklists, charts, forms, and other handy quality-and-safety tools** that you can use right now.
- **Brief case studies** to help you get a quick handle on solutions to the problems that your organization might be facing.
- **Interviews and commentaries** from dynamic experts in health care quality and safety. Get the latest on the hot topics that everyone is talking about—patient safety initiatives, the nursing shortage, pain management, performance measurement, and more.
- **Tool tutorials** that help you quickly understand and apply various quality-and-safety tools to your own projects. All the basics in easy-to-use detail. Perfect for educating staff!
- **Field notes** that detail quality and safety projects in progress. Learn from colleagues how to overcome common obstacles and find successes en route to your goals.

Subscription term: 1 year - 12 issues

Call Customer Service for Canada, Mexico, and international rates.

To order, and for subscription rate information, call 800/346-0085, ext. 558, or visit InfoMart at http://www.jcrinc.com/infomart.

NEW! *Joint Commission International Newsletter™*

Looking for authoritative information on international health care accreditation, patient safety, and quality improvement?

Turn to *Joint Commission International Newsletter*, the official online bimonthly newsletter of Joint Commission International. Rely on this essential source of information and networking for quality-minded health care organizations around the world.

With an international perspective, *Joint Commission International Newsletter*™ brings you news and information on:

- Patient safety
- Quality improvement
- Accreditation and accreditation preparation
- Evaluation system development
- Operations improvement

Subscribe now to *Joint Commission International Newsletter*™ for the following:

- **News and updates** on Joint Commission International initiatives, accreditation programs, events, and conferences
- **Global good practices**
- **Invaluable guidance** from international health care experts on quality improvement, patient safety, and international standards compliance
- **Profiles of health care organizations around the world** that are achieving new levels of quality and safety
- **Timely updates and tips** on how to avoid adverse events
- **Compliance tips** for international accreditation standards

Subscription term: online only, 6 issues per year

Call Customer Service for Canada, Mexico, and international rates.

To order, and for subscription rate information, call 800/346-0085, ext. 558, or visit InfoMart at http://www.jcrinc.com/infomart.

Celebrate Accreditation Products

Celebrate and promote your accreditation!

We know that Joint Commission accreditation requires a significant commitment, and the achievement of accreditation pays off in many ways. Joint Commission accreditation makes a strong statement to your community about your desire to provide services of the highest quality. But does the public really know about your accreditation status and what it means? We offer several products that help you display your accreditation to the public. Let them know that you're committed to the highest standards of quality health care. We Are Accredited products are available to Joint Commission–accredited organizations.

We Are Accredited by JCAHO Brochure

Display this elegant brochure in your patient reception areas, include it in patient handbooks, or use for media or fundraising activities. The brochure explains the rigorous evaluation, national recognition, and commitment to quality Joint Commission accreditation stands for, and bears the Joint Commission Gold Seal of Approval.

Available folded or unfolded (to add your own logo), and in English or Spanish. Folded, the brochure fits into a standard business envelope.

Quantity	Price per 100
100–400	$35
500–900	$32
1,000–1,400	$28
1,500 or more	$26

Order Code:

WB-30 (English, folded)
WB-30U (English, unfolded)
WB-40 (Spanish, folded)
WB-40U (Spanish, unfolded)

Banners

No one who walks into your reception areas or waiting rooms can miss the message of these highly visible 5' x 2' banners. Choose either horizontal or vertical designs. Each banner is imprinted in blue, gold, and burgundy on one side of indoor/outdoor white vinyl and has brass grommets to hang securely.

Price: $98 each
Order Code: WBV-200BDK (vertical)
WBH-200BDK (horizontal)

Decals

Put your quality commitment out front by applying these colorful 5" x 10" decals to all your entrance doors and office windows. The decal bears the Joint Commission Gold Seal of Approval. Easily applied with a peel-off backing, these decals are sure to be noticed.
Price: $20 for 5-pack Order Code: WD-200BDK

Stickers

Put your quality imprint on everything with these rolls of circular stickers bearing the Joint Commission Gold Seal of Approval! They're perfect to apply to stationery, business cards, brochures, and anywhere else you want to send a quality-and-safety message.
Price: $12 for 100-sticker roll Order Code: WS-200BDK

Enamel Pins

Everyone on your staff can reinforce your quality message by wearing one of these colorful 1 1/4" x 3/4" die-struck, enamel pins. Staff members will be proud to show off the Gold Seal of Approval to patients, peers, and the community.
Price: $18 for 5-pack of pins Order Code: WPE-200BDK

Mugs

This mug is high-quality, white porcelain with an elegantly-shaped handle.
Price: $7.50 Order Code: WM-200

Folders

Perfect for taking notes at quality improvement team meetings, this handsome 8 5/8" x 6" leather-look desk folder features rounded corners, padded front and back covers, an interior pocket, a business card pocket, a pen loop, and a 5" x 8" perforated memo pad.
Price: $20 Order Code: WPH-200

Audiotapes

Sentinel Event Policy and Survey Issues: An Overview

This 60-minute audiotape, which includes print materials, explains the definition of a sentinel event, which sentinel events fall under the Joint Commission's Sentinel Event Policy, confidentiality issues, and how sentinel events affect a survey. This audiotape package was produced as an educational supplement for Joint Commission surveyors and is now available to you!
2000. 60 minutes.
Price: $24.95 Order Code: A/9813

Reproductive Hazards, Toxicant Chemicals, and Drugs

Reduce duplication of efforts to comply with Joint Commission standard requirements and OSHA guidelines!

If toxicant chemicals and drugs are not prepared, handled, and administered properly, they can pose unique risks to health care workers, patients, families, and friends. The *Reproductive Hazards,*

Toxicant Chemicals, and Drugs audiotape, originally prepared as an educational tool for Joint Commission surveyors, provides a comprehensive overview of the scope and nature of problems associated with these drugs.

The audiotape and its companion workbook include the following:
- Applicable OSHA regulations and guidelines relating to hazardous drug use
- Relevant Joint Commission standards
- Information on how to recognize applicable OSHA regulations and guidelines and Joint Commission standards

1997. 45 minutes.
Price: $25 **Order Code: A/9701BDK**

Videos

Joint Commission Resources provides educational videos as valuable learning tools for organizations in all health care settings. This learning venue dispenses education in a format that can be used repeatedly to deliver the flexibility of learning when and where you need it.

Joint Commission Resources is dedicated to supplying you accurate, timely information to satisfy your organization's educational needs. Our videos examine current issues and innovative approaches in health care and give relevant, practical examples that you can easily adapt to your health care setting. Keep your organization educated on a variety of topics, including Shared Visions–New Pathways®, quality health care delivery, emergency department overcrowding, medication management, and disaster preparedness.

Why are JCR videos so unique?

JCR offers a diverse selection of videotapes and auxiliary learning materials. Every video includes guides for both the group leader and the viewers to enhance the learning experience.
- The Leader's Guide provides materials that help the discussion leader prepare for viewing the sessions and supplies questions and activities to enhance the learning experience.
- The Viewer's Guide contains sample reference documents, a list of applicable standards, and more!

NEW! *Improving Healthcare Quality Series*

Part I: Using Run Charts

As we move toward twenty-first century quality care, a simple quality improvement tool—the run chart—can make a huge difference in your ability to learn from your data. Yes, the run chart can help you monitor processes, establish whether an intervention has been successful, and increase your ability to bring about true quality improvement.

To introduce a wider audience to the uses and advantages of run charts, Washington Health Foundation's *The Learning Center* and Joint Commission Resources has joined with Raymond G. Carey, Ph.D, Principal R.G. Carey and Associates, an internationally recognized statistical thinking specialist. Dr. Carey has given countless successful seminars to thousands of quality professionals. As you will see in this presentation, he has the ability to make learning easy, no matter your current level of statistical skills.

A separate workbook is included with each part in this series that provides supporting material, additional exercises, and self-test questions to support understanding.

Part II: Using Control Charts

Wondering which measurement tools you should use to achieve a high level of quality? Run charts can be useful as a basic measuring tool. To take advantage of an even more sophisticated technique, you need to understand and use control charts, a powerful tool for analyzing variation and measuring process improvement.

Once again, the Washington Health Foundation's *The Learning Center,* Joint Commission Resources, and Dr. Raymond G. Carey, Principal R.G. Carey and Associates, an internationally recognized statistical thinking expert, have partnered to bring the classroom directly to you with a step-by-step learning approach.

The knowledge you will gain about data analysis will be helpful in preparing for Joint Commission surveys. In fact, Dr. Carey has been working with the Joint Commission and was appointed to its Council on Performance Measurement in 2000. Co-author of two industry standards, *Program Evaluation: Methods and Case Studies* and *Measuring Quality Improvement in Healthcare: A Guide to Statistical Process Control Applications,* Dr. Carey is a popular seminar leader for the American College of Healthcare Executives and the Institute for Healthcare Improvement. Both *Part I: Using Run Charts,* and *Part II: Using Control Charts,* are musts for your organization's learning library.

A separate workbook is included with each part in this series that provides you with supporting material, additional exercises, and self-test questions to support your understanding.

Improving Healthcare Quality Part I: Using Run Charts (CD-ROM)
Price: $209.00 Order Code: IHQ01BDK

Improving Healthcare Quality Part II: Using Control Charts (CD-ROM)
Price: $209.00 Order Code: IHQ02BDK

Improving Healthcare Quality Parts I and II (Both CD-ROMs)
Price: $349.00 Order Code: IHQ03BDK

Improving Healthcare Quality Part I: Using Run Charts (Video)
Price: $209.00 Order Code: VIHQ01BDK

Improving Healthcare Quality Part II: Using Control Charts (Video)
Price: $209.00 Order Code: VIHQ02BDK

Improving Healthcare Quality Part: I Using Run Charts and Part II: Using Control Charts (Both Videos)
Price: $349.00 Order Code: VIHQ03BDK

NEW! *Think Twice, Save a Life: The Pharmacy's Role in Medication Safety*

Use this learning program to increase pharmacist understanding and buy-in to your organization's performance improvement efforts to prevent medication errors. The video features real-life, hands-on vignettes to help pharmacists understand their role in preventing medication errors. The video is divided into learning modules and segments, with prompts indicating when to refer to the workbook for continued information on a topic.

The workbook includes information, strategies, and tips to help pharmacists prevent medication errors. The workbook gives pharmacists ideas for partnering with nurses, physicians, patients, and families to improve the medication-use process. It discusses and builds upon the Joint Commission's standards for patient safety and medication management as well as the National Patient Safety Goals.

The workbook also includes self-assessment exercises and additional resources lists for further study. This program is appropriate for individuals or a group of pharmacists as part of an in-service. CEU units are provided.
2004.
ISBN: 0-86688-867-5
Price: $295 Order Code: V-W0403

NEW! *Part of the Oath: The Physician's Role in Medication Safety*

Use this learning program to increase physician understanding and buy-in to your organization's performance improvement efforts to prevent medication errors. This program is appropriate for individuals or a group of physicians as part of an in-service. CME units are provided.

The video features real-life, hands-on vignettes to help physicians understand their role in preventing medication errors. The video is divided into learning modules and segments, with prompts indicating when to refer to the workbook for continued information on a topic.

The workbook engages the physician's interest with practical information, strategies, and tips to help prevent medication errors. The workbook also gives physicians ideas for partnering with nurses, pharmacists, patients, and families to improve the medication-use process. It discusses and builds upon the Joint Commission's standards for patient safety and medication management as well as the National Patient Safety Goals.

The workbook also includes self-assessment exercises and additional resources lists for further study.

This workbook/video learning tool is applicable to physicians who work in hospital, ambulatory, behavioral health care, long term care, and home care settings as well as office-based practices.
2004.
ISBN: 0-86688-867-5
Price: $295 Order Code: V-W0403BDK

NEW! *Shared Visions–New Pathways®: An Innovative Approach to Patient Safety and Quality Improvement*

This video defines the Joint Commission's new accreditation process, Shared Visions–New Pathways, and its key elements; compare and contrast the old and new survey processes, define the Priority Focus Process and its components, identify the tracer methodology and its role in the new survey process, and describe the implementation timeline for Periodic Performance Review.
Price: $275 Order Code: V03/01BDK

NEW! *Governance, Quality and Safety: The Impact of Joint Commission* Accreditation on Health Care Delivery

Governing boards have the critical responsibility of representing the interests of the patient and their communities when decisions have to be made. The scope of the Joint Commission's mission is similar in nature; to continuously improve the quality and safety of care provided to the general public. This unique video outlines for board members how the Joint Commission helps organizations reduce risk and develop processes that maximize quality and performance. In addition to providing a background on Joint Commission standards and the survey process itself, the video specifically outlines those standards that apply to the governing board.
Price: $275 Order Code: V02/03BDK

NEW! *Reducing Risks, Improving Care: Medication Management and the Joint Commission's Survey Process*

Medications are an essential component of care and the most common cause of sentinel events, significant adverse reactions, and medical errors. Medication use requires effective management and must be coordinated among the various services and health care professionals involved. *Reducing Risks, Improving Care: Medication Management and the Joint Commission's Survey Process* is a new video featuring the case study of a pilot survey. Viewers learn important information from surveyor interviews of staff regarding the following:

- Selection, procurement, and storage of medication
- Prescribing, ordering, and transcribing medication
- Preparing and dispensing medication
- Administration of medication
- Monitoring medication
- Special medication

Viewers will be able to identify the new and revised medication-use standards, describe the medication-use survey process, and apply the medication-use survey process to future Joint Commission surveys.
Price: $275 Order Code: V03/02BDK

Emergency Management: Plan for the Unthinkable

The need for effective emergency management against chemical, biological, or nuclear substances is well established. This timely new video enables health care organizations to consistently train new and veteran employees on the strategies necessary to successfully respond to and plan for emergencies. Key topics covered include: the role of health care organizations and staff, strengths and weaknesses in the health care delivery infrastructure, and promoting efficient planning within your organization.

Price: $275 Order Code: V02/02BDK

FMEA: A Proactive Approach to Reducing Errors

Health care organizations that encounter issues with care delivery often conduct a root cause analysis (RCA) to improve their processes in the future. (FMEA), Failure mode and effects analysis, provides organizations with a unique, proactive alternative to risk reduction. What are the strengths of each approach and in which instances should they be used? This video concisely communicates the pros and cons of each approach and outlines the key elements of FMEA. The specific steps of FMEA are described using a common household task (making a cup of coffee) as an example of how FMEA can be used in the assessment of a particular process.

Price: $275 Order Code: V02/01BDK

NEW! *Emergency Department Overcrowding: Managing Patient Flow, Long Term Success*

Is your emergency department (ED) overcrowded? According to an April 2002 American Hospital Association survey, the majority of hospital EDs perceive they are at or over operating capacity. These capacity constraints translate into longer waiting times for treatment, longer stays in the ED, and delays in being admitted to a general acute, critical care, or psychiatric bed. What can be done to solve this problem? *Emergency Department Overcrowding: Managing Patient Flow, Long Term Success* is a new video that helps health care organizations reduce their risks related to ED overcrowding. Included are discussions regarding:

- Joint Commission standards related to ED overcrowding
- Root causes of ED overcrowding, including communication, patient assessment process, and staffing-level issues
- Risk-reduction strategies for ED overcrowding such as orientation and training processes, transfer procedures, staffing plans, and triage procedures
- Joint Commission recommendations for ED overcrowding

Price: $275 Order Code: V03/03BDK

Pain Management in Special Populations

Special populations have special needs for pain management. This new series of videos helps your entire staff understand the management of pain in special populations, how care is specified for different patient types, and how the Joint Commission pain management standards are linked to caring for these different patient populations.

Pain Management in Special Populations: Pediatrics

Price: $195 Order Code: V01/01

Pain Management in Special Populations: Geriatrics

(Supported by an unrestricted educational grant provided by Purdue Pharma LP)

Price: $195 Order Code: V01/02

Pain Management in Special Populations: Disease Related Pain

(Cancer, HIV/AIDS, Sickle Cell)

Price: $195 Order Code: V01/03

Pain Management in Special Populations: Challenging Populations

(Cognitively Impaired, Non-English Speaking, Chemical Dependency)
Price: $195 Order Code: V01/04BDK

Purchase all 4 Pain Management in Special Populations videos for only $663!
(A savings of $117)
Order Code: V01/05BDK

Pain Management Across the Continuum of Care: The Patient's Experience

Supported by an unrestricted educational grant provided by Purdue Pharma LP.

On her way home from a weekend with friends, Amanda was run off the road by a motorist who failed to see her or the motorcycle she was riding. Jim, a middle-aged man with rheumatoid arthritis, suffered a heart attack in front of his house, fell and hit his head on the sidewalk. This video follows these two patients through the continuum of care at a local hospital as they are treated for injuries sustained in the accidents. From pre-entry through discharge, it takes you through the different levels of treatment and shows you how the new Joint Commission pain management standards are met.
2000. 42 minutes.
Price: $195 Order Code: V20/00BDK

Using Clinical Practice Guidelines Across the Continuum of Care

Caregivers can effectively implement Continuum of Care standards to create positive outcomes for patients in a variety of settings. This video focuses on how to perform important patient care functions while continuously improving an organization's performance and outcomes.
35 minutes.
Price: $195 Order Code: V20/02BDK

A Guide for Completing the Statement of Conditions™

Completing your Statement of Conditions (SOC) does not have to be an overwhelming task. The activities and information needed for the SOC are the same kinds of safety and engineering evaluations you probably have been doing all along as part of your ongoing building maintenance program. This video walks you through each section of the SOC, to show you how to translate your normal evaluation activities into the information needed to complete your SOC, while at the same time providing a safe, functional, and effective environment for staff, visitors, and patients. Also appropriate for long term care organizations.
60 minutes.
Price: $195 Order Code: V2001BDK

Technological Solutions to Standards Compliance: Automated Dispensing

Supported by an unrestricted education grant provided by Omnicell.
Do you have questions about the growing role of automated dispensing in health care or how it will be viewed during a survey? This 30-minute video is the solution you've been seeking to teach you how automated dispensing systems can be versatile and secure tools that comply with Joint Commission standards. It uses an investigative news documentary approach to illustrate an overview of decentralized automation implementation and use of automation for standards compliance.
30 minutes.
Price: $195 Order Code: V20/03BDK

When Bad Things Happen to Good Health Care Organizations: Sentinel Event Series

Introducing a new three-part video series that explains the Joint Commission's Sentinel Event Policy requirement, how to develop a methodology for responding appropriately to a sentinel event, and what can be done to help prevent a sentinel event.

Unexpected and unplanned adverse outcomes can happen to any health care organization. This new three-part video series discusses how to deal with these unexpected events and how the Joint Commission's Sentinel Event Policy applies to these occurrences. In part one, you learn the goals of the Sentinel Event Policy, what constitutes a reportable sentinel event, and how to report a sentinel event. In part two, you learn how to conduct a root cause analysis, effective risk reduction and measurement strategies, and how the Joint Commission processes root cause analysis reports. In part three you learn what proactive risk reduction is, how to identify the processes that carry the greatest risk, and how this strategy can be implemented in your facility.
Price: $195.00 Order Code: V9903BDK

SET the Standard Videos
Introducing two new videos to help home medical equipment, pharmaceutical, home health, and hospice organizations in educating staff on the proper handling, storage, transporting, and tracking of hazardous materials.

Delivering and handling hazardous materials in the home poses safety risks for patients, care givers, and home care staff. These videos are designed to help home care staff recognize and understand these safety issues and practice safe techniques when delivering and providing such services in the home. To promote learning, a SET the Standard acronym is used, which stands for Study the Regulations, Employ safe practices, and train patients and families. It provides a straightforward and structured approach to help staff remember how to provide these products and services safely and in accordance with the law and regulation as well as Joint Commission expectations.

After viewing the videos and completing the print-based exercises, staff will be better able to do the following:

- Describe how applicable hazardous material regulations, laws, and Joint Commission expectations relate to their organization and their job responsibilities
- Safely handle, transport, and dispose of hazardous materials
- Describe to patients and families how to handle these hazardous materials safely

40 minutes.
Price: $195 Order Code: V9901BDK

Web-Based Training
Web-based training offers a convenient way to receive continuing education credit at work or at home, at any time of the day. This flexible learning style comes with the satisfaction that you're receiving information from the reliable source on Joint Commission–related topics. The courses are self-paced and last for an average of one hour. They can be completed in one session or you may leave the program and come back at a later time. Registration, content evaluation, and assessment are all automated and paperless. When the course is finished, you can print a continuing education learning certificate.

Components of Patient Safety
This program focuses on hospital standards with processes applicable to all settings. It covers health care errors, failure mode and effects analysis, Joint Commission patient safety standards, and international patient safety standards.

Intended for health care staff and management.
Single Use Price: $149 Order Code: DEP-48BDK

Medication Management / Medication Use
This course describes the interrelated set of steps used to provide medication therapy to patients. Learn the components of the medication management process and preview the Joint Commission's new survey approach to evaluating this process.

Intended for health care staff and management.
Single Use Price: $149 Order Code: WBT0303BDK

OSHA/JCAHO Bloodborne Pathogen Safety Training

Meet OSHA requirements and Joint Commission standards in one course. Learn to reduce occupational exposure to infectious materials and minimize the transmission of bloodborne pathogens. Key topics include appropriate response to emergencies, acceptable labeling and recordkeeping, engineering, and workplace controls.

This program is designed for any employee who could encounter blood or other potentially infectious materials as a result of performing their job.

Single Use	**Price: $89**	**Order Code: DEP-40**
CD-ROM	**Price: $109**	**Order Code: BORNEPTH**
WBT Site License	**Price: $495 + $10 per user**	**Order Code: DEP-40S**

Patient Rights

This program covers the Joint Commission standards that relate to the considerations of patient preferences and values, informing patients of their responsibilities, a health care organization's responsibilities under law, and managing the health care organization's relationships with patients and the public in an ethical manner.

The training is designed for physicians, nurses, clerical, and administrative staff, as well as hospital and long term care executives.

Single Use **Price: $149** **Order Code: DEP-52**

Concepts in Staffing Effectiveness

This course covers critical topic areas helpful in improving staffing effectiveness. This includes new standards, indicators and measures, methods and tools, survey highlights, and frequently asked questions.

This training is intended for clinical and staff managers, administrative personnel and health care executives responsible for staffing.

Single Use **Price: $149** **Order Code: DEP-49**

Patient Confidentiality

This course covers the Joint Commission standards that relate to patient confidentiality, including sources of data, control of access, storage and security of paper and electronic data, HIPAA, and the human resources aspect of confidentiality.

This course is intended for health care staff and management.

Single Use **Price: $149** **Order Code: WBT0203**

Turning Data into Useful Information for Performance Improvement

Learn to monitor and improve organizational performance through data. Focus on performance measurement; transforming data into information; data collection, display, and analysis. A short case study is included.

This program is specifically designed for clinical managers, administrative personnel, and health care executives responsible for performance improvement.

Single Use **Price: $149** **Order Code: DEP-50**

New Survey Process Initiatives

Gain insights into the Joint Commission's new accreditation process. Learn the difference between old and new standards, and the revised agenda and implementation of the tracer methodology by surveyors.

This course is appropriate for health care executives, quality managers, and managers charged with preparing for accreditation.

Single Use **Price: $149** **Order Code: WBT0103BDK**

Risk Management

This program highlights the clinical and administrative risk management activities that apply to staff at all levels. Learn to help identify, evaluate, and reduce the risk of injury to patients, staff, and visitors and to minimize losses for your health care organization. Key to this program are the discussions about the Joint Commission's National Patient Safety Goals and the relationship between risk management, patient safety, and quality. Techniques to incorporate risk management awareness into daily performance are also highlighted.

This program is designed to help managers, health care professionals, and general staff who manage risks everyday.

Single Use Price: $149 Order Code: DEP-53BDK

Credentialing and Privileging: The Fundamentals

The process of credentialing and privileging is a critical element of a health care organization's quality assurance program. The Medicare Conditions of Participation and many state regulations require a process for credentialing and privileging. The Joint Commission's standards outline more specific requirements and expectations. The purpose of this program is to provide an overview of the credentialing and privileging process and how it supports your organization's quality program.

This program is intended for medical staff coordinators and persons responsible for Joint Commission compliance.

Single Use Price: $149 Order Code: WBT0403BDK

New Manager's Guide to Accreditation

This program is designed for those managers faced with the new responsibility of Joint Commission compliance. Learn how Joint Commission standards should be an ongoing part of the daily routine. The course provides available resources, explains the survey process, and demonstrates how incorporating standards requirements into routines can result in effective performance improvement.

Single Use Price: $149 Order Code: DEP-51BDK

Safety in the Environment

Health care organizations must be able to respond to incidents that create mass casualties. Communities turn to health care organizations to provide medical care to those injured following an emergency or disaster, when times the organizations themselves and their staff are also victims of the disaster. This program is designed as a practical guide to help health care organizations in mitigating, preparing for, responding to, and recovering from emergencies.

This course is designed for health care educators and other personnel responsible for the overall environment of care in a health care setting.

Single Use Price: $149 Order Code: WBTSE01BDK

eBooks

eBooks (electronic/online books) provide an alternative education vehicle providing timely and focused information. eBooks are accessed via the Internet using a secure login and password. You'll have the ability to find the information you need at any time, from any location that has Internet access. You'll receive your password immediately after purchase.

Additional Benefits:

Speed and convenience—You'll receive your online book faster than a traditional printed publication.

Links to more information—Online books have hyperlinks to additional information on the Joint Commission and JCR Web sites as well as other online resources.

Access—Available 24 hours a day via the Internet.

Strengthening Physician and Staff Partnerships

Successfully coaching a physician colleague through a period of disruptive behavior preserves and cultivates his/her sense of well-being while enhancing partnerships and teamwork throughout the organization. This online book helps you explore the background on disruptive behavior and discover effective solutions. Learn from the positive experiences of organizations like yours and compare their winning approaches while reviewing their policies, survey tools, and other helpful documents.

Price: $55   Order Code: EB-02PSBDK

Staffing: Interpreting and Analyzing Data

This online tool focuses on analyzing and interpreting data so that your organization can effectively evaluate its staffing needs and performance improvement areas. Also included is how the new Joint Commission staffing standards affect your organization's survey preparation.

Price: $55   Order Code: EB-02STBDK

Organizational Ethics

The recent corporate scandals that have shaken the business world place a new focus on how companies conduct business. This focus on ethics is also impacting the health care industry. Health care organizations must question whether all aspects of business are being conducted with methods that demonstrate organization. This online book helps organizations with this task by defining characteristics of an ethical organization, identifying processes for education and dissemination of information, and demonstrating how organizational ethics can influence the quality of care delivery.

Price: $55   Order Code: EB-0903BDK